'The most incredible book'

Delia Smith, *The F...*

'A calm, incisive dissection of veganism's salvationist claim to protect human health and the planet'

John Lewis-Stempel, *Country Life*

'A brave, well researched and highly readable book that confronts the many myths about meat, health and climate change. Buxton's deep dive into the science and politics of these questions makes this book a must-read for anyone who cares about their health – or the planet'

Nina Teicholz, science journalist and bestselling author of *The Big Fat Surprise*

'*The Great Plant-based Con* is absolutely exceptional. When you've read the works of Gary Taubes and Nina Teicholz, you'll need to add this to your essential reading list. I was ignorant of so much that is so elegantly explained'

Professor Tim Noakes, scientist and founder of The Noakes Foundation, and author of *Lore of Nutrition* and *Real Food on Trial*

'With incredible skill, Jayne Buxton captures the edifice of intellectual and cultural fraud behind today's mythology of the safety of plant-based eating. Everyone needs this important and timely book'

Sally K. Norton MPH, nutritional scientist and author of *Toxic Superfoods*

'[A] forensic examination of the evidence ... Buxton is brilliant at reminding us of some basic statistical truths, ones that are usually forgotten these days ... It's refreshing to read a book which recognises that life is complicated'

Mark Mason, *Daily Mail*, Book of the Week

'This book fills an important space in the currently highly polarised debate about which dietary approach is scientifically most appropriate for human health, ecosystem functionality and climate impact ... There will be those on both the pro-meat and anti-meat sides who pillory this book due to feeling threatened by it. I recommend you read it yourself for a genuine understanding of the biases and concealed agendas behind much of the mainstream narrative around diets today, the failings of mainstream nutritional advice, especially government dietary guidelines, and what science really says about diets and human health today'

Ian Davis MCIWEM C.WEM MIEnvSc.,
environmental professional and retired farmer

'How I have waited for this book! A much needed, fact-packed, lucidly argued demolition of pervasive, endlessly recycled, anti-animal-source food propaganda, and a very welcome, closely argued, well-reasoned defence of our traditional omnivore diet'

Joanna Blythman, investigative journalist and
author of *Swallow This* and *Shopped*

'Jayne Buxton's compelling read, *The Great Plant-based Con*, challenges the "plant-biased" narrative literally sweeping across the globe and embedding itself into the very fabric of our society. Incredibly, who decides what we eat, and why, has not been based on science. Jayne takes a deep dive into the vested interests and religious ideology shaping the plant-based con, leaving no stone unturned'

Belinda Fettke, https://isupportgary.com

About the author

Jayne Buxton was born in the UK and has lived in Canada, the US and the UK. She has an MBA from IMD Business School and a master's degree in creative writing from Kingston University. She spent fifteen years working as a management consultant specialising in business strategy and data analysis at a major international consultancy before publishing her first work of non-fiction, *Ending the Mother War: Starting the Workplace Revolution* in 1998. The book was called a 'fiercely intelligent' exploration of the entrenched positions and false choices faced by women wanting to combine motherhood and careers, and led to Jayne being recognised by the *Guardian* as one of the women writers driving a 'quiet revolution' in feminism. Like *Ending the Mother War, The Great Plant-based Con* challenges the dominant narrative about an important issue and proposes a compelling alternative perspective.

Why eating a plants-only diet won't improve your health or save the planet

The Great Plant-Based Con

JAYNE BUXTON

PIATKUS

PIATKUS

First published in Great Britain in 2022 by Piatkus
This paperback edition published in 2023 by Piatkus

3 5 7 9 10 8 6 4

Copyright © Jayne Buxton 2022

The moral right of the author has been asserted.

A CIP catalogue record for this book
is available from the British Library.

ISBN 978-0-349-42795-9

Typeset in Sabon by M Rules
Printed and bound in Great Britain by
Clays Ltd, Elcograf S.p.A

Papers used by Piatkus are from well-managed forests
and other responsible sources.

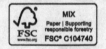

Piatkus
An imprint of
Little, Brown Book Group
Carmelite House
50 Victoria Embankment
London EC4Y 0DZ

An Hachette UK Company
www.hachette.co.uk

www.littlebrown.co.uk

Notice

The information in this book is not intended to be a definitive guide to what you should eat, but as a reference volume that provides a broad understanding of the health and ethical factors to consider, thereby enabling you to make your own informed decisions. The information given is not intended to replace any advice given to you by your GP or other health professional. If you have any concerns about your health, please contact the relevant health professional.

Mention of specific companies and organisations does not imply endorsement by the publisher, nor does mention of specific individuals, companies or organisations imply that they endorse all of the arguments presented in this book. All efforts have been made to assure the accuracy of the information contained herein, as of the date of publication.

*For the farmers around the world who will take
us towards a sustainable, real food future.*

Contents

PART THREE:
WHO IS ADVOCATING FOR THE PLANT-BASED DIET, AND WHY?

PART FOUR:
HOW SHOULD WE EAT?

Author's Note

About six months after I started doing the research for this book, I found myself sitting at a table in the tearoom of the Ham Yard Hotel in central London. Some of the tables around mine were laid with crisp white cloths, fine bone china and towers of scones and sandwiches, whereas others were occupied by lone urbanites tapping away on laptops, cappuccinos at the ready, or small gatherings of people huddled in discussion. The afternoon tea takers and those using the tearoom as a workspace were all dressed in some variation of fairly formal urban attire. A few immaculately coiffed ladies sported silk tea dresses with bows at the neck. It was all very English, and likely exactly what people around the world would imagine when asked to picture a modern-day tearoom in a smart hotel in London.

Into this scene strode a tall, broad-shouldered figure with a magnificent handlebar moustache and wearing a giant Stetson and cowboy boots. Heads swivelled and more than a few conversations were paused as this American cowboy made his way to my table.

This was Nebraskan rancher Trent Loos. Trent was in the UK visiting farmers and gathering information that he could share with the American Ambassador in connection with US–UK trade talks. After listening to one of his radio interviews, I had emailed him with some questions, and he had told me that, by coincidence, he would be in London and would be happy to meet.

Trent was accompanied by Englishman Andrew Henderson, who, I would soon discover, is managing director of Nemi Milk and a friend of Trent's. The three of us spent a couple of hours together, during which both Trent and Andrew enlightened me as to the realities of meat and dairy farming in both the US and the UK and shared their thoughts on everything from the misconceptions about US meat to their hopes for technologies and farming approaches that would both benefit the environment and deliver more nutrient-dense food.

At some point, I asked Trent how he had come to be a spokesperson for farmers and to have a radio show that was broadcast on one hundred stations across twenty-one states in the US. He told me that it all started in 1999 when he got 'really pissed off' by what he saw as increasing amounts of misinformation about farming and farmers. 'People were being misled,' he said. 'I wanted to be part of the solution. I thought, this false story that was being put about by animal rights activists is just going to dominate unless I and others tell the real story. We, who have first-hand experience, needed to share what was really going on.'

In May 2000, Trent walked into a local radio station and asked for his own show. Six months later he was producing *Loos Tales*, a Monday to Friday daily look at the people and places in rural America that truly make it what it is. He has been broadcasting ever since, in addition to speaking all over America and across three continents. His aim always is to send people away wanting to make a difference.

That meeting with Trent and Andrew was the first of many I had while I was researching and writing *The Great Plant-based Con*, but it was the only one in which I sat in a tearoom with a giant of a man in a Stetson and another man who'd brought a carton of his own milk for me to try. I met people who, like Trent, are concerned about the way the debate about food, health and the environment has been commandeered by plant-based advocates intent on pursuing a single solution to all our human and environmental problems. They shared their expertise, guided me through their work and towards the work of others, and gave generously of their time so that I could put forward the case for reframing that debate. It is not an exaggeration to say that I could not have written this book without them. A list of the individuals I interviewed, as well as others whose published work was invaluable to informing mine, is provided at the back of this book. If you are interested in knowing more about some of the topics that will be discussed over the next few hundred pages, you can go straight to the experts via their published works and the Web, podcast and Twitter addresses provided.

A note on terminology

Before we get started, a number of things need to be clarified, notably the term 'plant-based' itself, which seems to mean different things to different people. For some it means eating mostly plants with a bit of fish, meat or dairy thrown in occasionally, or even every day, whereas for others it means eating nothing but plants at all times. For yet another group of people it might mean including some plants in their mostly omnivorous diet. An Australian survey from 2010 confirms that people interpret the terms 'plant-based', 'vegan' and 'vegetarian' in significantly different ways.[1] A more recent study investigating the association between dietary patterns and Covid-19 evidenced similar levels of misunderstanding. Respondents who described themselves as eating a plant-based diet subsequently reported eating dairy twelve times a week, meat or seafood five times, and eggs twice. Their consumption of vegetables was only marginally greater than that of people who described themselves as not following a plant-based diet.[2]

Given this confusion around terminology, and the apparent mismatch between how people describe their diet and how they actually eat, it's important for me to clarify the terms that I'll be using in this book. I will use the term 'plant-based' to refer to diets containing very few or no animal foods, by which I mean vegetarian diets comprising mostly plants alongside some dairy and eggs but no animal flesh (meat or fish), and vegan diets containing no animal-sourced foods whatsoever. When differentiation between veganism and vegetarianism is helpful or necessary, I will use one or other of these terms rather than the more generic 'plant-based'. And when I talk about meat, I am referring to all meat (red and white), but I will discuss red meat – and, specifically, beef – more than any other type, since red meat has been the focus of so much research and public debate.

It's also important to establish that when I use the term 'plant-based advocate' I am referring to those people and organisations engaged in the active promotion of the idea that a strict plant-based diet should be rolled out across the globe. I am not referring to individual vegetarians and vegans who have chosen not to eat animal foods for personal reasons, and who quietly get on with the business of eating without imposing their beliefs and choices on other people.

I must also explain my use of the word 'con'. The Merriam-Webster dictionary defines a con as 'something, such as a ruse, used deceptively to gain another's confidence'.[3] But that is not the sort of con I have in mind here. There is no confidence trickster at the heart of a carefully honed plan, hell-bent on deceiving us and stealing our money. The con is the gradual conditioning of the public's thought processes by a constellation of individuals and organisations – who may well believe in the truth of the views they express – such that things which are far from certain are accepted as established fact. It is the cumulative effect of the over-arching, all-pervasive message that the plant-based diet will improve our health and save the planet, and our collective failure to challenge the accuracy of that message.

I should say that I agree with those who say that current meat consumption patterns are unsustainable, and that factory farming must be consigned to history. Where I part company with them is in the nature of solutions proposed. Where they advocate drastic reductions in the levels of meat consumption – and even the elimination of meat from restaurant and household menus – I, and many of those whose work is featured in this book, are proposing something different: a radical change in the way we view meat and animal foods, and a wholesale shift to producing them in the manner currently deployed by the best and most sustainable systems. That may well take us towards a reduced level of consumption by many in the big meat-eating nations – but our journey will be driven not by the belief that meat is intrinsically bad for health and bad for the planet but rather by the belief that meat and other animal foods are essential to human health, and that the problem is not with the foods themselves but the way they are produced.

A call for nuance

Each of us has an emotional connection to the food we eat, and individual decisions about food are always taken within specific emotional, health, social, religious and cultural contexts. These days, arguably more than ever before, decisions are also being taken within a specific political context – one that increasingly demonises animal foods and advocates the plant-based diet as a global imperative. Because food has become a political issue, we must bring more facts and less emotion to the table. We must also bring nuance, as writer Nicolette Hahn Niman has argued:

> today's debate over meat is characterised by polarizing, oversimplified rhetoric, pitting an implacable, defensive agribusiness in one corner against equally intractable vegan activists for abolition of all animal farming on the other. What has really fostered my interest in the debate ... is not a desire to encourage meat consumption but a longing for some nuance in the discussion.[4]

Hahn Niman – an environmentalist, lawyer, cattle rancher and long-term vegetarian recently turned omnivore[5] – is the personification of the kind of nuance we need in the debate. In her book, *Defending Beef*, she puts forward a passionate but balanced argument for the inclusion of beef and other animal foods in our diets, alongside a plea for the wholesale reform of industrial animal agriculture. Building on Hahn Niman's work and that of other farmers, scientists, writers and medical practitioners working in the field, I hope to do the same.

Dismantling the engine of plant-based advocacy

An early reader of this book, whose input was invaluable, described it as being akin to 'opening the bonnet of a car and dismantling the engine in order to understand how it works'. Like the parts of an engine, the arguments in support of the plant-based cause are connected in ways that are not immediately obvious. And much as those unfamiliar with engines might wonder about the role played by a particular component of an engine, some readers of this book may wonder why I'm delving into a particular, seemingly unconnected, topic.

But, as all parts of the engine are critical to its functioning, so all aspects of the arguments in favour of plant-based diets are critical to the overall message we are being conditioned to accept. So, please bear with me while I dismantle the engine. It will be a long and messy process, but hopefully it will also be a rewarding one, and by the time we've been through it, you'll be able to put the engine back together yourself.

Introduction

How an Emergency Became a War

On 16 January 2020, the BBC news featured a long segment on climate change. Science editor and presenter David Shukman first showed us a rotating globe lit with bright yellow patches, 'the blaze of lights evidence of the many impacts we're having on the globe'. These impacts included whole forests in Madagascar being cut down to create farmland, huge mines in Germany gouging out coal for power stations, and cities sprawling into natural habitats. And this was 'all on a scale so large it's even changing the climate, and the world now faces crucial decisions,' he said. Then came David Attenborough, imploring us to recognise that 'the moment of crisis has come'. 'As I speak, Southeast Australia is on fire. Why? Because the temperatures on the earth are increasing. That is a major national – international – catastrophe. To say that it's nothing to do with the climate is palpably nonsense.'[1]

Sir David was not completely despondent, however. He was encouraged by the huge change in public opinion that he had witnessed in the previous year. 'People can see the problem, young people in particular can see the problem, and that must force governments to change.'

Sir David was correct in his observation that 'people can see the problem' and are demanding change. (Whether he was right about the Australian fires being entirely the result of climate change is a question that was much debated in the months afterwards.) During the two years leading up to the BBC programme, Greta Thunberg and Extinction Rebellion (XR) had helped to force the issue of climate change centre stage, generating a surge in public awareness and a desire for change. More and more people became convinced that they needed to take personal action to avert the climate crisis. Grappling for solutions, many settled on one that seemed to be a no-brainer, which was to change their diet. In this manner a crisis engendered a war: the war on meat and other animal foods.

A key aspect of both Thunberg's and XR's message was, and continues to be, the demonisation of meat and dairy. In her 2018 TED talk, Thunberg asked 'why are we all still eating meat and dairy?'[2] During the London protests, XR staged a dramatic blockade of Smithfield's market and called for the UK to transition to veganism. Others have echoed the Thunberg–XR call to reduce or eliminate meat consumption. In November 2019 we saw the mayors of fourteen cities around the world, including London's Sadiq Khan, commit their citizens to the near-vegan Planetary Health Diet.[3] Prue Leith, the esteemed British cook and doyenne of *The Great British Bake Off*, called for all UK schools to serve vegetarian meals twice a week in order to improve students' health and to save the planet.[4] Students at three UK universities banned beef from campus bars and shops.[5] Property development firm Igloo Regeneration sought to reduce meat consumption among their staff by banning meat from expense claims.[6]

The call to reduce or even eliminate red meat consumption continued unabated in 2020 and 2021, with the publication of two reports, one by the UK Health Alliance on Climate

Change, and another by UK FIRES.[7] The UK FIRES report recommended that beef and lamb be phased out of our diet by 2050 in order for the UK to reach its goal of delivering net-zero emissions. A week after the report's publication, it was reported that the UK government was considering imposing taxes on meat and cheese as part of the drive to achieve its net-zero carbon pledge.[8] A few months later, UK cabinet minister Kwasi Kwarteng urged people to go vegan to save the planet.[9] And during the period in and around the Cop26 meeting in Glasgow, the idea of a meat tax was revived and much discussed.

Large sections of the media jumped on board the bandwagon, taking every opportunity to paint a negative picture of animal agriculture and animal foods. It was regularly asserted that animal farming was the biggest factor in climate change. In her piece titled, 'The Green Pages', Lucy Siegle, *The Times* Magazine environment editor, wrote 'Do give up meat', explaining that 'going straight for the plants puts you on the eco fast-track'.[10] Another journalist asserted (incorrectly) that a single hamburger generated the same greenhouse gas (GHG) emissions as a flight from New York to Los Angeles. (I'll provide evidence that this and other claims noted here are erroneous in Chapter 7.) A woman's magazine claimed (again, incorrectly) that livestock farming was responsible for a quarter of all emissions.[11] An article in *The Economist* concluded with the ludicrously inaccurate assertion that 'die-hard leaf eaters can claim to have knocked 85% off their carbon footprint'.[12] (The claim was either a misinterpretation of the data or a simple misprint; either way, it left readers believing that they could virtually eliminate their carbon footprint by becoming vegan.)

A BBC documentary, titled *Meat: A Threat to Our Planet*, which encouraged viewers to think about whether to eat any meat at all, was followed, in the space of one week during

January 2020, by four programmes with a pro-vegan slant. One of them, _Apocalypse Cow_, claimed (erroneously) that livestock farming was responsible for more GHG emissions than the entire transportation sector.* Restaurant critic Giles Coren, having adopted a vegan-till-6pm diet, stated: 'Greenhouse gas emissions from animal farming now comprise 51 per cent of the total global output [emissions] ... dwarfing the problem caused by cars, planes, power plants and Harry and Meghan put together.'[13] However, his number – 51 per cent – was more than three times the actual global percentage and more than ten times the relevant percentages for the UK and US. At a climate-change protest in the UK in February 2020, young protesters carried banners emblazoned with the same entirely false 51 per cent statistic. And in early 2021, Didier Toubia, co-founder of Aleph Farms, cited the same statistic while promoting his company's lab-based meat product (without any apparent challenge or correction from the journalist who interviewed him).[14]

From the other side of the Atlantic there came a much-publicised documentary titled _The Game Changers_, which purported to demonstrate that athletes could perform at a high level while eating a plant-based diet, and even insisted that men on vegan diets would enjoy longer and more frequent erections. Also in America, vegan activist director James Cameron (one of the executive producers of _The Game Changers_) and his wife Suzy persuaded Oprah Winfrey to urge Americans to join her in eating less meat.[15] (Oprah reportedly said that the idea of starting with one vegan meal per day was 'graspable'.) Jonathan Safran Foer penned an opinion piece for the _New York Times_ titled 'The end of meat

---

* This is untrue both at a global level and for the US. In the US, for example, livestock is responsible for around 3.9 per cent of emissions, whereas transport generates 29 per cent: www.epa.gov/ghgemissions/inventory-us-greenhous-gas-emissions-and-sinks.

is here'.[16] In the run up to the US election in November 2020, Kamala Harris said that she would support a change in the US dietary guidelines to reduce the consumption of meat.[17] In early 2021, *Epicurious* magazine announced that it would no longer feature recipes containing red meat, and one of New York's finest restaurants announced that it would no longer serve any meat or fish.[18]

People around the world heard the call to reduce or eliminate meat consumption. 'Many consumers perceive that plant-based foods are a healthier option and this notion is the key driver behind the reduction in meat consumption in recent years,' said research company Mintel's global food and drink analyst. The proportion of UK meat eaters who reported having reduced or limited the amount of meat they consume rose from 28 per cent in 2017 to 39 per cent in 2019. In 2021, it was reported that sales of meat had fallen in many parts of the world (down 12 per cent on the previous year in the US, and 4 per cent in Argentina, and predicted to fall by 1 per cent in Europe).[19] (The World Health Organization nevertheless predicted a small rise in global meat consumption in 2021, driven largely by growth in low- and middle-income countries.)[20]

The proportion of those declaring themselves to be fully vegan, both in the UK and worldwide, remains tiny but is increasing. (According to the Vegan Society, in the UK, the number of declared vegans quadrupled between 2014 and 2019, from 0.25 per cent to 1.16 per cent of the population, and veganism is more popular in the UK than in any other country.) Worldwide sign-ups for Veganuary (where people eat vegan for the month of January) have been steadily climbing, rising from 59,500 in 2017 to 250,000 in 2020 and 582,000 in 2021. According to the Vegan Society, around ten times as many people try Veganuary as sign up for the official programme, meaning that some five million people may have tried Veganuary in 2021.[21]

Of those who tried UK Veganuary in January 2020, 87 per cent were female. Men might not have signed up for the official programme in the same numbers as women but that didn't mean they weren't giving vegetarian and vegan diets a try. The young, whatever their gender, were particularly persuaded of the benefits of eating a plant-based diet. It was reported that 5 per cent of people aged between sixteen and twenty were vegan, versus 1.6 per cent of the general population.[22] It seemed to me that every other person under the age of thirty that I spoke to in 2020 had either given up animal foods or was contemplating doing so.

Some saw patterns in the vegan trend. Glen Burrows, a former vegetarian and the founder of The Ethical Butcher, observed that the highest take-up of veganism was among the white, urban middle classes. 'These are people who have the luxury of buying foods from all over the world and to remain totally disconnected from how they are produced.'[23] Farmer Joe Stanley remarked that disconnection from the land and the systems of production also allowed urban plant-based advocates to call themselves conservationists, while never having to do any of the actual conservation work in which farmers are engaged every day.[24]

The pro-vegan message is everywhere, although it now benefits from being wrapped up in the eminently softer and more widely acceptable term 'plant-based'. In an interview about the vegan stuffing balls that her family ate at Christmas, Mary McCartney (daughter of Paul and Linda) said, 'plant-based sounds more beautiful and natural'.[25] Clearly, many agree with her. The term 'plant-based' has become, in the words of one commentator, 'the marketing balm that soothes every conscience', prompting corporations to promote ultra-processed foods such as 'plant-based nuggets' as being good for health, and allowing consumers to feel good about eating them.[26]

Farmers are reeling in the face of this challenge to their way of life and the denigration of their contribution to society.[27] UK dairy farmer Abi Reader reported feeling 'nervous for the safety of the farm' after George Monbiot's *Apocalypse Cow* made her the centre of attention from vegan activists.[28] Farmer James Rebanks wrote that 'farmers are taking a bashing. You can't go on social media, turn on the TV or radio, or read a newspaper without someone telling you earnestly that farming is more or less the devil's work.'[29] In the US, Europe and Australia, too, farmers report feeling as though they are under siege. Some 84 per cent of UK farmers under forty now believe that mental health is the biggest problem facing the industry.[30]

A group called Farmers Against Misinformation tweeted that 'farmers everywhere are just shaking their heads', retweeting a comment made by a frustrated livestock farmer: 'As a livestock farmer ... I imagine an "environmentalist" surveying the landscape. There is rampant urbanisation, thousands of houses being built everywhere, there's a busy airport and high-speed rail link under construction. Container ships are docked in ports full of goods made in China, with power derived from burning coal, some of which is hauled from Australia. Fleets of lorries carry the containers on ever more congested roads to huge distribution depots, where swarms of vans are leaving to make deliveries. The environmentalist's attention is drawn to a distant hillside, where sheep are grazing. They make an announcement, "I've seen the solution – the sheep have GOT to go!"'[31]

'Farmers are shocked that the media has turned on them in this way,' said Roland Bonney, a farmer and co-founder of FAI Farms.[32] Patrick Holden, CEO of the Sustainable Food Trust, insisted that there needed to be a 'differentiation between livestock systems and meats that are part of the problem, and those that are part of the solution'.[33] Holden went on to say that sustainable agriculture represented one of the most 'significant opportunities to mitigate irreversible climate change, primarily through the regeneration of our soils'.[34]

There is no shortage of people arguing for a more balanced and fact-based debate. In the wake of the airing of Monbiot's *Apocalypse Cow*, two academics – Professor Myles Allen of the Oxford Martin School, a lead author on the Intergovernmental Panel on Climate Change (IPCC) Special Report on 1.5 degrees, and Dr John Lynch, from Oxford University's Department of Physics – sought to counter misconceptions about the impact of methane from livestock.* In their podcast discussion with FAI Farms, it was revealed that current methods of accounting for emissions can exaggerate the methane emissions of individual livestock farms by 70 per cent and whole farm emissions by 50 per cent.[35] Allen and Lynch warned that the focus on methane from livestock could divert attention away from the main culprit in the climate-change problem: fossil fuels. The authors of a study published in *Nature* share that worry, asserting that 'public policies need to place far more importance on directly cutting back the use of fossil fuels or removing their emissions through CCS (Carbon Capture and Storage)'.[36]

Award-winning investigative food writer Joanna Blythman stepped up to emphasise the importance of livestock farming to both human and environmental health.[37] Alice Stanton, Professor in Cardiovascular Pharmacology at the Royal College of Surgeons in Ireland, and director of human health at Devenish Nutrition, told me that the public have been let

* CO_2, often referred to simply as carbon, is one of three main greenhouse gases, the other two being methane (CH_4) and nitrous oxide (N_2O). The overall carbon impact of all these gases combined is calculated in terms of CO_2 equivalents, or CO_2e. Some of these gases are produced and consumed by natural processes. While burning coal and other fossil fuels releases new carbon into the air, the carbon that is produced by rotting plants and animals returns to the soil and is part of a natural carbon cycle.

down by a failure to properly discuss the alternatives to eradicating meat: 'It's like saying, cars are bad for the environment, so let's get rid of them. But we're not saying that with regard to cars. We're saying let's move to electric cars. Let's change the process. We should be saying the same about animal agriculture.'[38]

Farmers and environmentalists, such as Nicolette Hahn Niman and Matthew Evans, have written books that make a convincing case for sustainable meat production. Twitter was, and remains, awash with links to research provided by nutritionists, medical practitioners, scientists and farmers, all attempting to stem the tide of false information in the media and to generate awareness of the positive impact that livestock farming can have on both health and the environment. Scientists Dr Frank Mitloehner (professor and air-quality specialist at UC Davis) and Professor Frédéric Leroy (professor of food science and biotechnology at Vrije University, Brussels) have consistently been at the forefront of the social media debate, fighting the onslaught of misinformation with fact-based refutations.

One basic fact is this: 85 per cent of global emissions (and more than 95 per cent of US and UK emissions) are generated by sources *other than* animal agriculture. (I'll discuss these numbers in detail in Chapter 7.) So why are we vilifying farmers and the meat and dairy products they produce? Is it because meat and dairy represent easy targets? Or could it be because the idea of changing the way we eat seems somehow doable – or to use Oprah's word, *graspable* – whereas taking on the fossil fuel-producing giants, and our dependence on their product for our way of life, seems impossible? Could it be down to the simple fact that people feel guilty about the damage they are doing to the planet, and giving up meat makes them feel a little less guilty? This would seem to be the case for the actor Joaquin Phoenix, who used his 2020

Oscars speech to urge the world to go vegan. Later, having suspended himself from a London bridge alongside a banner that urged Londoners to 'Go vegan' he said, 'We all struggle with what the right thing to do is and we make mistakes. The [film] industry does consume a lot of power and a lot of resources so the way to mitigate that for me is to maintain a vegan lifestyle.'[39] Many people have expressed a similar sentiment to me: giving up meat makes them feel that they are doing *something* positive in the context of a situation over which they feel they have little influence or control. Bafflingly, during one Twitter exchange about how the leaders at Cop26 ought to lead by example, one individual insisted that leaders ought to go vegan, even if the evidence did not support it, just to show that they were doing *something*.

If the disparaging of animal agriculture within the environmental debate makes little sense, the campaign to convince people that a plant-based diet is best for health makes even less. For while plant-based advocates and their sympathisers in the media extoll the virtues of diets devoid of fish, meat, milk, butter, eggs or cheese, evidence of the importance of animal foods to human health is there for anyone who chooses to seek it out. Nutritionists regularly note the many vitamins, minerals and essential amino acids provided by meat that are often missing from plant-based diets, and they also point to the fact that the nutrients in plants are, in any case, less bioavailable than those in animal products. Others have demonstrated that a meat-inclusive, low-carbohydrate diet can be successful in reversing type-2 diabetes, and people with autoimmune diseases and depression have transformed their health by eating nothing but meat. (I'll cover the evidence for these health benefits in chapters 2, 5 and 6.)

The science is compelling; so are the stories. Standing in stark contrast to the positive messages about veganism propagated by Veganuary, the Vegan Society, PETA (People for the Ethical

Treatment of Animals) and the vegan community on social media, there are the health horror stories recounted by former vegans. And yet, despite the evidence that animal foods are good for health and have a much smaller impact on climate change than many other sectors of the global economy, the anti-meat message continues to ring loud and clear. Why is that?

Dr Mitloehner believes that much of the responsibility lies with a 2006 report by the Food and Agriculture Organisation (FAO) of the United Nations. This report, 'Livestock's long shadow: Environmental issues and options', made the claim that livestock is responsible for 18 per cent of global GHGs, making it a greater emitter than the global transportation sector.[40] The report generated a flood of headlines like this one in the UK's *Independent*: 'Rearing cattle produces more greenhouse gases than driving cars'. Although the FAO eventually reduced their 18 per cent number, revising it down to 14.5 per cent, based on a successful challenge by Dr Mitloehner, he believes that 'the consequences of that particular report continue to play a significant role in the climate quagmire that global agriculture finds itself in today'.[41] The idea that livestock generates more emissions than transportation seems to be entrenched in popular consciousness.

The other problem, says Mitloehner, is that emissions from animal agriculture are highly variable around the world, but the global number is the one that is most often cited.

'The problem is that there are people out there with an anti-agriculture agenda, and they like to use the global numbers – because they are so high – to make people stop eating animal-sourced foods.' Those who have a beef with livestock 'may have worked on the animal-welfare front or the food-safety front. But those subjects didn't resonate widely enough with the public to get people to stop eating animal-sourced food. However, they found that the climate angle really resonates well,' says Mitloehner.[42]

The climate angle, in combination with the insistent voices of all those who stand to gain from a plant-based revolution, means that the plant-based message has been amplified to a decibel level far higher than that which you would expect based on the small numbers of declared vegans around the world. The radical voices are so loud that, listening to them you would think that we were a few short years away from eradicating livestock from the face of the earth and enforcing a plant-based diet for all.

Among the radical voices is that of Pat Brown, founder and CEO of Impossible Foods, who has made it his mission to eliminate all animal agriculture.[43] Top UK scientist Sir Ian Boyd, a 'facultative vegan', has also warned us that farming is in its last decades.[44] George Monbiot is convinced that factory-produced protein will replace that from farming whether we like it or not.[45] Vegan entrepreneur Jonathan Petrides said, 'I strongly believe that rearing animals for food and dairy products will become obsolete in the coming decades.'[46] Tony Seba, co-founder of think tank RethinkX echoes this view, predicting that the meat and dairy industries will completely collapse, destroyed by the combined power of plant-based advocates and the corporations rushing to profit from supplying them with meat alternatives.[47] Christiana Figueres, former head of the UN Framework Convention on Climate Change, has gone on record to claim that meat eaters should one day be treated like smokers: 'if they want to eat meat, they can do it outside the restaurant'.[48]

It's easy to see the appeal of the radical anti-meat message, particularly for those invested in a thriving economy, because the corollary of 'eat less meat' is 'eat more of something else', namely plant-based and lab-grown foods. There is no implied economic contraction or sacrifice. Other solutions to the environmental crisis – build less, buy less, drive less, fly less – are obviously less attractive, since they necessarily imply

economic contraction. No wonder, then, that corporations and politicians seem to favour a switch to a plant-based diet over other, potentially more impactful, solutions.

Add immense amounts of power and money to the intent and certainty of the radical voices and the economic appeal of the anti-meat message, and what do you end up with? Ordinary citizens being conditioned to think that the universal adoption of a plant-based diet is the only option if we're to save ourselves and the planet. As I stressed in the note at the beginning of this book, this is not to say that plant-based advocates are acting together in a fully coordinated and directed effort, but rather to propose that the alignment of their beliefs and interests leads to actions that have the effect of a coordinated effort. No matter that the data do not support their cause, as Ivor Cummins, a researcher specialising in the root causes of modern chronic disease, commented: 'Plant based advocates are massively motivated ... it's like a religion. And they've been successful over the past 30 years, setting up corporations and huge non-profits and now we're seeing it really come home with the billionaires backing it. The narrative sounds beautiful to the vast majority of bureaucrats in these large international organisations. They don't look at the data. The data get in the way of the narrative, which has already been accepted and is believed in. Data is awkward.'[49]

What's an ordinary citizen to do if they don't like this picture? If they've harboured suspicions that we might all be victims of a conditioning effect that puts money in the pockets of the pea-protein suppliers and creates an out clause for fossil-fuel producers, or if they fear that removing animal foods from the diet might have negative, unintended consequences for their own health and the health of the planet?

Some, too busy to dig beneath the surface of the headlines and false claims, will climb aboard the plant-based bandwagon with varying degrees of reluctance or enthusiasm.

Others will continue to eat animal foods while feeling guilty about it. Parents will face enormous quandaries: what should they feed their children, and how should they respond to their children's anxiety about climate change and the eating of animal foods?

There is an alternative. That alternative is to engage with the 'awkward' data. You might not have time to challenge the headlines yourself, or to dissect the studies behind the headlines, but you *can* seek out the work of the scientists, doctors and nutritionists who *have* spent the time. This book is the culmination of my two years spent doing just that. What I have found has disturbed and shocked me, but I feel better equipped to go into battle in this war on meat and stand up to those who are waging it.

My aim is to equip you, too. This book will give you everything you need to know to help you to counter the plant-based dogma that's ringing in your ears, and to make more informed decisions about the food you choose to eat. It tells a story in four parts:

1. Is a plant-based diet better for your health?
2. Will a plant-based diet save the planet?
3. Who is advocating for the plant-based diet, and why?
4. How should we eat?

As we explore these questions, it will be necessary to discuss not just meat and plants but also sugar, fat, protein, lectins, processed foods, cholesterol, vegetable oils, diabetes, cancer, heart disease, soil health and more. Why? Because it isn't possible to understand why we need animal foods in our diet, and why the plant-based diet is no answer to our own or the planet's health, without discussing these things. It isn't possible, for example, to understand why removing animal foods from the diet and replacing them with grains, beans and pulses is

ill-advised unless we understand how excess consumption of these replacement foods can do harm to health and the environment. We can't have a conversation about the health benefits of eating meat, without addressing the long-standing controversy about the links between saturated fat, cholesterol and heart disease. We can't fully understand why cooking with animal fats is optimal, unless we understand why vegetable oils are bad for us. We can't know why removing animals from the land will be a disaster unless we understand their role in replenishing our denuded soils.

It will also be necessary to discuss the vast array of corporations and organisations that have a monetary interest in persuading us to eat a plant-based diet replete with processed food. We'll look at Big Food, Big Pharma and organisations whose business it is to advise us about our diets. We'll delve into the workings of the Seventh-day Adventist Church, an organisation little known in the UK that has exerted a worrying amount of global influence over dietary science and advice for more than a hundred years.

The fact that we must discuss these things is part of the problem, of course, as environmentalist and former vegan Lierre Keith has written:

Vegetarians can sum up their program in neat sound-bites – Meat Is Murder – and self-evident solutions, like those compelling sixteen pounds of grain. I could come up with my own slogans – Monocrops are Murder? The Million Microbe March? – but they aren't understandable to the general public. I have to start from the beginning, from the first proteins self-organising into life, moving to photosynthesis, plants, animals, bacteria, soil, and finally agriculture. I call this chat 'Microbes, Manure, and Monocrops,' and I need a good thirty minutes for the back-story, which is essentially a basic education in the nature of life. And yes, this is information – material, emotional, and spiritual – we should all have been given by the time we were four ... But it's not just the amount of information that makes the discussion hard. Often, the listener doesn't want to hear it, and the resistance can be extreme.[50]

Unable to fall back on soundbites, we have no choice but to embark on a magical mystery tour of everything from sugar and heart disease to the Seventh-day Adventists and soil. Our tour will also take us around the world, drawing on research and examples from the UK, the United States and elsewhere. You will read about ranches in North Dakota and Virginia, as well as farms in Devon and Lincolnshire.

Before we set off, however, let me be clear about something. This book is not anti-plants. I love fruit and vegetables and subscribe to the view expressed by human nutrition scientist Stephan van Vliet, which is that plant and animal foods work synergistically to generate maximum nutritional benefits for human health. 'Ironically,' says van Vliet, 'you could argue that the reason we are even able to engage in this ethical debate about whether we should be eating animals is precisely because our brains have the sophisticated capabilities that came from eating both plants and animal foods for millions of years.'[51]

Neither is this book anti-vegetarian or anti-vegan. If an individual chooses to follow a plant-based diet because eating animal products conflicts with their religious beliefs or their values, or because they simply do not like meat, that is their prerogative. Comedian and popular philosopher Russell Brand asserted this prerogative in early 2021 when he explained that he was vegan because he 'couldn't get his head around eating animals', but that he had always tried to stay clear of the political and evangelical aspect of veganism. Essentially, he wants to eat a vegan diet for personal reasons but isn't trying to convince anyone else to do so.

'People can eat however they want,' said Ivor Cummins, 'but the trouble is that some very powerful interests are driving an ideology that will hurt people, and that makes it my business.'[52] That individual dietary choices are being exploited in the name of an ideology that is then being propagated based on vast amounts of misinformation is something that should concern us all. The extent of the misinformation certainly concerns many working in the health and nutrition space. Nutritionist Tim Rees said that he was worried 'about people who are suckered into veganism because they think it's healthier – which it's not, it's a disaster – or because they think it's better for the environment, which it's not'.[53] Health and fitness professional, author and filmmaker Vinnie Tortorich confessed to being concerned to the point of being angry: 'I'm mad at the people who are lying to the people who are turning to veganism, the doctors who use so-called studies and misrepresent the results to make them fit what people want to hear.'[54]

If this book is neither anti-plant nor anti-vegan, what is it? It's a plea for us to take a hard and honest look at the plant-based diet in the context of the facts about human and environmental health. It's also a call for an end to mudslinging between omnivores and plant-based advocates. Less mud, more facts. Like farmer and author Matthew Evans, I have no interest in converting vegans to omnivory. But I support his plea for a 'more honest, intellectually rigorous debate about what we eat, how it is produced, and what is affected in the process'.[55]

Another point on which I must be clear: industrial, factory farming is abhorrent, and the wholesale clearing of the Amazon's forests for the raising and feeding of livestock must be halted. We need to be eating animal-sourced foods that have been sustainably and humanely reared. As individuals wanting to make a difference, we could do worse than to follow Joanna Blythman's advice: 'if you want to eat meat, poultry, eggs and dairy foods, buy less of them but maintain your spend by trading up to buy higher welfare, more extensively farmed, free-range, grass-fed products'.[56] Those who place environmental concerns and animal welfare at the heart of their purchasing choices will find, as Matthew Evans has, that they have more in common with those who abstain from eating meat than many who consume it.[57]

We must reframe the debate. The problem is not with meat in the diet per se but what farming system the meat comes from. Or, to put it more simply, it's about the how, not the cow. And this is a critical moment. If we continue to allow the debate to be dominated by those with a vested interest in eradicating animal foods from our diets and from the planet, we will, one day, reach the point of no return. In the process, we will have sacrificed our own health and the health of future generations and squandered the power of regenerative agriculture to heal our planet. Armed with knowledge, we stand a chance of halting the plant-based juggernaut before it's too late.

Part One

Is the Plant-based Diet Better for Your Health?

'For the last 50-plus years, we've been told that meat, eggs and animal fats are bad for us and that we'll live longer and enjoy superior health if we minimize or avoid them. The idea has been so drilled into our heads that few people even question it any more. In fact, if you asked the average person on the street whether a vegetarian or vegan diet is healthier than an omnivorous diet, they'd probably say yes.'

CHRIS KRESSER, M.S., L.Ac, author and co-director of the California Center for Functional Medicine

'The drive to promote plant-based diets and to demonise animal-based diets continues. The nutritional facts continue to support the opposite.'

DR ZOË HARCOMBE, PhD, researcher and author in the field of diet and health

'As for the idea that a healthy diet must be mostly plants, that it must include fruits, vegetables, whole grains, pulses and legumes, we have no meaningful clinical trial evidence to support this idea.'

GARY TAUBES, science journalist and author, *The Case for Keto*

Part One

Is the Plant-based Diet better for Your Health?

1

Why Do We Think Meat is Bad for Us?

One evening in 2019 my husband and I met friends Will and Julie for supper. Will announced that he had followed Julie's lead and decided to stop eating meat. 'I find that I don't even want it any more,' he said. 'And, let's face it, plant-based is so much better for you.' My expression must have told Will that I didn't necessarily agree with him. 'What? You don't think so?' he said. My husband shot me a look from across the table. The look said: *Don't get into this now. It's not the time.* And he was right, so I shrugged in a non-committal way and started perusing the menu. The conversation moved on. I never mentioned to Will that my study was piled high with research materials, all of which had persuaded me that a plant-based diet was definitely not 'so much better for you'.

Will's casual assertion that a plant-based diet is better for health than a diet that includes animal foods is far from unusual. Personal health is the second most frequently cited reason for people trying Veganuary.[1] Writing about an interview with Bill Bryson, the author of *The Body*, the journalist said, 'you might expect that the healthily informed Bryson would turn vegan', thus making the automatic link between being informed about health and veganism.[2] In some academic papers, scientists have based their complex models and arguments on weak – and therefore far from definitive – epidemiological evidence from other papers that purport to show that eating meat is harmful.[3] (I'll come on to why epidemiology can be weak and misleading later in the chapter.) Interviewed for a BBC Future article, psychologist Hank Rothgerber said, 'There's more and more evidence, more and more arguments, and more and more books about how eating meat is bad ... but still, our behaviour hasn't changed significantly.'[4] Translation: meat is definitely bad for us and our failure to reflect that in our behaviour is a problem.

How did we get here? How did so many people come to believe that meat is bad for us and plant-based diets are best for health? Dietitian Jillian Ceasrine, a former vegetarian turned omnivore, has said that the fault lies with mainstream nutrition advice and its bias against saturated fat. 'It was a natural choice for me to study dietetics in school. I learned a lot in school, but one of the key takeaway messages I gathered through my formal education was to limit red meat consumption. The logic being that the high consumption of red meat is bad for health because it contains a high amount of saturated fat. Consumption of too much saturated fat increases your LDL cholesterol, which in theory increases your chance of heart disease.'[5]

Where, then, did these theories about meat, saturated fat and cholesterol come from and how did they come to dominate thinking about what constitutes a healthy diet? To answer this question, we need to go back to the 1950s and understand the work of the now infamous biologist and pathologist, Ancel Keys.

Ancel Keys and the diet–heart hypothesis

Ancel Benjamin Keys hypothesised that saturated fat caused heart disease. His hypothesis became known as the diet–heart hypothesis (sometimes called the cholesterol hypothesis, or the diet–heart–cholesterol hypothesis). The fascinating story of how this hypothesis came to dominate thinking about diet and heart disease, and became embedded in the dietary advice given to Americans and populations all around the world, has been recounted at length by two science journalists and authors, Gary Taubes (*Good Calories, Bad Calories*) and Nina Teicholz (*The Big Fat Surprise*).

Keys, who began thinking about fat and heart disease in the 1930s, initially became persuaded that cholesterol was 'one of the main culprits in the development of coronary disease'.[6] Years later, in 1953, Keys hypothesised that it was the consumption of fat that caused cholesterol to rise. His 'Six Country Study' (of Japan, Italy, England and Wales, Australia, Canada and the US) showed a strong correlation between fat intake and death rates from heart disease. Later, in 1957, researchers Jacob Yerushalmy and Herman Hilleboe addressed the limitations of this study, primary among them that it had studied just six countries. Yerushalmy and Hilleboe mapped the data from twenty-two countries and produced a graph showing a much less convincing correlation between fat and heart disease.[7] They noted, for example, that 'in the narrow band between 30 per cent and 40 per cent dietary fat [calories from fat as a percentage of total calories], there appears the entire gamut of heart disease mortality, ranging from less than 300 per 100,000 for Austria, West Germany, Sweden, Norway, Denmark, and the Netherlands, to 600 or more for Australia, Canada, and Finland and as much as 739 for the United States'. They maintained that 'the selection of the original six countries, for whatever reason, greatly exaggerated the importance of the association'.[8] Moreover, there were problems with definitions of food consumption and groupings of 'cause of death' data, and, when other dietary factors were examined, they were found to have an equally strong correlation with deaths from heart disease.

Yerushalmy and Hilleboe concluded that 'the apparent association in itself cannot serve as supporting evidence for the theory that dietary fat plays a role in heart disease mortality'. They noted, however, that by the time of writing the causal link between fat intake and death from heart disease had already 'assumed the stature of a proved fact'.[9] Keys' original caution regarding the conclusions that might be drawn on the basis of his study was subsumed by interpretations that 'gave the association greater stature and definitiveness'.[10]

In 1958, Keys and his fellow researchers embarked on the 'Seven Countries Study', a more extensive analysis that tracked results at intervals over many years. However, as with the Six Countries Study, this study omitted results from countries that might have disproven the original hypothesis. Several practical reasons for certain countries being omitted were given, including the unwillingness of some countries to participate.[11] The fact remains, however, that the associations between dietary fat and deaths from heart disease that appeared convincing for the seven countries chosen would have been much less convincing had other countries also been studied.

A few years ago, Dr Malcolm Kendrick compared Keys' original seven country analysis (based on Italy, Greece, the former Yugoslavia, the Netherlands, Finland, the USA and Japan) with his own analysis (based on data from Finland, Israel, the Netherlands, Germany, Switzerland, France and Sweden), noting that his own list would have 'demonstrated the exact opposite result' to that from the Keys study.[12]

Dr Zoë Harcombe took Dr Kendrick's analysis a step further in 2010 and looked at the relationship between cholesterol and heart disease. (Cholesterol being the middle-man in the diet–heart hypothesis, supposedly being linked to saturated fat intake.) Analysing up-to-date WHO data for 192 countries, Dr Harcombe found an inverse relationship between cholesterol levels and deaths from cardiovascular disease (CVD), and an inverse relationship between chol-esterol levels and deaths from any cause.[13] Dr Harcombe updated her analysis in 2020, plotting non-communicable diseases (the data on CVD was no longer available) and all-cause mortality against average country cholesterol levels for 181 countries. All associations were, as before, inverse; the higher the cholesterol levels, the lower the death rates.[14]

Of course, regardless of which countries were selected by Keys and his fellow researchers, both the Six and Seven Countries Studies were epidemiological (observational) in nature, and could therefore only show association, not causation. It's worth taking a brief detour to consider these terms – epidemiology, association, causation – because they're going to crop up again and again in this book.

The imperfect science of epidemiology

Often referred to as 'observational science', epidemiology is based on the formulation of hypotheses that are then tested by the tracking of specified data, or outcomes, over a period of years. In nutrition science, these outcomes are most often reported in terms of risk factors for the occurrence of a cer-tain disease: eating X gives you a 15 per cent increased risk of contracting Y. Epidemiological studies consistently suffer from three flaws:

Firstly, they can show **association but not causation**. A study might show that two factors increase – the consumption of a particular food and the incidence of a particular disease outcome – but that doesn't mean that the first factor is a cause of the second. The two factors are merely associated within the same study, and the 'cause' of the disease outcome might well be any one of a number of different factors not being measured. It has been shown, for example, that the number of people who drowned by falling into a pool between 1999 and 2009 correlated almost perfectly with the number of films in which Nicolas Cage appeared. This does not mean that Nicolas Cage films cause people to drown in pools.[15] A website called Spurious Correlations (tylervigen.com) provides dozens of examples of this sort of spurious correlation, even allowing people to invent their own. I mapped the number of people who die falling down the stairs with per capita cheese consumption and found an almost perfect – yet entirely spurious – correlation.

Relative and absolute risk A second flaw with epidemiological studies is that their results tend to be reported in terms of *relative* as opposed to *absolute* risk because the relative risk always sounds more newsworthy: for example, it has been claimed (by the WHO) that each 50g portion of processed meat eaten daily increases the risk of colorectal cancer by 18 per cent. But this is a *relative risk* number. If you look at the incident rate for bowel cancer in the UK, for example, it is around 47 people per 100,000. An increased relative risk of 18 per cent takes this up to 55 people per 100,000. But your *absolute risk* is still low, because 55 in 100,000 represents a risk of much less than 1 per cent. And that's if the association being claimed can be said to translate directly into causation, which it cannot since epidemiology cannot, on its own, prove causation.

Confounding variables Then we have the problem of confounding variables, as with the 'healthy person confounder'. For example, if a study finds that vegetarians live longer than meat eaters, this might have nothing to do with the fact that vegetarians don't eat meat and everything to do with the fact that they practise other health-enhancing behaviours such as exercising, watching their alcohol intake and not smoking. (This is the case with one frequently cited study comparing Seventh-day Adventist vegetarians with Americans eating a standard diet.)

Similarly, if a study finds that eating red meat is associated with higher rates of cancer, how can we be sure that it's the red meat that's at fault, and not the bun, fries and cola consumed alongside it, or the lifestyles of the people who eat more meat in an environment when people generally think that they should eat less? Sorting out cause and effect amidst so many imperfectly controlled variables becomes virtually impossible, as has been acknowledged by several prominent epidemiologists, including John Bailar and John Ioannidis. In his paper titled 'Why most published research findings are false', Ioannidis wrote that, 'for many current scientific fields, claimed research findings may simply be accurate measures of the prevailing bias' and that 'false findings may be the majority or even the vast majority of published research claims'.[16]

How Keys' epidemiological research became gospel

Epidemiology's greatest success was the discovery that cigarettes caused lung cancer. In that case the difference between smoking and non-smoking populations was so large (ten to thirty-fold) that causation could reasonably be inferred, and any other weaknesses in the observational approach discounted. Keys could claim no such undeniable causation, however. Compounding the essential weakness of the correlation was the fact that, like most epidemiology applied to nutrition, the research relied upon retrospective food frequency questionnaires (FFQs) that required participants to recall exactly what they ate over an extended period.

Despite what Dr Kendrick calls the 'crippling flaws' of his study,[17] Keys continued to assert its main take-home point: that saturated fat intake leads to high cholesterol and high cholesterol leads to heart disease. And most people, writes Gary Taubes, believed that he had proved it beyond doubt.[18]

There have always been scientists who disagreed with Keys' hypothesis. They included Peter Ahrens, whose experiments linked carbohydrate intake and resulting high triglyceride levels to heart disease, and John Yudkin, a British doctor who posited the hypothesis that sugar was the real culprit in heart disease.[19] Yudkin's work was ignored by the majority of the medical profession. George Mann, whose work showing that saturated fat intake was not related to heart disease, was similarly sidelined. Mann later described the diet–heart hypothesis as 'the greatest scam in the history of medicine' and accused the 'heart mafia' of supporting the dogma and hoarding research funds, meaning that for a generation 'research on heart disease has been more political than scientific'.[20]

As time went on, Keys' hypothesis was belied by the emerging facts about many small communities around the world. Studies of the Navajo Indians, Irish immigrants to Boston, African nomads, Swiss Alpine farmers, Benedictine and Trappist monks, the Maasai of Kenya and the Italian Americans of Roseto, to name but a few, all suggested that dietary fat was unrelated to heart disease.[21] In addition, several studies carried out in the 1950s and 1960s provided compelling evidence that the diet–heart hypothesis was wrong about the links between saturated fat, cholesterol and heart disease. One study directed by Keys himself – the Minnesota Coronary Experiment (1968–73) – showed not only that the diet–heart hypothesis was wrong but also that polyunsaturated fats (vegetable oils) were the bigger risk to health. The data was so inconvenient that it was buried, and it was not until 2016 that the original data was discovered and re-analysed. One of the lead authors on the 2016 paper was Daisy Zamora, who said, 'had this research been published forty years ago, it might have changed the trajectory of diet–heart research and recommendations'.[22] Commenting on the data, Professor Tim Noakes said that had it been revealed at the time of the study's conclusion 'the 1977 [dietary] guidelines might never have come into being and the subsequent obesity and diabetes epidemics might have been avoided'.[23]

Another early study that disproved the diet–heart hypothesis was the Sydney Diet Heart Study (1966–73). As with the Minnesota Coronary Experiment, the data was not fully revealed until Dr Christopher Ramsden and his colleagues (including Dr Zamora) recovered it and re-analysed it. Ramsden and his colleagues found that 'substituting dietary linoleic acid [found in polyunsaturated vegetable oils] in place of saturated fats *increased* risk of death from all causes, coronary heart disease and cardiovascular disease' (italics mine).[24]

With important data from studies like these having been buried, and data from various populations around the world ignored or explained away, the diet–heart hypothesis established a firm stranglehold over scientific and medical opinion. Keys reportedly used his forceful personality and connections to persuade the American Heart Association (AHA) to accept the findings of his flawed studies and join him in vilifying butter, eggs and anything other than small quantities of lean meats. The AHA became, said Nina Teicholz, an 'ocean liner, steaming the diet–heart hypothesis forward'.[25] The National Institute of Health (NIH) in the US soon jumped on board that ocean liner. Saturated fats became the enemy, and so-called heart-healthy polyunsaturated fats were the new darlings of the nutritional world.

The healthy-eating guidelines are born

In 1977, all debate about saturated fat was quashed and the fat issue seemingly settled when the McGovern Committee issued the first Dietary Goals of the United States.[26] Vinnie Tortorich's film, *Fat: A Documentary*, tells the story of how these guidelines were pushed through despite the grave reservations of many scientists who said that there was insufficient evidence to support them. Philip Handler, then president of the National Academy of Sciences, questioned the right of the federal government to conduct such a 'vast nutritional experiment' with the American people as subjects 'on the strength of so little evidence'.[27]

Handler's warnings were ignored, and a vast nutritional experiment began. The Dietary Goals report recommended that Americans eat fewer calories, less fat, less saturated fat, more polyunsaturated fat, less cholesterol, less sugar, less salt, more fibre and more starchy foods.[28] The combination of the 'eat less fat' and 'eat more starch' recommendations were picked up by food manufacturers, who began to churn out highly processed, low-fat, carbohydrate-rich foods that were like rocket fuel for the ensuing diabetes and obesity epidemics. Fat was deemed guilty as charged, and the theory that saturated fat literally clogged the arteries became ubiquitous, as did crude images of those clogged-up arteries. This theory made its way into formal dietetics programmes around the world, influencing thinking about diet and health for the next fifty years and becoming what Teicholz has called the 'acorn that grew into the giant oak tree of our mistrust of fat today'.[29]

Despite the fact that there was no evidence to support dietary fat limits, they were incorporated into the dietary guidelines that were rolled out in the US, the UK and other countries, becoming the basis of simple eating guides, or plates.[30] In the UK the plate is called the Eatwell Guide; in the

US they have the My Plate Guide, which is itself a version of the old US Food Pyramid. Recently, another form of plate – the Planetary Health Diet – has come to us via the EAT-Lancet Commission. All these eating guides advocate diets loaded with bread, rice, potatoes and pasta (all carbohydrates) but light on meat, fish and dairy. They also advise the consumption of vegetable oils rather than saturated fats.

If you wonder why dietary guidelines like these matter, consider this: the USDA guidelines directly influence one in four Americans via school lunches, food-support programmes, prison cafeterias and the military. They exert wider influence via the national curriculum for dietitians and other professionals, as well as the guidelines rolled out in other countries, including the UK, where a similar cascade of influence is replicated.[31] Evidence from both the US and the UK indicates that actual food consumption mirrors the guidelines closely, and has done since they were introduced in 1977, which also marks the moment that obesity and diabetes rates began to skyrocket.

In the UK, GPs use the Eatwell Guide template to provide dietary guidance to their obese and diabetic patients. Enlightened GPs who have seen the evidence for low-carbohydrate, high-fat (LCHF) diets as effective tools for treating these conditions cannot openly challenge the official Eatwell guidelines, which are supported by NHS England and its National Diabetes Prevention Programme, for fear of falling foul of the General Medical Council.

The mounting evidence against the diet–heart hypothesis

Over many years the pro-carbohydrate, anti-fat message became firmly embedded in the guidelines, despite findings that countered the diet–heart hypothesis continuing to roll in. The 1980s saw results from the Helsinki Businessmen study, the Framingham study, the MRFIT trial, the CPPT trial and studies in Honolulu, Puerto Rico and Chicago, all of which punctured holes in the diet–heart hypothesis. (Gary Taubes provides a good, layperson friendly summary of all these trials in *Good Calories, Bad Calories*.)[32] Some trials showed that the risks of cardiovascular disease and mortality were greater among those with low serum cholesterol levels (that is, low levels of cholesterol in the blood), particularly for women and for men aged over fifty.

Faced with this flood of troublesome findings, diet–heart enthusiasts used all manner of means of dismissing them. Sometimes they simply buried the data, as was the case with the Minnesota and Sydney studies. Another tactic, says Dr Kendrick, was to explain away some results as paradoxical. The Maasai, the French, the Israelis, the Swiss, the citizens of Malmö, the Aboriginals, older men and all women were deemed to be paradoxes. In 2015, another 'paradox' came to light when it was discovered that there had been a decline in mortality from coronary heart disease in Japan despite a marked rise in total cholesterol. Dr Kendrick commented that this should have been yet another nail in the coffin of the diet–heart hypothesis but researchers chose, instead, to assert the possibility that there may be 'some protective factors unique to the Japanese'.[33]

Yet another tactic was the proposal of what Dr Kendrick calls 'ad-hoc hypotheses'.[34] These were like sub-clauses of the diet–heart hypothesis designed to explain away inconvenient results. These ad-hoc hypotheses, and other tactics designed to keep the diet–heart hypothesis alive, led Dr Harcombe to call the hypothesis 'a slippery fish – always changing and moving'.[35] She wrote:

Over time, therefore, the hypothesis has mutated from: dietary cholesterol raises blood cholesterol and causes heart disease; to saturated fat causes heart disease (no mention of cholesterol); to saturated fat and blood cholesterol and heart disease 'tend to be related'; to lots of variants of a form of cholesterol hypothesis ... We seem to have ended up with the hypothesis that 'saturated fat raises LDL-cholesterol and causes heart disease', although there are variants of this.[36]

The hypothesis might have been a slippery fish, but one thing has continued to be clear: the data does not support it. In addition to the data from the Minnesota and Sydney studies being brought to light, new studies, such as the 700-million-dollar Women's Health Initiative Randomized Controlled Dietary Modification Study (sometimes referred to simply as WHI) showed no connection between fat intake and heart disease. It also suggested that those women who had previously suffered a heart attack and who ate the 'heart-healthy' low-fat diet during the trial period were at a 26 per cent increased risk of experiencing further heart problems. (This finding was not reported in the study's abstract but was buried deep in the text.)[37]

A 2014 study concluded that 'current evidence does not clearly support cardiovascular guidelines that encourage high consumption of polyunsaturated fatty acids and low consumption of total saturated fats'.[38] In 2017, the Prospective Urban Rural Epidemiology (PURE) study of over 135,000 people in eighteen countries found that those who ate animal protein and fat had fewer heart attacks than those who ate more cereal grains.[39] Total fat intake and types of fat eaten were not associated with cardiovascular disease, heart attack or death from cardiovascular disease, but saturated fat intake did predict a lower risk of stroke.[40] More recently, a 2020 review of the evidence by the Cochrane Collaboration concluded that:

There was little or no effect of reducing saturated fats on non-fatal myocardial infarction [heart attack] ... or CHD mortality ... but effects on total (fatal or non-fatal) myocardial infarction, stroke and CHD events (fatal or non-fatal) were all unclear as the evidence was of very low quality. There was little or no effect on cancer mortality, cancer diagnoses, diabetes diagnoses, HDL cholesterol, serum triglycerides or blood pressure, and small reductions in weight, serum total cholesterol, LDL cholesterol and BMI.[41]

The 2020 report by the Cochrane Collaboration was the fourth since 2011. Reviewing all of the reports, Dr Harcombe concluded that none of them 'has ever found anything for any dietary fat intervention (reduced or modified, total or saturated) for anything related to mortality. Not all-cause mortality, or cardiovascular disease (CVD) mortality, or coronary heart disease (CHD) mortality, or fatal heart attacks.'[42] Nor had the reports found anything linking reductions in total or saturated fat to reductions in CHD events, strokes or non-fatal heart attacks. In fact, she says, 'there have been no findings against total fat ever, and there have been no findings against saturated fat that have withstood scrutiny (as reported in the Cochrane publications themselves)'.[43]

In September 2021, having reviewed the totality of the data on saturated fats and cardiovascular outcomes, a group of esteemed researchers echoed the Cochrane findings, writing that there is 'a lack of rigorous evidence to support continued recommendations either to limit the consumption of saturated fatty acids or replace them with polyunsaturated fatty acids'.[44]

Dr Kendrick writes that he could 'fill an entire book of studies that have been done contradicting the diet–heart hypothesis' and that 'there are even studies showing, quite clearly, that reducing saturated fat is harmful'.[45] As the studies mounted, and the work of people like Gary Taubes, Nina

Teicholz, Stephen Phinney, Jeff Volek, Dr David Ludwig and Dr Eric Westman penetrated public consciousness, the tide started to turn. Parts of the media seemed willing to challenge the diet–heart hypothesis. In 2014, butter appeared on the front cover of *Time* magazine, accompanied by an article stating that contrary to popular belief, fat and cholesterol in the diet have no effect whatsoever on cholesterol and heart disease. And statements issued by the 2015 USDA Dietary Guidelines Committee confirmed that 'available evidence shows no appreciable relationship between consumption of dietary cholesterol and serum cholesterol ... Cholesterol is not a nutrient of concern for overconsumption.'[46] Dr Dariush Mozaffarian and Dr David Ludwig wrote that the committee's position was 'concordant with scientific evidence demonstrating no appreciable relationship between dietary cholesterol and serum cholesterol or clinical cardiovascular events in general populations'. (The emphasis on general populations is important – those with specific existing conditions such as type-2 diabetes may be at risk from excess cholesterol consumption[47] and the National Lipid Association recommends that those with established hypercholesterolemia limit dietary cholesterol.[48])

Cholesterol and saturated fats were beginning to be relieved of their pariah status; furthermore, red meat itself was exonerated by a series of reviews published in the *Annals of Internal Medicine* in 2019.[49] These large-scale meta-analyses (systematic reviews of available studies) led researchers to conclude that the evidence linking meat consumption to heart disease and cancer is of 'low to very low certainty'. They advised the continued consumption of red and processed meat. Not all scientists accepted the study's findings, and some reacted with positive outrage (I'll discuss this at length in Chapter 12), but many highly respected scientists all around the world attested to the high standard of the research. As to the accusation that the study's authors had neglected to consider much of the epidemiological and short-term studies,[50] these omissions were entirely transparent and intentional. The authors had applied the rigorous GRADE method to assess the quality of research, and much of the epidemiological research was simply too weak to qualify. As Professor Frédéric Leroy and Nathan Cofnas pointed out in 2020, so much of the epidemiological research about the effects of meat consumption *has* been weak, being based on notoriously unreliable food frequency questionnaires, beset by confounding variables and showing relative risks that are much too small (that is, much below two) to imply causation.[51]

Fred Provenza and colleagues point out that epidemiology as applied to meat consumption also fails to account for many important factors:

Epidemiological studies that find inverse associations between eating red meat and health do not distinguish between meat from livestock fed high-grain diets in feedlots and livestock foraging on phytochemically rich mixtures of plants. Nor do they address how herbs, spices, vegetables, and fruits eaten in a meal with meat can enhance health.[52]

Other research supports the *Annals* conclusions regarding meat consumption. The most recent PURE study (2021) concluded that higher unprocessed meat consumption (250g versus 50g) was not significantly associated with mortality or CVD. Similarly, no association was observed between poultry intake and health outcomes.[53] (However, the researchers did find an association between higher intake of processed meat and a higher risk of mortality and major CVD.) A 2019 study published in the *Lancet* compared the risks associated with fifteen different aspects of diet (including, for example, the risks from diets high in trans fats or diets low in fruits and vegetables).

Diets high in red meat came last in terms of being risks for both deaths and disability-adjusted life years (DALYs).[54] In other words, reducing red meat consumption is the last thing we should be thinking about when trying to improve long-term health outcomes. Another 2019 meta-analysis of randomly controlled trials (RCTs) of red meat in comparison with various other diets, by Marta Guasch-Ferré and colleagues, found that 'there were no significant changes in blood concentrations of total, low-density lipoprotein, or high-density lipoprotein cholesterol, apolipoproteins A1 and B, or blood pressure'.[55]

Moreover, there is evidence to suggest that eating some red meat can be good for us and may even be protective against heart disease. A 2021 study with over 18,000 participants set out to assess the association between adherence to the Paleo diet (which promotes the consumption of fruit, nuts, vegetables, eggs, meat and fish) and the risk of CVD in a Mediterranean cohort. Findings suggested that the Paleo diet may have cardiovascular benefits, particularly in the context of a Mediterranean cohort and low consumption of ultra-processed foods. Moreover, those who ate the most red meat (104g per day) had a significantly lower risk of CVD than those who ate the least (81g per day).[56]

How might meat offer protection against heart disease? Perhaps by improving nitric oxide synthesis. 'It is impossible to overstate the importance of nitric oxide (NO) on cardiovascular health,'[57] says Dr Kendrick. Meat – along with a few other things like sun exposure, red wine and certain vegetables – has been shown to increase nitric oxide synthesis. A substance called L-arginine, itself known to increase nitric oxide synthesis, is found in abundance in animal-sourced foods but is scarce in vegetarian and vegan diets.[58]

Another explanation for the inverse association between red meat intake and CVD incidence has been suggested by research showing that one type of gut bacteria associated with meat consumption can metabolise TMA – trimethylamine – and its precursors without producing TMAO, which is a type of gut bacteria that has been associated with inflammation. This means, say the researchers, that these bacteria are 'in effect severing a key link in the cardiovascular disease chain'.[59]

Having reviewed the evidence on meat consumption and health, Professor Alice Stanton maintains that eating moderate portions (around 120g) of red meat between two and four times a week appears to be protective against heart attacks, strokes and cancer,[60] and that adverse health impacts are only significantly associated with very excessive consumption of red meat (more than 120g per day or 900g per week).[61] Data on stunting rates (rates of impaired growth and development) around the world also suggest that meat has a positive impact on health.[62] The highest stunting rates correlate with those places where less meat is eaten, with as many as one in three children suffering. Although the link between meat consumption and stunting is only an association, the health benefits of meat are supported by an RCT, which tracked a group of Kenyan children over two years. It found that the children who were fed meat as part of their diet consistently outperformed the other children in terms of intellectual attainment and academic results.[63]

Still, old theories about saturated fat and meat die hard, and the fear of cholesterol remains acute, despite the evidence that has been thrown at it. In the next part of this chapter, I want to dig a little deeper into the topic of cholesterol: what it is, how it works, and why we shouldn't be afraid of it. But before we leave Dr Keys and his diet–heart hypothesis behind, it's worth remembering that although he was adamant that we should all be avoiding animal fats and foods, his nightly dinner ritual often included steak, chops and roasts. As early as 1954, says Dr Harcombe, Keys was recorded as having admitted that the evidence indicated that the cholesterol content of natural diets had no significant effect on either the cholesterol level or the development of atherosclerosis in man.[64] In the late 1970s Keys also publicly acknowledged that there may have been no basis to make the claim that trends in heart disease mortality in the US reflected changes in the consumption of any particular item of food.[65] And in the late 1980s he cast further doubt on his original hypothesis, stating, 'I have come to think that cholesterol is not as important as we used to think it was.'[66]

This admission came too late to save us from the impact of his original hypothesis, which had been enshrined in dietary policy since the publication of the 1977 McGovern report and given further credence by the so-called 1984 consensus conference. The message from that conference and the ensuing expert reports was that the benefits of low-fat diets were indisputable and that saturated fat was unwholesome, despite the fact that the evidence for these beliefs was already becoming progressively less compelling.[67]

New thinking about cholesterol

If Keys eventually conceded that cholesterol was perhaps *not as important* as he had once believed, genetic epidemiologist and author Tim Spector is less equivocal, stating that the idea that 'cholesterol in food was to blame for heart disease by increasing levels of cholesterol in the blood ... has been disproven, and no serious scientist believes it today'. Moreover, says Spector, 'no study has successfully shown that switching from a normal or high-fat diet to a low-fat or low-saturated fat diet can reduce heart disease or mortality'.[68] Dr Kendrick is less equivocal still. Stealing a phrase from *Blackadder*, he says that the diet–heart hypothesis 'is wronger than a very wrong thing'.[69] 'We have been sold a pup,' he says, 'and a rather large one at that.'

There are many hundreds of doctors and researchers who agree that the diet–heart–cholesterol hypothesis is bunk. Many keep their counsel, but others have spoken out and been stomped into silence. Some of those doctors and researchers who agree that the cholesterol hypothesis is bunk are members of an organisation called The International Network of Cholesterol Skeptics (THINCS). The members of this group 'represent different views about the causation of atherosclerosis and cardiovascular disease, [and] some of them are in conflict with others', but what they all oppose is that animal fat and cholesterol play a role.[70] The THINCS website is full to the brim of research about cholesterol, to be perused at your leisure should you be interested.

Here, I'm going to call upon the work of a biochemical engineer, Ivor Cummins, who now dedicates his life to exploring the science behind cholesterol and heart disease, and software engineer Dave Feldman, whose mission is to get to the bottom of the cholesterol story. What can engineers add to our understanding of cholesterol and the body? A lot. Engineers are systems-and-design thinkers who excel at identifying the root causes of problems. They are also experts at manipulating inputs and outputs so as to better understand data. Cummins and Feldman have used all these skills to turn the cholesterol story inside out.

Cummins first started to question conventional theories about cholesterol in 2012 when his own blood tests gave results that doctors were unable to explain. He realised that something was 'enormously wrong in the medical world'. By going back to all the relevant scientific papers and delving into the biochemistry he worked out that it was carbohydrate metabolism (the inability of the body to effectively process carbohydrates and convert them into energy) that was the problem and that 'we were all being told the wrong thing'.[71]

In his book, *Eat Rich, Live Long*, written with Dr Jeremy

Gerber, Cummins sets out to correct widespread misunderstanding about cholesterol. The first thing he urges us to appreciate is that cholesterol is vital for life. It is a critical building block for the many hormones that are central to the control systems of our bodies, a key part of the immune system, and central to the body's tissue-repair apparatus.[72] Without cholesterol, there would be no cell renewal, and no life.[73]

Nature has evolved ways for cholesterol to travel around the body – Gerber and Cummins call them 'boats'. These are lipoprotein particles: HDL (high-density lipoprotein) and LDL (low-density lipoprotein). There's a third carrier of cholesterol packed inside these lipoprotein particles: a type of fat called triglycerides. Too many triglycerides in the blood *is* a major issue, and the most common driver of these blood fats is excessive carbohydrate in the diet.

The small, dense form of LDL, called sdLDL, is the real bad boy in the cholesterol story: it's the result of LDL becoming distorted (oxidised) in an inflammatory environment. The best way to create that inflammatory environment and make your LDL turn into the sdLDL variety is to become insulin resistant. (I'll talk in more detail about insulin resistance later in this chapter.) As with triglycerides, carbohydrate intake plays a role here. (Nutritional psychiatrist Dr Georgia Ede writes, 'chances are: if you have "high cholesterol" you do not have a cholesterol problem – you have a carbohydrate problem'.[74])

If your LDL value is high, it might be that your blood is full of damaged LDL particles (sdLDL) that are inflaming your arteries. And this would be a cause for concern. On the other hand, it might not mean this at all. It's important to examine LDL in the context of other values – HDL, triglycerides, insulin levels and blood glucose – that provide indications as to whether or not your blood is full of sdLDL. Yet the vast majority of doctors draw meaning from LDL values alone. This is, say Cummins and Gerber, 'beyond tragic'.[75]

Tragic – and absurd. The absurdity of using LDL on its own as a measure of health is highlighted by a 2009 study of 137,000 people who presented in hospitals with vascular disease. More than 75 per cent of these atherosclerosis-afflicted people had LDL levels well below the average.[76] The reliability of LDL as a predictor of heart disease was further undermined by a study published in 2020 called 'Hit or Miss: the new cholesterol targets'. This review of thirty-five randomised controlled trials had shown that achieving new target levels of LDL (below 180 mg/dl)* 'did not confer any additional benefit'. In the press release for the study it was asserted that 'setting targets for "bad" (LDL) cholesterol levels to ward off heart disease and death in those at risk might seem intuitive, but decades of research have failed to show any consistent benefit for this approach'.[77]

Cummins and Gerber advocate the use of key ratios to assess risk and metabolic health instead of the simple LDL measure. The best of these ratios is triglycerides:HDL, which is 'vastly more predictive than the LDL value' on its own. This ratio should be below 1.2 or even 1.0.[78] The total cholesterol to HDL (total:HDL) ratio is also a good measure and should be lower than 5. The power of this ratio has been demonstrated again and again across many studies whereas LDL has been shown to be 'irrelevant by comparison'.[79]

Like Cummins, Dave Feldman has helped to shape a more nuanced understanding of LDL cholesterol. He began reverse-engineering cholesterol himself when he saw his own levels

---

* In the UK and much of Europe, cholesterol is measured in millimoles per litre of blood (mmol/L), whereas in the US it is measured in milligrams per decilitre (mg/dL). Current international guidelines for total and LDL cholesterol are as follows: Total cholesterol of 5.2mmol/L (200–239 mg/dL) is borderline high; >6.2mmol/L (240mg/dL) is high. For LDL, optimal is lower than 2.5mmol/L(100mg/dL), high is 4.1–4.8mmol/L (160–189mg/dL) and very high is over 4.9mmol/L (190mg/dL).

rising after adopting a low-carb lifestyle. Through a series of self-experiments he found that he could change his lipid levels substantially, and now many who follow his work have replicated this in kind. He suggests that this rise in cholesterol can be due to the fact that it 'ride shares' with the fat we use for fuel in the same protein carriers. He calls this the 'lipid energy model' and it is now widely discussed in the low-carb community. (You can find out more about this at his site, www.cholesterolcode.com.)

Feldman's model helps to explain why one might see LDL cholesterol rise when being 'fat adapted' (that is, burning fat for fuel, as one does on a low-carbohydrate diet). It also helps to explain why so many who follow a low-carb lifestyle can see their HDL rise and triglycerides fall. He regularly refers to this as the lipid 'triad' (high LDL-C, high HDL-C and low triglycerides) and points to studies showing that this combination is associated with a low risk of cardiovascular disease. A recent paper looked at 3,590 men and women from the Framingham Heart Study and found the odds ratio was nearly identical between the low- and high-LDL groups where HDL was high and triglycerides low.[80] Another paper with nearly three thousand participants from the Copenhagen Male Study concluded that men with conventional risk factors for IHD (ischemic heart disease), including an LDL level higher than 4.40mmol/L (which is 170 mg/dL) have a low risk of IHD if they have low TG (triglyceride) and high HDL-C levels.[81] In other words, a low triglycerides:HDL ratio is protective even in the presence of high LDL.

Dr Georgia Ede has written that the formerly simplistic way of thinking about cholesterol and heart disease is 'changing before our very eyes'.[82] There is a large and growing community of medical professionals around the world who subscribe to the more nuanced theories about cholesterol put forward by the likes of Cummins and Feldman, including cardiologist Dr

Aseem Malhotra, Professor Tim Noakes, Dr Robert Lustig, Dr Nadir Ali, Dr Eric Westman and Professor Ben Bikman. Type any of these names into YouTube and you will find a treasure trove of lectures explaining advanced thinking about cholesterol in layperson friendly terms. All these experts maintain that high LDL is not an issue in and of itself in the context of other indicators of metabolic health. LDL can indeed be raised by certain diets, such as low-carb high-fat, but those LDL levels tell you little about whether or not you're going to die of heart disease.[83]

Insulin resistance and metabolic syndrome: the bigger threats to health

In a 2012 paper Tim Noakes concluded that 'cholesterol is not an important risk factor for heart disease, and the current dietary recommendations do more harm than good'.[84] Cardiologist Dr Aseem Malhotra published a study in the *British Medical Journal* (*BMJ*) titled 'Saturated fat is not the major issue'.[85] If saturated fat and high LDL do not cause heart disease, what does? Many experts in the field are agreed that a major risk factor is insulin resistance, which is associated with metabolic syndrome. Dr Malhotra explained this in an interview with health and nutrition podcaster/filmmaker Brian Sanders:

> If you look at the web of causation of heart disease, insulin resistance is at the root of it. It's number one. And most cardiologists do not know this. And the best way to explain it, in terms of a cluster of risk factors, is metabolic syndrome. So, if you have any three of high triglycerides, low HDL cholesterol, increased waist circumference, pre-diabetes or type-2 [diabetes], and hypertension, that is basically metabolic syndrome.[86]

In his book, *A Statin Free Life*, Dr Malhotra refers to the research (considered on page 42) showing that while 75 per cent of people admitted to hospital with heart disease have normal cholesterol and lower than average LDL levels, 66 per cent 'fulfilled criteria for having insulin resistance syndrome, known among medical professionals as "metabolic syndrome"'.[87] 'Optimising metabolic health is the best way to reduce heart disease and heart attacks,' he says.

Insulin resistance

What is insulin resistance? Simply put, it is a condition whereby blood levels of insulin are raised and the insulin doesn't work as well.[88] Dr David Harper, research scientist with the BC Cancer Research Centre in Vancouver, views insulin resistance as one of three points on an 'axis of illness', the other two being obesity and inflammation. These three things are closely linked to one another, and together they could be responsible for 70 per cent of chronic disease, including cardiovascular disease, cancer, diabetes and Alzheimer's.[89] In his book, *Why We Get Sick*, Professor Ben Bikman puts forward a similar case. He explains that insulin resistance is implicated in many conditions, including heart disease, brain and neurological disorders, reproductive ill-health, cancer, ageing and skin disorders, gastrointestinal disorders, metabolic syndrome and obesity.[90]

As early as 2001, research established insulin resistance as a predictor of age-related diseases. A study published in the *Journal of Clinical Endocrinology & Metabolism* found that insulin resistance was an independent predictor of all clinical events (such as hypertension, diabetes, heart disease and cancer), and that age-related clinical events developed in one out of three individuals with high levels of insulin resistance (at the start of the study), whereas no clinical events were observed in those who were not insulin resistant.[91]

GPs in the UK are gradually waking up to the importance of insulin and insulin resistance. At a gathering of UK GPs and other health practitioners that I attended in 2020[92] all were in agreement that insulin resistance was a root cause of metabolic syndrome, commonly manifested as obesity and type-2 diabetes. 'The trouble is, we've missed the damage that insulin does because we haven't been measuring it,' said one GP. Indeed, insulin levels are rarely measured. The ratio between triglycerides and HDL (trig:HDL), which, as we discovered earlier, has been shown to be vastly more predictive of heart attack risk than the LDL value, is sometimes noted, but has not displaced LDL as the primary measure of metabolic health used by general practitioners and cardiologists.[93]

Cummins and Gerber posit several reasons for this; significant among them is the fact that no patented drugs have been shown to work to impact the key ratios. What *does* work is changing the diet to lower your ingestion of carbohydrates, but no drug company is going to make money from people pursuing a diet-based strategy to improve their metabolic health.

On the other hand, drug companies do make money – lots of it – from selling statins. Pfizer's Lipitor alone earned nearly two billion dollars of revenue in 2019, and prior to patent loss in 2011 it was earning north of ten billion dollars a year.[94] With the threshold for diagnosing high cholesterol getting ever lower,[95] it will not be long before every human on the planet will meet the criteria for taking a daily cholesterol pill. We are already seeing policy moving in this direction, with calls to prescribe statins to children,[96] and the National Institute for Health and Care Excellence (NICE) recommending that statins automatically be made available to all patients with a 10 per cent risk of having a heart attack. Many clinicians, including Dr Malhotra, believe this is wrong.

Statins: how effective are they?

The evidence for the efficacy of statins to prevent heart attacks and deaths from heart disease is far less conclusive than the public has been led to believe. Even the study that was heralded as having provided definitive proof that more people should be taking statins – the British Heart Foundation's Heart Protection Study (HPS) – delivered no such proof. In 2004, the lead investigator on this study, Sir Rory Collins, said that the HPS 'shows unequivocally that statins can produce substantial benefit in a very much wider range of high-risk people than had been thought . . . If, now, as a result, an extra 10 million high risk people were to go onto a statin treatment, this would save about 50,000 lives a year.'[97]

But how impressive a result is this, really? Ten million people must take a drug to benefit 50,000? That's one person in 200 who's life will be 'saved'. But that person's life won't in fact be saved: death will merely be postponed, and not for very long. As Dr Kendrick points out, it would be more accurate to state that 'if ten million people (at very high risk of heart disease) took a statin for a year they would all live on average two days longer'.[98]

Another study came to a similar conclusion as Dr Kendrick. Statins do not benefit many people very much. For primary prevention (people who have not yet had a heart attack), the median postponement of death was 3.2 days (during the period of the trial). For secondary prevention (people who have already had one heart attack), the median postponement of death was 4.1 days.[99]

Dr Malhotra asserts that 'the overwhelming majority of patients taking a statin with heart disease, or who have suffered a heart attack, will receive no benefit whatsoever'. The NNT (number needed to treat) data illustrates why. 'For those with heart disease, taking a statin every day for 5 years results in a 1-in-39 chance of preventing a non-fatal heart attack and a 1-in-83 chance of delaying death. So the NNT for statins in those with heart disease is 39 for preventing a non-fatal heart attack and 83 for preventing or delaying death.'[100] In other words, eighty-three people need to be treated in order for one to benefit in terms of delaying death.

Such limited benefits in terms of life extension might be acceptable if statins were harmless drugs. But they are not. Statins interfere with the body's ability to produce cholesterol, thus reducing the amount of cholesterol available for the body to use.[101] They may also disable something called the mevalonate pathway, without which human cells cannot rejuvenate properly, as proposed in a book by James and Hannah Yoseph titled *How Statin Drugs Lower Cholesterol: And Kill You One Cell at a Time*.[102] The possible immediate side effects of this include balance issues, severe muscle pain and memory loss.

The fine print of the leaflet for a leading statin, Lipitor, says that the more common side effects might affect 10 per cent of people,[103] but anecdotal evidence suggests that this is an understatement. Dr Malhotra has accused NICE of siding with the drug companies and relying on industry-sponsored statistics, which consistently under-report the risk of side effects.[104]

Health campaigner Marion Holman first began investigating the effects of statins when her father, who'd been prescribed Lipitor, suffered rapid memory loss, balance issues and acute muscle pain. She read every independent study and book on the topic and joined two Facebook forums, Side Effects of Lipitor and Atorvastatin, and Stopped Our Statins. She felt as though she had opened Pandora's box: 'Hundreds of forum members suffering in just the same way as my father. Some had more severe damage which led to necrotizing myopathy. Others had the same memory loss issues and balance problems, and several had more severe autoimmune diseases, such as Parkinson's disease, ALS (Motor Neurone Disease), Lupus, and Rheumatoid Arthritis.'[105]

The types of concerns raised by Marion Holman led Fiona Godlee, editor-in-chief of the *BMJ*, to call for independent third-party scrutiny of the statins trial data. Godlee cited Richard Lehman, who wrote that adverse effects of statins are much more common than the trials suggest and that 'muscle pain and fatigability are not a figment of misattribution and public misinformation . . . they are too prevalent and recurrent in people who desperately want to stay on statins'.[106]

In addition to these commonly noted side effects, a number of meta-analyses have demonstrated an association between statin therapy and diabetes, although causality has not yet been proven. What is known is that statin therapy can cause significant increases in both blood glucose and blood insulin levels.[107]

But the most insidious side effect of statins could well be the false sense of security that they provide. Many will think that by reducing their LDL with statin therapy they are taking the most effective action (or even the only necessary action) to prevent a heart attack and will be disincentivised from taking more impactful measures to improve their underlying metabolic health. Why bother to lose that spare tyre or address an insulin resistance problem with a low-carbohydrate diet and exercise when you can simply take a pill to reduce your LDL level and get a gold star from your doctor?

In November 2020, a study published in the *New England Journal of Medicine* (*NEMJ*) poured cold water on the idea that the side effects of statins were serious, claiming that 90 per cent of the side effects reported could be explained by what they called the nocebo effect – that is, they're all in the mind. People expect to experience side effects, therefore they do. The study was found to be seriously flawed, however, as was pointed out by three doctors who wrote to the *NEMJ*.

The study's small sample size (49) and extensive exclusion criteria served to limit the applicability of its findings for the general population. (An in-depth discussion of this study can be found at www.zoeharcombe.com.)[108]

Pharmaceutical companies have every reason to play down the harm that statins can do, while continuing to promote the cholesterol hypothesis and, in particular, the demonisation of LDL. LDL is what statins are designed to lower, therefore LDL must be regarded as a thing to be feared. Those who question the link between LDL and heart disease and the efficacy of statins are pressured to conform. Take, for example, the publication (in 2019) by the *Mail on Sunday* of an article in which it was claimed that Drs Harcombe, Malhotra and Kendrick were 'statin deniers' (as opposed to, say, doctors with an alternative point of view) peddling 'deadly propaganda' (rather than, say, alternative interpretations of the data) about cholesterol and statins. The article cited a joint open letter from the editors-in-chief of thirty major heart journals (all cardiologists) who claimed that lives were at stake due to the 'wanton spread of misinformation'. It suggested that the doctors were conspiracy theorists, and addressed only a small amount of the (extensive) evidence that they have amassed, failing, for example, to explain why Dr Harcombe's analysis of WHO data for 192 countries had found higher cholesterol – not lower cholesterol – to be associated with lower rates of death.[109]

It is not unreasonable to wonder whether dissent is discouraged partly because pharmaceutical companies – and the scientists whose research they fund – have an obvious interest in the perpetuation of the notion that LDL is a problem requiring treatment with statins. Another factor is the intransigence built into the medical system: health agencies have invested money in, and staked reputations on, the diet–heart hypothesis and the ensuing anti-saturated fat, anti-cholesterol messaging, and they cannot change their tune without losing face. Moreover, outdated notions are not easily relinquished by ordinary doctors. Those who have not kept up with the latest research, or who are too busy or afraid to challenge the status quo, continue to dispense the same old advice. The US doctor Ken Berry, author of *Lies My Doctor Told Me*, describes this with reference to what he calls the eggs-are-bad-for-you lie:

> Even after researchers had quietly backed away from the eggs-are-bad-for-you lie, it kept getting repeated by the media and doctors for years. When the scientists and most of the media (but not all) had stopped telling this lie, it was still repeated by primary care doctors, spouses, parents and know-it-all neighbours for many more years. To this day, I still have the occasional patient who will argue with me that eggs are full of cholesterol.[110]

Outdated theories and the war on animal foods

All those primary-care doctors, spouses, parents and know-it-all neighbours spouting outdated theories, emboldened by erroneous reporting by large sections of the media and flawed notions of healthy eating, such as the Eatwell Guide, have led us to where we find ourselves today: in the midst of a war on meat and other animal foods. Most people still believe that LDL cholesterol is inherently bad, and that eating meat, dairy and saturated animal fats contribute directly to high LDL. It is not uncommon to hear journalists and plant-based advocates calling upon that tired old image of arteries clogged with saturated fat to make their point, or extolling the virtues of this or that plant-based food on the basis that it has less cholesterol and saturated fat than the animal food equivalent.

Let's recap here, because there's been a lot to take in: the diet–heart hypothesis has been roundly rejected by many within the medical community. Most of the evidence used to support it has consisted of epidemiological studies with weak associations. High LDL cholesterol, on its own, has been shown to be a poor predictor of risk for heart disease, and the widespread prescription of statins to reduce LDL, while lucrative for the drug companies, has not been proven to be warranted – certainly, there are many in the medical profession who question it. What we should be concerned about is insulin resistance, a condition far more likely to be improved by reduced carbohydrate intake than by the avoidance of the cholesterol and saturated fat in meat and other animal foods.

If cholesterol and saturated fat do not constitute good reasons to avoid meat and other animal foods, you might still be wondering about the other big charge against these foods: that they cause cancer. We'll look at this charge now.

Meat and cancer: does the evidence stack up?

A 1997 report by the World Cancer Research Fund (WCRF) and the American Institute of Cancer Research concluded that there is neither 'convincing' nor 'probable' reason to believe that fat-rich diets increase the risk of cancer. A decade later Arthur Schatzkin, chief of the nutritional epidemiology branch at the National Cancer Institute, told Gary Taubes that the accumulated results from the trials designed to test the hypothesis (linking fat intake to cancer) were 'largely null'.[111]

This message is entirely lost amidst the content of a website often referenced by plant-based advocates on social media: eatingourfuture.com. The site lists hundreds of studies and opinion pieces about the harm to health caused by saturated fat and meat, with cancer being high on the list of the alleged side effects of a meat-rich diet. Just looking at the sheer volume of articles might be enough to make you clear your freezer of meat and adopt a plant-based diet post-haste. But these studies and articles are reliant on the same type of weak epidemiology as that used to justify the diet–heart hypothesis, with tiny hazard ratios well below two. (Remember that thirty-fold risk of contracting lung cancer if you were a smoker? It makes a risk of 1.2 look like a mere blip in the data, or, what Dr David Klurfeld has called, 'noise in the system'.)

Tiny hazard ratios are just one of many problems with the research concerning meat and cancer. A team of researchers led by Mina Händel reviewed the evidence base relating to processed meat and cancer and concluded that 'there are severe methodological limitations to the majority of the previously published systematic reviews and meta-analyses that examined the consumption of processed meat and the risk of cancer' and that 'the primary studies included in the reviews had the potential risk for the misclassification of exposure, a serious risk of bias due to confounding, a moderate to serious risk of bias due to missing data, and/or a moderate to serious risk of selection of the reported results'. All of these factors, they said, 'may have potentially led to the overestimation of the risk related to processed meat intake across all cancer outcomes'.[112]

Several studies by Professor Walter Willett, chair of the Department of Nutrition at the Harvard School of Public Health from 1991 to 2017 (and a well-known advocate of vegetarian diets), are referenced at eatingourfuture.com. One of them, 'Dietary protein sources in early adulthood and breast cancer incidence: prospective cohort study',[113] was published in the *BMJ* in 2014 and was still doing the rounds on Twitter in 2020, despite its having many methodological flaws and showing only very weak associations between red meat intake in early adulthood and breast cancer.

Professor Willett's work is frequently cited by other researchers seeking to build the case linking animal proteins to cancer. The authors of a study published in the *Journal of the American Heart Association* in February 2021 ('Association of Major Dietary Protein Sources With All-Cause and Cause-Specific Mortality: Prospective Cohort Study') referenced six of Willett's studies, including the *BMJ* study noted above, in their introduction.[114] The authors went on to conclude that 'a higher plant protein intake and substitution of animal protein with plant-protein were associated with lower risk of all-cause mortality, CVD mortality, and dementia mortality' and that nuts are a healthy alternative to red meat, eggs, dairy products and legumes. (The Mail Online reported the study results under the headline 'High protein vegan diet can slash the risk of early death in older women by almost 50%'.[115]) There are many reasons to be cautious about the conclusions of this study, including the fact that it failed to account for differences in carbohydrate intake and the fact that the FFQs (food frequency questionnaires) used were deemed, by the authors, to be less than 60 per cent accurate when tested against actual food intake. As with many studies of its type, it relied on relative risk numbers, rather than absolute risk, and even the relative risks (as represented by hazard ratios) were very low indeed: of 180 hazard ratios associating the levels of consumption of different plant and animal protein sources with all-cause and specific mortality rates, there was not a single hazard ratio above 1.23 or below .77, and most hovered close to 1.0. (A hazard ratio of 1.0 signifies no association; a ratio above 1.0 signifies an increased risk, and a ratio below 1.0 signifies a decreased risk.) Moreover, the various hazard ratios did not increase or decrease consistently or logically between different levels of consumption of each type of protein. For example, eating a small amount of red meat was deemed to increase the risk of dying from cancer by 1.02, but eating a very large amount had no effect on cancer mortality at all; similarly the hazard ratio pertaining to chicken consumption and CVD mortality was lower at the highest level of consumption (0.99) than it was at the lowest level of consumption (1.02).

Most astonishing of all, in a study claiming that substituting animal protein with plant protein would reduce the risk of mortality was the following statement (not found in the abstract): 'After adjustment for age, race/ethnicity, socioeconomic status, dietary and lifestyles factors, and baseline and family history of diseases, animal protein intake was *not* associated with all-cause or cause specific mortality, comparing the highest with the lowest quintile.' (Italics mine.) In other words, the amount of animal protein eaten, whether it is a little or a lot, has no effect on your risk of dying from any cause or from the specific causes studied (CVD, cancer and dementia).

All of the complex substitution analysis (a theoretical substitution of nuts for meat, or legumes for eggs, for example) carried out by the researchers, which served to generate the study's reported conclusions and the media headlines, could not erase or explain these two basic findings – animal food consumption is not associated with higher mortality and eating more plants in place of animal foods will not reduce your risk of dying of cancer. Stuck for a definitive explanation the authors noted that 'dietary proteins are not consumed in isolation, so that *interpretation of the findings could be difficult* and should be based on the overall diet'. (Italics mine.) This and other acknowledged limitations of the study did not prevent the popular press from reporting on the study's results as though they constituted irrevocable proof that a plant-based diet is a sure-fire route to longevity.

This study on protein sources and disease will likely make

its way to eatingyourfuture.com to sit alongside all the other studies with weak hazard ratios and glaring inconsistencies that plant-based advocates often use to bolster the case against animal foods. But what the study *actually* tells us, despite newspaper headlines to the contrary, is that the health risks from eating animal proteins are insignificant. Given that the study was based on a re-analysis of data from the Women's Health Initiative, this is not surprising. Previous analysts of WHI data found that those who were eating what most would consider to be a healthy diet – low in fat, high in fruits, vegetables and whole grains – had no less breast cancer than those who ate a typical American diet. As Gary Taubes has pointed out, not only was this result significant, but it 'confirmed those of every study that had been done on breast cancer since 1982'.[116]

How statistics can mislead

Like many others involved in nutrition research, the researchers involved in the 'Association of Major Dietary Protein Sources' study are not making intentionally false statements, but the statistics emerging from their studies can nevertheless mislead. Peter Attia MD calls this kind of research 'a kind of unwitting chicanery; interpreting and promulgating statistics in a manner that often exaggerates associations, making things appear more meaningful than they are ... the statistic allows one to be truthful, but at the risk of fooling people.'[117]

Many of us are both fooled and confused by the daily onslaught of articles that make the results of studies appear more meaningful than they are. In a now famous 2018 article, Professor John Ioannidis illustrated the absurdity of taking the reported results of such studies at face value:

Assuming the meta-analysed evidence from cohort studies represents lifespan-long causal associations, for a baseline expectancy of 80 years, eating 12 hazelnuts daily (1oz) would prolong life by 12 years (i.e., 1 year per hazelnut), drinking 3 cups of coffee daily would achieve a similar gain of 12 extra years, and eating a single mandarin orange (80g) daily would add 5 years of life. Conversely, consuming 1 egg daily would reduce life expectancy by 6 years, and eating 2 slices of bacon (30g) daily would shorten life by a decade, an effect worse than smoking.[118]

A *Times* editorial later cautioned against the naive interpretation of studies in the context of one that purported to show that swapping meat for nuts could cut your risk of dying of a heart attack by 17 per cent:

> other reports in recent years have suggested that the risk [of dying of a heart attack] can also be reduced by statins, drinking the right amount of coffee, losing weight, beta blockers, aspirin, gene therapy, fibre, fruit and vegetables, ghee, more testosterone, less testosterone, moving to a warmer climate, having cold baths, dark chocolate, tea, folic acid, omega-3 fatty acids, not living in Scotland, losing weight, being religious, having a dog, laughing, exercise, sleep, stopping drinking, drinking red wine, and stopping drinking altogether. Simple logic suggests that doing all of these things at once, if it were possible, would reduce the risk by several hundred per cent.[119]

The inanity of weak observational science – and the media headlines on which it is based – is thus laid bare. A strategy for cutting through the inanity is suggested by Dr Attia. Regarding epidemiological (observational) studies that come to his attention, he says, 'the first thing I do is look at the strength of the association. If it's less than 2, I ditch it (with very rare exceptions). Most studies meet this ditchable criteria.' [120]

Like Peter Attia, researchers Frédéric Leroy and Nathan Cofnas urge caution when interpreting studies delivering hazard ratios below 2, pointing out that 'such low RR (Relative Risk) levels in isolation would not be treated as strong evidence in most epidemiological research outside nutrition'.[121] 'It is not good practice,' say the authors, 'to infer a causal connection to meat-eating from such weak and confounded associational data.' Observational data should be viewed only as hypothesis generating, particularly 'when results are so counterintuitive, as is the case for meat-eating, given its long record as an essential food within our species-adapted diet'.[122]

As consumers of research studies, we need to be alert to the ways we can be misled. This is true even when the research is carried out by esteemed institutions we might wish to regard as the ultimate authorities, the WHO being no exception.

The WHO's verdict on meat and cancer: a case of bad science amplified

In 2015 a twenty-two-strong working group within the WHO's International Agency for Research on Cancer (IARC) completed an evaluation of the carcinogenic risk to humans of red and processed meat consumption. The working group took into consideration all the relevant data showing a positive association between consumption of red meat and cancer. Looking at the studies involving humans, they concluded that 'there is *limited* evidence in humans for the carcinogenicity of the consumption of red meat' and that 'there is *sufficient* evidence in human beings for the carcinogenicity of the consumption of processed meat'. Looking at the studies based on animal experiments, they concluded that 'there is *inadequate* evidence in experimental animals for the carcinogenicity of consumption of red meat and *of processed meat*'[123] (all italics mine). Despite the profusion of limiteds and inadequates, the working group produced a summary report in which it was claimed that the 'consumption of red meat is probably carcinogenic to humans' and that the 'consumption of processed meat *is* carcinogenic to humans'.[124]

The leap from the assessments of the evidence to the overall conclusions is baffling. What's worse, the authors placed processed meat in Group 1 of known carcinogenic substances, alongside tobacco and asbestos, a fact that was widely reported in newspapers across the world.[125] In a Q&A paper, the WHO explained that 'this [classification] does NOT mean that they are all equally dangerous'.[126] But this Q&A paper did little to publicly clarify matters. The more dramatic proclamations made headlines worldwide and had a major impact on how people think about meat and health.

Medical professionals and scientists came forth to critique the WHO findings, emphasising that the statistical risks associated with eating red and processed meat are very small. The day after the WHO report came out, Dr Harcombe wrote an article pointing out its many weaknesses, including the facts that it was based mostly on observational studies that had deployed unreliable dietary questionnaires, had failed to account for confounding variables, and had greatly overstated the risks by using relative rather than absolute risks numbers (see page 26).[127] One of the founders of the GRADE system issued a public warning that the scientific case against red meat by the IARC panel of the WHO had been overstated, doing 'the public a disservice'.[128]

Nutritional psychiatrist Dr Georgia Ede dug deep into the WHO–IARC report to expose its many weaknesses. (Among

them is the fact that it relies heavily on epidemiological studies, which are 'not experimental and should not be viewed
as conclusive evidence'.[129]) She concluded that 'the WHO
report is not a scientific document. It is a political document.
Politicians can get away with making sweeping statements to
the general public that stand on shaky ground. Scientists are
held to a higher standard. They are supposed to show their
work and defend their positions as objectively and honestly
as possible. After reading the studies upon which the WHO's
anti-meat proclamations are made, I concluded that there
is simply no scientific evidence that meat causes cancer in
humans.'[130]

Dr Ede pointed out that she was not alone in this view.
Twenty-three cancer experts from eight countries had previously gathered in Norway to examine the science related to
colon cancer and red/processed meat (the very same science
that the WHO had considered) and concluded that the data
was inconsistent and the underlying mechanisms linking meat
to cancer were unclear.

Dr Ede proceeded to detail the many failings of the WHO–
IARC report.[131] (Thirty minutes spent reading her critique,
'WHO says meat causes cancer?' at www.diagnosisdiet.com,
would be a good investment of your time.) Her bottom-line
assessment was this:

the only plausible evidence to suggest that red meat might
be risky to human colon health is contained in two, that's
two, human studies, both of which were very small and
poorly designed, and therefore unable to give us useful
information about the effects of red meat on cancer risk.
These studies are inconclusive at best, and worthless at
worst ... trumpeting to the world that meat causes cancer
on the basis of these two studies is ridiculously irresponsible
and makes a mockery of the WHO.

Dr David Klurfeld, national programme leader for human nutrition at the Agricultural Research Service of the USDA, served on the IARC committee that reviewed the research and delivered the anti-meat conclusions. He described the experience as 'the most frustrating professional experience' of his life, revealing that its conclusions were based on extremely poor science. Although the committee claimed to have based its conclusions on eight hundred studies, only eighteen studies were actually considered. Only twelve of the eighteen studies concluded that there was a risk associated with processed meat, and just seven out of fourteen studies looking at red meat showed a risk associated with eating red meat. 'And the risk is only an association,' Dr Klurfeld reminds us. The committee declined to consider two important clinical trials put forward by Dr Klurfeld (one study by the National Cancer Institute and the WHI study mentioned earlier in this chapter) that had shown red meat and saturated fat intake to be unassociated with the incidence of cancer. And the relative risks shown by the associational studies that the committee did consider were too small to be significant.[132] A 'significant number of us did not agree' (with the committee's conclusions) says Dr Klurfeld. 'It was essentially a majority vote.'

Echoing the view of Dr Attia, Dr Klurfeld maintains that it is impossible to say with any certainty that any particular foods or diets can cause cancer because most studies show extremely small risks. 'With risks of 1.1 or 1.2, you can't be confident if that's a real risk or noise in the system, and you certainly can't ascribe it [the risk] to a single factor,' he has said. (There are rare exceptions. The risks associated with eating mouldy corn or peanuts, for example, has been associated with six times the risk of stomach and liver cancer.)[133]

The researchers who published their reviews in the *Annals of Internal Medicine* would reach the same conclusion as those who were critical of the WHO report, namely that the evidence linking meat consumption to heart disease and cancer is insufficient to warrant telling people to cut back on meat.[134] Similarly, Leroy and Cofnas have asserted that 'the current epidemiological and mechanistic data have not been able to demonstrate a consistent causal link between red meat intake and chronic diseases, such as colorectal cancer'.[135]

That there is no reliable, conclusive evidence that meat is bad for us should come as no surprise. Meat is an old-fashioned food, part of the human diet for millions of years. As Surgeon Captain Peter Cleave, a former director of Royal Navy medical research, is reported to have said, 'For a modern disease to be related to an old-fashioned food is one of the most ludicrous things I have ever heard in my life.' Dr Klurfeld says you have 'everybody lining up and saying ... meat's killing us, from all of these different directions. It's really not plausible, if you think about it objectively. We've been eating meat since before we became humans. Meat contributed, it's thought by anthropologists, to our becoming humans.'[136]

There is plenty of evidence not only that eating meat is what made us human, but that it still plays a vital role in sustaining human health. This is why it really matters when weak evidence is amplified to discourage us from eating it, as one team of researchers led by Marije Oostindjer has warned:

Strong media coverage and ambiguous research results could stimulate consumers to adapt [sic] a 'safety first' strategy that could result in abolishment of red meat from the diet completely. However, there are reasons to keep red meat in the diet. Red meat (beef in particular) is a nutrient dense food and typically has a better ratio of N6:N3 poly-unsaturated fatty acids and significantly more vitamin A, B6 and B12, zinc and iron than white meat ... iron deficiencies are still common in parts of both developing and industrialised countries, particularly pre-school children and women of childbearing age … red meat also contains high levels of carnitine, coenzyme Q10, and creatine, which are bioactive compounds that may have positive effects on health.[137]

Of those who tried Veganuary and intend to keep up plant-based eating for the foreseeable future, how many are aware of these facts about vitamins, minerals, fatty acids, carnitine and creatine? Likely too few, but the facts are there for the taking. Which leads us nicely on to the next chapter: a discussion of the relative nutritional value of plant-based and omnivore diets.

2

The Nutritional Scorecard – Plants Versus Animal Foods

Among the well-known health and nutrition experts whose work I consulted while doing research for this book are a number of former vegetarians who were prompted to become omnivores when they started digging into research about nutrition. Nina Teicholz recalls having her view of food and health turned upside down once she started the research for her book *The Big Fat Surprise*. 'You suddenly realise that everything you believed to be true is just a house of cards,' she said.[1] Dr Zoë Harcombe remembers having a light-bulb moment during a talk about nutrition given by the Weston A. Price Foundation. She texted her husband to say that she would be coming home a meat eater.[2] Chris Kresser and Chris Masterjohn favoured plant-based diets until research, undertaken partly to resolve personal health issues, convinced them that their own health would be better served by an omnivore diet.

The more vociferous among today's plant-based advocates, on the other hand, seem to be impervious to both the facts about nutrition, and the recounted experience of those whose health has suffered from years spent avoiding animal foods, continuing to promote the health benefits of a diet that is based entirely on plants. In a recent interview with a BBC journalist, senior researcher of environmental sustainability and public health at Oxford University (and a vegan) Marco Springmann asserted that, 'we've found that the vegan diet could be one of the healthiest diets ... the vegan diet is higher in fruit, vegetables and legumes and the health benefits of these compensate [for] anything else'.[3] The reader was left in the dark as to what the 'anything else' might be and whether it was a cause for concern. Moreover, Springmann failed to cite a single study to support his bold assertion.

The fact is that few reliable studies have been done, and those that have been done cannot be viewed as being definitive. According to Faidon Magkos, associate professor at Copenhagen's Department of Nutrition, Exercise and Sports, most available studies are purely observational (that is, epidemiological) and have failed to account for the fact that vegans tend to exercise more, and smoke and drink less, and that these factors might make vegan diets appear to be better for health than they actually are.[4] (When data pertaining to Seventh-day Adventists – who neither smoke nor drink alcohol – is omitted, for example, the beneficial associations of vegetarian diets with cardiovascular health are less pronounced or are absent.[5]) Professor Magkos states that 'there are still uncertainties around the vegan diet, particularly when it comes to long term effects'.[6]

One large-scale randomised clinical trial (RCT) that can shed light on the question of whether a plant-based diet is better than an omnivore diet is the aforementioned Women's Health Study. This eight-year study of almost 50,000 women found that those who ate more fruit, vegetables and grains and less fat experienced *no significant reduction* in coronary heart disease (CHD), stroke or cardiovascular disease (CVD).[7]

Even Michael Pollan, who has written extensively (and beautifully) about food, and who brought us the mantra 'Eat food. Not too much. Mostly plants' (*In Defence of Food*), was unable to summon much convincing evidence that eating 'mostly plants' is better for us. He wrote that while scientists might disagree about what's so good about eating plants 'they do agree that plants are *probably* really good for you' (italics mine).[8]

Award-winning science journalist and author Gary Taubes, commenting on the notion that we should be eating 'mostly plants', said that 'we have no meaningful clinical trial evidence to support this idea'.[9] Yet people believe it, he said, 'and Pollan argues for it, not because they have compelling experimental evidence (i.e., clinical trial results) that it is true, and not because they've seen obese and diabetic patients switch from omnivorous or meat-rich diets (without sugar and food-like substances) to mostly or all-plant diets (without sugar and food-like substances) and get healthier for doing so, but because they, well, all seem to believe it. This is what cognitive psychologists would call a "cascade" or "groupthink", and it's exceedingly common in this kind of soft science.'[10]

The nutrition question

If there is a scarcity of clinical evidence in favour of diets that are either 'mostly' or 'all' plants, how should we evaluate these diets? One way is to look at how plant-based diets deliver on the key nutrients that humans need to survive and thrive.

There have been many attempts to evaluate and compare the nutrient density of different foods, some of them documented by Adam Drewnowski in the *American Journal of Clinical Nutrition* in 2005.[11] He found most of them to be flawed. Four years after writing this critique of previous scoring systems, Drewnowski put forward another approach, based on the Nutrient Rich Foods (NRF) index.[12] The data generated by this approach was used to create a bubble chart that made the rounds on Twitter in 2019, lauded by vegans as showing that plant foods were the hands-down winners in the nutrition stakes. Fruit and vegetables were way over on the right of the chart (high nutrients-to-calories ratio) whereas meat, fish and dairy were placed much further to the left (lower nutrients-to-calories ratio).

The NRF index has its limitations, however. It is based on nine nutrients to encourage in the diet (protein, fibre, vitamins A, C and E, calcium, iron, potassium and magnesium) and three nutrients to limit (saturated fat, added sugar and sodium). Having read Chapter 1, you've probably spotted the first problem: saturated fat is deemed to be an anti-nutrient, despite the evidence that our bodies need it, and that it could be better for us than the polyunsaturated variety found in seed oils. (I will discuss the problems with seed oils in Chapter 4.) Moreover, the list of nine nutrients considered excludes many critical nutrients, including vitamin B12, vitamin D, vitamin K and omega-3. Had these nutrients been factored in, that bubble chart would have flipped.

A more recent study by Professor Dariush Mozaffarian and colleagues at Tufts University[13] featured the Food Compass nutrient profiling system (an extensive critique of which can be found at www.zoeharcombe.com[14]). The system ranked over 8,000 foods, giving them scores between 1 (least healthy) and 100 (most healthy). Alarm bells rang for me – and for many others – on seeing that a cereal had scored 100, and that meat, poultry and eggs, as a group, scored just 32.7 and were deemed to be less healthy than beverages. A number of the choices and assumptions underlying the model were also concerning: by measuring nutrients per 100 calories, placing artificially fortified foods on a par with foods naturally high in nutrients, deciding not to differentiate between the forms of nutrients best absorbed by the body and less bioavailable versions (of which much more later), and deeming saturated fat to be less healthy than unsaturated fat, the researchers had skewed the system against meat, poultry and eggs and in favour of plants.

Another recent study, conducted by GAIN (the Global Alliance for Improved Nutrition, launched at the UN in 2002), generated different conclusions by focusing on a different set of nutrients and taking the saturated fat factor out of the equation. GAIN looked at the calories and grams of different foods that are required to deliver an average of one-third of the recommended intakes of six nutrients deemed essential for optimal health (folate, calcium, iron, zinc and vitamins A and B12). The study concluded that the 'top sources of priority nutrients are organs, small fish, dark leafy vegetables, bivalves [a type of mollusc], crustaceans, beef, goat, eggs, milk, cheese, and canned fish with bones. Lamb, mutton, goat milk, and pork are also good sources, and to a lesser extent, yoghurt, fresh fish, pulses and teff [a type of grain].'[15] Of the twenty foods mentioned, seventeen are from animal sources. Many of the foods deemed to be of moderate or low nutrient density are whole grains, seeds, nuts and root vegetables, all of which must be consumed in enormous quantities to meet the criteria of delivering one-third of the RDAs for the six nutrients. (For whole grains, for example, one must consume 803 grams, at a calorie cost of 1640!)

What this quick tour through a handful of nutrient profiling systems should tell you is that the assumptions underlying any system and the nutrients selected for measurement matter very much and can skew an outcome in one way or another. Profiling systems cannot tell us everything, and sometimes they can even tell us the wrong thing. How, then, can we gain a better understanding of how different foods impact human health? And by that I mean, how they *actually* impact human health as opposed to how they have been associated with broad health outcomes in epidemiological studies. We need to dive in and get granular.

The basics of nutrition

Let's get some essential nutrition terminology out of the way. Human diets must provide both macronutrients and micronutrients. There are three macronutrients (four if you count water): proteins, fats and carbohydrates. There are many more micronutrients, including both fat-soluble vitamins (such as A and D) and water-soluble vitamins (such as B12 and C), in addition to more than fifteen minerals (including iron and magnesium).

Proteins (one of the three macronutrients) provide nine essential amino acids (EAAs). Fats provide two essential fatty acids, omega-3 (omega-3 EPA and omega-3 DHA) and omega-6 (linoleic acid). Both proteins and fats contain essential nutrients, however, according to the USDA, 'the lower limit of dietary carbohydrate compatible with life apparently is zero, provided that adequate amounts of protein and fat are consumed'.[16] This is an important fact to hang on to when we dig into the topic of carbohydrates in Chapter 5.

Another term that's critical to any evaluation of the nutritional quality of any particular diet is *bioavailability* (variously referred to as digestibility, absorption or conversion). Even though a food might contain a high amount of a certain nutrient that does not mean that our bodies have full access to that nutrient.

Armed with this basic understanding, we can look at animal foods and plant foods with a critical eye, assessing how much nutrition they deliver. In 2014, Dr Harcombe undertook such an analysis, looking specifically at five highly nutritious foods, three animal foods (chicken liver, sardines and eggs) and two plant foods (sunflower seeds and kale). When combined, these five foods would provide all the nutrients that an individual needs and could therefore be considered to be a complete diet.[17] She compared them in terms of their provision of essential fatty acids, complete protein (that is, containing all EAAs), twelve vitamins, and eight minerals. For eleven of the twenty-three nutrients considered, one or another of the plant foods delivers the highest level per 100g. For the other twelve, the animal foods deliver the highest level. Critically, the combination of animal and plant foods is what delivers the full nutritional profile.

Dr Harcombe went on to analyse the nutritional content of 100g each of five popular fruits and vegetables – apples, bananas, oranges, carrots and peas – all of which, incidentally, scored highly on that bubble chart based on the NRF index. Her analysis revealed the fruit and vegetable list to be nutritionally incomplete: 'The fruit and veg five-a-day has traces of essential fats; no complete protein; no retinol (the form in which the body needs vitamin A – don't assume carotene can be converted); no B12 and no vitamin D (note also that D3 is only available in animal foods – D2 is the plant version). Not one nutrient RDA/AI can be provided by 100g of any fruit and veg – not even vitamin C.'[18] Put another way, these fruits and vegetables, on their own, do not deliver the most or even *enough* essential nutrients. And they do not deliver anywhere near as much nutritional value as the combination of liver, sardines, eggs, seeds and kale.

In another analysis of the eighteen most nutrient-dense foods published by Michael Joseph of Nutrition Advance (a website that aims to provide accurate, simple information about food and nutrition), there were many animal foods and a few varieties of nuts and seeds on the list, but just two fruits and vegetables: dried seaweed and dried shiitake mush-rooms.[19] Not a great performance from the fruit and vegetable team, and yet the five-a-day rule, a foundation of the plant-based-is-best philosophy, is something that few people now question, even if they don't manage to apply it consistently in their own lives.

The origins of 'five-a-day'

Where did this slogan, in which we have all invested such faith, actually come from? According to Dr Harcombe it had its beginnings in California in 1991 as a public–private partnership between the National Cancer Institute (NCI) and the Produce for Better Health Foundation, the sponsors list for which included specialist fruit and vegetable companies, general produce farms and chemical companies producing seeds, fungicides and insecticides. Five-a-day was, essentially, a marketing campaign. A 2010 study that might have provided retrospective evidence to back up the campaign failed to do so. The EPIC study, involving half a million people across Europe over eight years concluded as follows: 'The possibility that fruit and vegetables may help reduce the risk of cancer has been studied for over 30 years, but no protective effects have been firmly established.'[20]

There is no clear evidence for the positive effects of eating a particular number of a random selection of fruit and veg-etables on any medical condition. What's more, the vitamin content of fruits and vegetables is often exaggerated relative to that of animal-sourced foods.[21]

Dr Harcombe maintains that eating five portions of fruits and vegetables a day is only beneficial to health (and for addressing obesity) if the fruit and vegetables are eaten in place of processed junk rather than instead of meat, fish, dairy, eggs and other highly nutritious foods. Because we have put fruit and vegetables on a nutrition pedestal, we tend to ignore the immense nutritional value of these animal foods. An apple a day is said to keep the doctor away, but a weekly serving of liver is probably what the doctor should be prescribing. It provides vitamins A and B12 (not provided by an apple), four times as much vitamin C, and between twenty-four and three-hundred times as much of other nutrients (phosphorus, iron, zinc, copper, vitamins B2 and B6).[22]

The much-maligned egg can give liver a run for its money in the all-round nutrition stakes. A single egg contains omega-3 essential fatty acids in DHA form, vitamins A, B6, B12, E, D and K, calcium, iron, zinc, thiamine, folate, folic acid, phosphorus, protein, potassium, choline, lecithin and phospholipids, copper, manganese and selenium. That's quite the list for a food that has, at certain times in history, been banished to the list of diet no-nos.

Red meat – a more maligned food than the egg – boasts an equally impressive nutrient profile. 'A major asset of meat is of course its high protein value,' say researchers Leroy and Cofnas, but red meat also delivers B vitamins (with B12 being restricted to animal sources only), vitamins A, D and K2, various minerals (with iron, zinc and selenium being particularly important), and bioactive components such as taurine, creatine, conjugated linoleic acid, carnitine, choline, ubiquinone and glutathione.[23] And, as discussed in Chapter 1, red meat intake encourages nitric oxide synthesis. This nutrient profile is completely at odds with the portrayal of red meat as a threat to health. And, news for the fat-phobic: red meat needn't be a major source of saturated fat. A 100g sirloin steak comprises just 6g of saturated fat, the remainder of the fat being the monounsaturated variety found in olive oil.[24]

Even butter – a food eaten sparingly and guiltily by

many – has nutritional value. It provides nutrients such as vitamins A, D, E and K, DHA, choline, calcium, phosphorus and proteins.[25] But when was the last time you heard anyone urge their children to 'finish up all your butter'?

Of course, liver, eggs, steak and butter are all banned on a plant-based diet, along with many other highly nutritious foods. This should give us pause for thought the next time we hear someone claim that the 'vegan diet could be one of the healthiest diets'.

A deep dive into the vegan diet

One way to get a sense of how misleading are the claims about the healthfulness of the vegan diet is to look at Dr Harcombe's dissection of the diet advice featured on the Veganuary.com website. She found the diet being endorsed by the site to be deficient in vitamins A, B12 and D, iodine, iron, omega-3, protein, selenium and zinc.[26] Although the Academy of Nutrition and Dietetics (AND) is quoted as having said that 'all of the major dietetics societies have published papers stating that a vegan diet is nutritionally adequate for all stages of human health', accompanying this statement is a list of all the nutrients that need to be obtained via fortification and supplements, an admission that a vegan diet is not, in and of itself, safe or complete.

Functional medicine clinician Chris Kresser did a similar analysis and concluded that 'if you want nutrient-dense foods, you need to eat animal products'.[27] Dietitian Valerie Burnazov specifies the many nutrients that are lacking in plant foods: 'Nutrients that are only found in animal foods include: preformed vitamin A, B12, D3 and K2 (MK4 subtype), haem iron, taurine, carnosine, creatine, CLA, EPA and DHA. Nutrients that are low in plants include: zinc, iodine, methionine, leucine, choline, and glycine. Furthermore, plants often have different forms of the same nutrient that are less bioavailable and are metabolized differently.'[28]

Let's take a closer look at some of these nutrients and see why we need them and where we can find them.

Vitamin A

A fat-soluble vitamin, vitamin A is important for many aspects of bodily function including protein and calcium assimilation, bone growth, eyesight, immune system function, thyroid function and the production of stress and sex hormones. Our bodies require vitamin A in the form of retinol, the best sources of which are animal foods generally, and particularly liver, mackerel, salmon, butter, eggs and some cheeses.[29] Plants contain the precursor to vitamin A, which is beta-carotene, but conversion rates are very poor. (A precursor is a substance that can be converted to the actual vitamin according to the body's needs.)[30] It takes twelve times more carotenoid in a plant to get the same amount of vitamin A as that from an animal source.[31] Conversion and storage are difficult or impossible for some groups of individuals, including babies and children, diabetics and those with poor thyroid function. Vegetarian and vegan diets have been shown to suffer from a 'near total' lack of this vitamin.[32]

The Global Burden of Disease (GBD) report lists vitamin A as a nutrient of concern, particularly in developing countries, estimating that a third of children in the world are deficient.[33] There is a simple way to fix this and other deficiencies, writes farmer and author Matthew Evans, and that is to give people access to animal foods: 'Meat can't fix all of the world's malnourishment problems, but it can go a damn long way to cutting those numbers drastically.'[34]

Vitamin D

Another fat-soluble vitamin, vitamin D promotes strong bones, a healthy immune system, reduced inflammation, mineral metabolism, calcium absorption, muscle tone, healthy glucose metabolism, cell function and longevity.[35] It comes in two forms: D2 and D3. The body naturally wants D3, which the body makes when exposed to the sun and can obtain from animal foods, including shellfish, fish liver oils, egg yolks, organ meats, butterfat and the fat of birds and pigs. D2 (from plants) is vastly inferior, the D3 from animal foods being considerably more bioavailable and more potent.[36] Conversion from D2 to D3 is poor, so vegans must supplement.

The importance of vitamin D was brought home during the Covid-19 crisis, when it came to light that those with blood vitamin D levels greater than 30ng/ml (nanograms per millilitre) had a 95 per cent chance of survival from the virus and a minute chance of death, whereas someone below these limits had a 90 per cent chance of a critical or fatal illness. It has been suggested that vitamin D deficiency could be responsible for the high incidence of Covid-19 deaths among black, Asian and other ethnic minorities. These populations' pigmented skin is 'inefficient at producing vitamin D by the action of the sun. As a result, these populations have on average blood vitamin D levels only half that of the white population, and even they have levels that are lower than desirable.'[37]

Cholesterol

As discussed in Chapter 1, cholesterol is vital for life. Its main function is to maintain the integrity and fluidity of cell membranes – every cell in our bodies has cholesterol as part of its structure and needs cholesterol to function.[38] Cholesterol also serves as the precursor for the synthesis of vital substances, including bile acids, vitamin D and steroid hormones. It has been called the 'mother of all hormones' because it plays a critical role in the conversion of ACTH (adrenocorticotropic hormone) into other important hormones such as pregnenolone, progesterone, cortisol and testosterone.[39]

All animal foods contain cholesterol, whereas plant foods contain a form of cholesterol called 'phytosterols' which the body cannot absorb. Although cholesterol is vital, you do not need to get it from food, however. 'Cholesterol is so important that the body can make it out of anything – fats, carbohydrates or proteins' and 'even if you eat a cholesterol free diet, as vegans do, your body will still make cholesterol,' explains Dr Georgia Ede. Most cholesterol from food, she says, 'does not get absorbed unless body levels are low'. And 'it is virtually impossible for cholesterol from food to cause "high cholesterol"'.[40]

What this means is that a desire to avoid consuming cholesterol should not be a reason to shy away from animal foods, and the absence of cholesterol in a vegan diet does not make it better for your health. Unlike the other nutrients discussed in this section, you do not need to ensure that you eat it, but neither do you need to fear it. (For an excellent in-depth but digestible discussion of cholesterol, I suggest reading Dr Ede's article, 'Cholesterol is Good for You', at www.diagnosisdiet.com.)[41]

Vitamin B12

It would be difficult to find any qualified medical practitioner or nutritionist who doesn't single out B12 as a key nutrient of concern for vegans. The vitamin is an essential nutrient that plays a role in DNA synthesis, myelin formation, red cell production and the maintenance of the central nervous system.[42]

Long-term B12 deficiency can have serious consequences for health. Registered nutritionist Maria Cross describes the four stages of deficiency. In stages one and two, serum depletion (a reduced amount of B12 in the blood) is evident, but there are no discernible outward symptoms. In stage three, levels of an amino acid called homocysteine begin to rise. By the time someone reaches stage four, symptoms can include fatigue, depression, anxiety, poor memory and numbness or tingling in the hands and feet. Additional symptoms develop over time, including balance problems, vision deterioration, mental confusion or memory loss, and severe depression. The most severe outcome is a form of myelopathy (damage to the spinal cord). And 'peripheral neuropathy (damage to nerves in the body's extremities) is seen in 25% of patients with vitamin B12 deficiency'.[43] Often, symptoms develop gradually, over several months to a year, before being recognised. (Since the adult liver can store enough vitamin B12 to last five years, symptoms may take even longer to materialise.) Infants will typically show a more rapid onset of symptoms and are more vulnerable to permanent damage.[44]

Statistics suggest that 7 per cent of vegetarians and 52 per cent of vegans are B12 deficient.[45] The statistics are misleading, however, says Chris Kresser, because B12 deficiency is underdiagnosed – serum B12 tests that most doctors use pick up only a small fraction of people who are actually B12 deficient. And serum B12 levels don't tend to go out of range until stage three or four has been reached. (An even bigger problem is that many doctors don't even use the conventional serum B12 test. Kresser reports having seen many patients that he diagnosed with a B12 deficiency in their forties, fifties or sixties who had never been tested for B12.[46])

There are more sensitive markers for B12 deficiency, Kresser explains, including the measurement of methylmalonic acid (MMA), homocysteine, or holotranscobalamin 11 (holoTC).

The latter can detect B12 deficiency at the earliest stage. A study using more sensitive markers showed that a whopping 83 per cent of vegans and 68 per cent of vegetarians were B12 deficient.[47]

Although rates of B12 deficiency are much higher in vegetarians and vegans than in omnivores, around one in twenty omnivores are also deficient,[48] and the elderly are particularly susceptible to B12 deficiency, something that can easily be overlooked when the symptoms of dementia become apparent. It is estimated that 10–15 per cent of people over the age of sixty have a B12 deficiency. And B12 deficiency drives high levels of homocysteine, which in itself is a risk factor for vascular dementia and Alzheimer's disease.[49]

An association between B12 deficiency and mental health has been demonstrated in populations other than the elderly. In one study comparing vegetarians and omnivores, vitamin B12 levels were significantly lower in the vegetarian group, and the frequency of depression was 31 per cent compared to 12 per cent in the omnivore group.[50] (It's important to note, however, that the direction of causation in such studies is not proven. Did the diet precede the mental illness, or was the mental illness a factor influencing the choice of diet?)

The reason vegetarians and vegans exhibit such high levels of B12 deficiency is that there are no reliable plant sources of B12. A common myth is that it's possible to get enough B12 from plant sources such as seaweed, fermented soya,* spirulina and brewer's yeast. But these foods actually contain B12 analogues (imitations), which have no vitamin effect and, furthermore, block the intake of, and increase the need for, true B12.[51] (Serum levels of the analogue are often what is

---

* Soy and soya are the same thing, with soy being the term generally used in North America and soya being more common in Europe. I generally use the word soya except when referring to specific organisations or sources who use the word soy.

being picked up by the serum B12 test, since these tests cannot differentiate between real and analogue B12.)

Only two types of algae – chlorella and nori – can be considered as B12 sources, according to Dr Schweikart, author of the website Vitamin B12 & Health. Both have significant weaknesses, however. Since B12 is not produced by the algae itself, but rather by the micro-organisms that live on the plant or in the soil, the actual B12 content depends heavily on the growing conditions. 'No definitive statement can be made about the exact B12 content of these algae. Even in the same location, levels can rise and fall from one year to the next quite dramatically.'[52]

The Vegan Society's resources section contains an acknowledgment of the fact that algae are unreliable sources of B12. An open letter written by a Vegan Society trustee states that 'algae and some other plant foods contain B12-analogues (false B12) that can imitate true B12 in blood tests while actually interfering with B12 metabolism'. The letter goes on to state that claimed sources of B12 – such as human gut bacteria, spirulina, dried nori, barley grass and most other seaweeds – are in fact inadequate, and that supplements and fortified foods are essential.[53]

Supplements are also advised for some omnivores, particularly the elderly; however, as with all artificial supplements, there are concerns about the tissue-retention rates from human-made B12 when compared to naturally occurring forms. In addition, human-made forms are not protein bound and are thus subject to more degradation, which might make them less effective.[54]

For omnivores, the advice is obvious: to optimise health and ensure against B12 deficiency, you are better off eating small amounts of foods such as sardines, tuna, clams, trout, meat, liver or kidneys several times a week than taking supplements. (B12 is best absorbed in small amounts.) For plant-based eaters, unfortunately, there is no simple solution to the B12 problem other than supplementation.

Omega-3 fatty acids

Omega-3s are important components of the membranes that surround each cell in the body.[55] They have many functions in your heart, blood vessels, lungs, immune system and endocrine system (the network of hormone-producing glands). Research has indicated that they may also play a role in preventing cardiovascular disease, promoting infant health and development, preventing cancer, and mitigating risks for Alzheimer's disease, dementia and cognitive dysfunction.[56]

There are two essential derivatives of this fatty acid: EPA and DHA.[57] The best sources are oily fish. Plants such as pumpkin seeds and blueberries can deliver only ALA (the precursor to EPA and DHA), and conversion is poor to non-existent (often under 1 per cent).[58] Moreover, conversion efficiency 'depends on the presence of co-factors such as selenium, zinc, iron and vitamin B6, which are less bioavailable from plant foods. For these reasons, vegetarians can have lower levels of DHA and EPA when compared to omnivores.'[59] Only 20 per cent of the world's population report consumption of the recommended daily amounts of EPA and DHA, which is 250–500mg.[60]

Another potential problem is that omega-6 fatty acids 'compete with ALA for enzymes involved in elongation and desaturation, which further diminishes the ability to obtain DHA and EPA from ALA'. This is particularly problematic in the context of the modern Western diet, which is characterised by a high ratio of omega-6 to omega-3 (about 16:1, versus a historic ratio of between 1:1 and 4:1).[61]

Naturopath Lucinda Miller advises clients that a healthy, nutritionally replete woman can convert a maximum of 10 per cent of plant-based omega-3s into DHA, and some males might only convert as little as 1 per cent. 'You really have to get your omega-3s from oily fish or carefully chosen grass-fed meat. You just can't do it with flax or chia seeds. They help a little but are not an easy replacement,' says Miller.[62]

Essential minerals

'There are 17 essential minerals, 7 macrominerals (of which you need rather large amounts per day) and 10 trace minerals (of which you need small amounts per day),'[63] explain Dr James DiNicolantonio and Siim Land in their book, *The Mineral Fix*. (A weighty tome indeed, with more than four thousand references, but a superb resource for anyone wanting to fully understand how mineral intake impacts health.) A significant proportion of the population (one in three people in the US for example) has at least 10 minerals in which they are deficient.[64] Why does this matter? It matters, say the authors, because 'mineral deficiencies drive, or contribute to, nearly all chronic diseases'.[65] Minerals are also 'necessary for all bodily processes, starting with energy production and ending with hormonal balance'.[66] It has also been found that deficiencies in some minerals (selenium and zinc, for example) are associated with poorer Covid-19 outcomes.[67]

Getting the right amount of the right combination of minerals is important, since some work synergistically, and others have an antagonistic relationship both with each other and with other nutrients.[68] But it's challenging to get the right amount and combination from a diet that's exclusively plant based. The food charts for thirteen minerals in DiNicolantonio and Land's book illustrate why. For most of the minerals, there are both animal foods and plant foods in the top ten food sources. But animal foods dominate the top ten list for five of the minerals, and plant foods dominate for six. (There are an equal number of plant and animal foods in the top ten for two.) From this we might surmise that the best way to ensure an optimal level of intake of all essential minerals is to eat a mix of plant and animal foods. It should be noted, however, that even where plant-food sources provide the most of a given mineral for a given serving, this may not translate into the body's absorption of that mineral. Spinach and kale, for example, while rich in calcium, actually inhibit calcium absorption due to their oxalic acid or oxalate content (of which more in Chapter 4).[69]

If we look at what we might call the mineral superfoods – those foods that provide the most of any given mineral (and in some cases more than the RDA in a single serving) we see a similar pattern. For the thirteen minerals covered, an animal-sourced food (yoghurt, sardines, molluscs, scallops, mussels, beef liver or oysters) takes the top spot (often delivering more than the RDA) in eight cases, while plant foods (pumpkin seeds, Brazil nuts, carrots, nori seaweed or blackeyed peas) take the top spot in five cases. (For iron provision, fortified cereals actually take the top spot, but I discounted this on the basis that artificially fortified cereals are not real foods comparable to the others on the list.)

A closer look at three essential minerals – calcium, iron and zinc – provides further illustration of why you might not want to put all of your mineral eggs into one plant-based basket.

Calcium

Calcium has several important functions including building strong bones and teeth, regulating muscle contractions such as the heartbeat, and ensuring that the blood clots normally.[70] The recommended daily intake is between 800mg and 1,200mg per day. You can obtain 1,000mg of calcium from two glasses of milk, a 30g serving of cheese and a serving of sardines. To get the same amount of calcium from plant foods, however, you'd have to eat around 1 kilo (raw weight) of broccoli, 1.5 kilos of white beans (cooked), 2.5 kilos of oranges, or 83 slices of wholemeal bread.[71] Soya drinks with added calcium can provide calcium, but there are many problems with soya, which I'll discuss in Chapter 4. Calcium supplements are discouraged since calcium in this form can be harmful.[72]

A 2020 study by Tammy Tong and colleagues found vegans to be more than twice as likely to suffer from hip fractures, as well as being significantly more at risk of other fractures.[73] The authors said that the higher risk of fracture could be owing to several dietary factors, such as lower intakes of both calcium and protein among both vegetarians and vegans.

Iron

The body uses iron to make haemoglobin (a protein in red blood cells that carries oxygen from the lungs to all parts of the body) and myoglobin (a protein that provides oxygen to muscles) and some hormones.[74] There are two types of iron: haem and non-haem. The body prefers the haem iron found in meat, which is five- to ten-fold more bioavailable than non-haem iron.[75] Foods that provide iron include beef, pork, oysters, clams, dark chocolate, beans, lentils, beetroot and spinach,[76] but plants are a relatively poor source of iron. Spinach, touted as being an iron-rich food, contains much less iron than people might think. (The iron content of Popeye's favourite food was exaggerated by ten times when a German chemist misplaced a decimal point, estimating the iron content of 100g of spinach at 35mg versus 3.5mg.)[77] Fortified cereals can provide sufficient iron but if you're eating those cereals as part of a vegetarian diet you'll need almost twice as much iron as someone who eats meat.[78] The reason for this is that absorption of iron from non-meat, non-fish sources is poor, being limited by several plant compounds such as phytates and polyphenols.[79] (I'll cover these compounds in Chapter 4.) 'Vitamin C and meat are the main enhancers of non-heme iron absorption, which is why adding meat to plant-based meals improves uptake of non-heme iron from plants,' say Stephan van Vliet and fellow researchers Kronberg and Provenza.[80]

Van Vliet and his colleagues state that 'iron deficiency remains one of the most common nutrient deficiencies in both developed and developing countries, and population groups such as children, adolescent females, and older individuals are particularly at risk for deficiency'.[81] Globally, more than 1.7 billion people could be affected.[82] The latest GBD (Global Burden of Disease) report estimates that iron deficiency is responsible for more than thirty-one million global disability-adjusted life years (DALYs) annually.[83] Iron deficiency is particularly harmful to women of menstruation age, and it is more common for vegetarians and vegans to be iron deficient.[84] The WHO notes that deficiency 'may occur throughout the lifespan where diets are based mostly on staple foods with little meat intake', and attributes one-fifth of perinatal mortality and one-tenth of maternal mortality in developing countries to iron deficiency.[85]

Zinc

In *The Mineral Fix*, the list of functions for zinc is longer than that for almost any other mineral, and includes immune system function, antioxidant defence, wound healing, glucose metabolism, brain development and plasticity, sex hormone production and DNA damage repair.[86] Deficiencies, say DiNicolantonio and Land, 'cause growth retardation, hormonal imbalances, impotence, delayed wound healing, frailty, hair loss, diarrhea, skin lesions and increased susceptibility to infections'.[87] 'Severe deficiency in the US is currently not considered common but many are likely subclinically zinc deficient.' (That is, they are ingesting a suboptimal amount for optimal health.)[88]

Globally, zinc deficiency is widespread, sufficiently so for zinc to be a nutrient of concern noted in the GBD report. Deficiency is thought to be responsible for around 16 per cent of lower respiratory tract infections, 18 per cent of malaria, 10 per cent of diarrhoeal disease and almost 3 per cent of loss of healthy life years.[89]

Red meat, fish, oysters, poultry and other animal foods are the best sources of zinc.[90] Plant food sources are legumes, nuts, seeds and oats, leafy green vegetables and sprouted beans. However, it is acknowledged that the best sources of zinc are animal foods, since plant sources are high in phytic acid, an inhibitor of zinc bioavailability.[91] This makes getting enough zinc from plant sources a challenging business, leading the WHO to state that zinc requirements for dietary intake are adjusted upwards for populations in which animal products are limited.[92]

A clear demonstration of the impact of phytic acid on zinc bioavailability was afforded by one study which showed that if you eat 120 grams of zinc-rich oysters with black beans, you will absorb just 50 per cent of the zinc in the oysters. If you eat the same oysters with a corn tortilla, you'll absorb virtually none of the zinc.[93] The absorption problem is reflected in a meta-analysis which found that both zinc intakes and serum zinc concentrations were lower in vegetarians than non-vegetarians.[94] Another study found that 47 per cent of vegans are zinc deficient versus 10 per cent of omnivores.[95] A study of Indian adolescents concluded that 'adolescents from developing countries such as India may be at risk of zinc deficiency because of unwholesome food habits and poor bioavailability of zinc from plant-based diets'.[96]

It's clear that a plant-based diet cannot match an omnivore diet when it comes to providing zinc and other minerals.

Next, we're going to consider protein. Can a plant-based diet live up to its billing as 'one of the healthiest diets' when it comes to delivering this important macronutrient?

Protein

Protein is found throughout the body – in muscle, bone, skin, hair and most other body parts and tissues. It also makes up the enzymes that power many chemical reactions, and the haemoglobin that carries oxygen in the blood. It is made from about twenty different amino acids, nine of which must come from food (histadine, isoleucine, leucine, lysine, methionine, phenylalanine, tryptophan, threonine and valine) and are thus deemed essential amino acids (EAAs).[97]

It is sometimes claimed that we eat too much protein. This is a spurious statement, firstly because there is no firm agreement on how much protein we require; for example, the WHO recommends 0.83g of protein per 1kg of bodyweight for all adults, whereas the US Dietary Reference Intakes (DRIs) recommend that men and women aged between nineteen and fifty consume 0.66g per 1kg. Critically, these allowances are the minimum requirement, not the optimum levels from which to thrive.[98] 'Protein researchers agree, pretty unanimously, that the protein RDA is too low for optimal health,' says nutrition scientist Stephan van Vliet. 'Ideally we would see intakes of 1–1.2g per kilogram of bodyweight, especially in older individuals.'[99] It's important to remember, too, that grams of protein are not the same as grams of food: for example, 100g of roast beef contains 27.2g of protein. Someone who eats 200g of beef every day could therefore not be accused of consuming too much protein, if that is their main protein source. Such claims are nevertheless frequently made.[100]

Absolute levels of protein vary widely between plant and animal foods, with the calorie cost of plant sources of protein being significantly higher than for animal foods. To get 30g of protein from potato or peanut butter, for example, you would have to consume 1,155 and 705 calories respectively. To get the same amount of protein from eggs or steak you would have to consume around 350 calories.[101]

Plant and animal proteins differ in other significant ways. 'People talk about protein and lump all proteins together as if they are the same,' says van Vliet. 'But they are entire foods that differ in so many ways – digestibility, amino acid profile, vitamins, minerals, and bio peptides for example – all of which have an impact on protein synthetic response [the ability of the body's cells to make new proteins].'[102] Two of these terms – digestibility and amino acid profile – are particularly important to the understanding of how plant and animal proteins function differently. The first, digestibility, is a measure of how much of a given protein is actually absorbed by the body, and thus determines bioavailability. Taken as a group, plant foods have lower digestibility ratings than animal foods.[103] The digestibility rating means that when you consider the amount of protein in any given food, you need to apply the multiplier as a percentage. Doing such calculations, it quickly becomes apparent that animal foods such as eggs and meat are more efficient than plant foods at delivering protein for a given weight of food or amount of calories.[104]

The second criteria for evaluating proteins is the amino acid profile – the extent to which they deliver all nine essential amino acids (EAAs), also referred to as completeness. Animal proteins are rich in EAAs and, unlike plant proteins, have been shown repeatedly to optimise protein synthesis.[105] Professor Tim Noakes quipped that when he was a medical student, he was told that plant proteins were second-class proteins, 'but you're not allowed to say that any more because it is offensive to vegetarians'.[106] That said, the fine print of the EAT-Lancet report, whose recommended diet is largely plant-based, contains an admission that 'animal sources of protein are of higher quality than most plant sources'.[107]

Several studies, including one by Stephan van Vliet and fellow researchers, suggest that the ingestion of the plant-based proteins, such as those in soya and wheat, results in a lower muscle protein synthetic response when compared to animal proteins, and that this might be the result of the lower levels of amino acids in plant protein.[108] Stephan van Vliet suggests that this could be because when some EAAs are missing, synthesis in vital organs such as the liver are prioritised over synthesis in the muscles: 'Suppose you were driving a car that was running out of fuel, and the car could sense this and stop you from driving over 60 miles an hour so as to conserve that fuel. Something like this could be happening in the body.'[109]

Since the proteins in plant food are incomplete, plant foods must be combined very carefully to ensure adequate levels of EAAs. Frances Moore Lappé, the author of one of the first popular books urging us to give up meat for the sake of the environment (*Diet for a Small Planet*, 1971) and who went on to write more than twenty books and founded the Small Planet Institute, nevertheless admitted that it is a challenge to achieve the right amino acid profile by eating only plant foods. This is because 'our bodies need all of the EAAs simultaneously in order to carry out protein synthesis. If one EAA is missing, even temporarily, protein synthesis will fall to a very low level or stop altogether.'[110] And if one EAA is present in a food in too small an amount, or not at all, it becomes 'limiting', meaning that it prevents proper synthesis of all the EAAs.[111] Plants tend to be low in either lysine, methionine or leucine, says Stephan van Vliet. 'These are essential amino acids that cannot be synthesised in the body and can only be obtained through the diet.'[112]

To achieve a complete EAA profile from plant proteins you need to know exactly which EAAs are in each food and to eat the right amounts of each food in the same meal or within a few hours. It can be done, but it's far more complicated than if you are eating animal foods containing complete proteins. And, as Dr Harcombe commented, 'I bet I could line up one-hundred vegetarians and vegans on Oxford Street today, and none of them would know this.'[113] Even creating a complete amino acid profile by blending various plant sources might not be sufficient. A 2019 study by Brennan and colleagues also found that plant-based proteins are not bio-equivalent to animal-based proteins, even when those proteins are blended to maximise EAA content.[114]

If you eat enough plant protein (around 1.6g per 1kg of body weight), the impact of limiting EAAs disappears. 'But then you have this very high intake of protein, which is not feasible for children and the elderly, for example,' says van Vliet. You also run the risk of consuming too many calories and too much carbohydrate in the process. Say you set out to get all your EAAs from a single plant source such as chick-peas, you could do so by eating 700g of boiled chickpeas in a single meal. But that's a veritable chickpea mountain, and it comes with a price tag of 1,200 calories[115] and over 140g of carbohydrate.[116] (I'll discuss why eating large quantities of carbohydrate is not advised later in the book.) Or you could get all your EAAs by eating quinoa, but you'd have to eat around 1.1 kilos (6 cups) in one sitting, which is six times as much as you would consider to be a normal serving.[117]

Soya is another popular plant protein. But, like all legumes, it is low in sulphur-containing amino acids, such as methionine, which are crucial for aspects of physiological function.[118] The methionine shortfall in soya has been known about for a long time, so much so that steps have been taken to genetically engineer soya to correct it.[119] DiNicolantonio and Land assert that sulphur-containing amino acids are 'easily found in the western food supply with the exception of vegan diets'.[120]

Pea protein isolate, that ingredient on which several plant-based meats rely, can provide most of the essential amino acids, but because it is a relatively inefficient provider, people would end up exceeding even the higher levels of protein intake recommended by some experts while trying to meet amino acid requirements, says van Vliet.[121] As for jackfruit, advertised as a good meat substitute with the texture of pulled pork, it delivers just 0.9g of protein per 100g. You would have to eat more than sixty tins of the stuff to fulfil your daily requirement for protein.

The internet is awash with information about protein that is misleading or even inaccurate. One article set out to provide sixteen complete protein pairings with wholewheat bread (combinations of foods that would provide all nine EAAs). Examples of the combinations included bread and carrots, bread and spinach, and bread and mustard. An astute reader would notice, however, that while the combinations did indeed provide complete protein in the sense that all EAAs were present, they were present in such small quantities that you would have to eat insane amounts of the foods to obtain the required daily amount of each EAA. Would you fancy eating thirty-nine carrots with seven slices of bread, or more than thirty-five cups of spinach with four slices of bread?

If the protein pairings article did not tell the whole story of plant proteins, a visual that was circulating on twitter in 2021 was, in the words of Diana Rodgers, 'just WRONG'. The visual positioned broccoli as a better source of protein than beef, the text claiming that beef delivers 6.4g of protein per 100 calories while broccoli delivers 11.1. In fact, beef contains 13g of protein per 100 calories as compared to 7g for broccoli. Moreover, the protein in beef is complete and more easily digested.[122]

An article in *The Times* (January 2022) served to mislead on the protein issue by failing to mention it at all. In answer to the question posed by the headline, 'Are mushrooms the new meat?', the article seemed to be saying yes: 'They're better for the planet than steak and taste as good.'[123] But how can mushrooms be the new meat when they provide just 3g of protein per 100g, compared to steak's 25g? And when that protein is less complete and bioavailable than the protein in steak?

Protein and overeating

Overeating is a possible consequence of trying to meet protein requirements from plant sources. The protein leverage hypothesis suggests that humans will continue to eat food until their protein needs are met. If protein-rich foods are insufficient in the diet, people might keep eating foods that are high in both calories and carbohydrates in an attempt to finally achieve the protein levels (in terms of EAAs) that they need, says Chris Kresser.[124] Nutritionist Tim Rees has observed that those on plant-based diets who try hard to meet their protein requirements can end up eating so many carbohydrate-rich plant foods such as grains, beans and pulses that they end up overweight, even if it's what he calls skinny-fat: skinny on the outside, fat on the inside. This skinny-fat condition is characterised by a build-up of fat in and around the organs, as is the case with NAFLD, or non-alcoholic fatty liver disease.[125]

What are the consequences of not getting enough protein? 'Consistently low intake of protein over time will result in lower muscle mass, lower bone mass, suboptimal immune functionality and even reduced cardiovascular health,' says Stephan van Vliet. 'These things develop over a long period of time, so you might not notice. It's easy for people to feel complacent and neglect protein for this reason.'[126]

Quality protein is particularly important as we age. The amino acids in protein tell the muscles and bones of the body to make new protein, which is essential in all stages of life but particularly for the elderly. We know that protein deficiency is a problem with older people, and this deficiency, combined with a sedentary lifestyle, creates big risks for osteoporosis, falls and fractures.[127] A 2021 study by Tomás Meroño and colleagues demonstrated a small association between animal protein intake by older people and lower levels of mortality. (The association was not found with plant-based proteins.)[128]

Although popular discourse, and films such as *The Game Changers*, have tended to focus on protein in relation to men's health, quality protein is critical for women. Obstetrician Dr Jamie Seemen emphasises that women need adequate amounts of both protein and fat to optimise hormonal health.[129] Red meat can provide not only the protein but also some of the essential fat alongside it. Diets without red meat, on the other hand, have been shown to be particularly damaging to women, with low red meat intake being associated with deficiencies in zinc, iron, vitamin B12, potassium and vitamin D.[130]

Phytochemicals[131]

For animals, 'Grasses, forbs, shrubs and trees are nutrition centers and pharmacies with a vast array of phytochemicals,' write Fred Provenza, Cindi Anderson and Pablo Gregorini. 'Historically, we did not appreciate that the nutritional and pharmacological properties of these minor components of the diet – best eaten in small doses – enable health.'[132] Historically, we have also failed to appreciate how important these same phytochemicals could be to human health. But this is changing. Dr Mark Hyman recently acknowledged that 'The most important parts of food may be the tens of thousands of medicinal compounds embedded in plants and even animal foods.'[133]

A large amount of research has been done to try to establish just how critical these compounds are to human health. The accumulating evidence is exciting, but much of it is preliminary, and the field of phytochemical research is relatively young. One team of researchers who reviewed the evidence that phytochemicals might play a role in protecting and repairing DNA and preventing cancer cautioned that 'in spite of the large number of publications much remains to be done'. They also warn that the potential benefits of supplementing with concentrated forms of phytochemicals must be 'evaluated in each case since a safe phytochemical at physiological concentrations could be toxic at higher concentrations'.[134] (I'll talk more about the downsides of ingesting excessive amounts of some phytochemicals in Chapter 4.)

It was previously thought that phytochemicals could only be found in plants. But recent research by Stephan van Vliet, Fred Provenza and Scott Kronberg has demonstrated that phytochemicals can also be found in some animal-sourced foods. The authors write: 'the contribution of phytochemicals from pasture-raised meat and milk to overall dietary intake should not be underestimated. While total phenolic levels ... in fruits and vegetables are generally 5 to 20-fold higher compared to pasture-raised meat and milk, various individual phytochemicals are abundant in pasture-raised meat and milk.'[135] The richer and more diverse the pasture, the higher the phytochemical content of the meat.

Van Vliet, Provenza and Kronberg stress that their findings should not be interpreted 'as "evidence" that animal foods negate a need for obtaining phytochemicals from plant foods' but rather that they serve to illustrate that 'plant and animal foods arguably improve human health in synergistic ways' and that 'pasture-raised animal foods can contribute substantially to phytonutrient intake in the human diet'.

If you chose never to eat pasture-raised animal foods or any other animal-sourced foods again, but you ate a wide variety of plant foods grown in nutrient-rich soil, you would certainly be able to tap into the potentially health-enhancing properties of phytochemicals. However, you would be doing your brain a disservice, as we'll see now.

Nutrients and the brain

In a presentation titled 'Our descent into madness: Modern diets and the global mental health crisis' (available on YouTube and well worth a half-hour of your time),[136] Dr Georgia Ede details the link between diet and mental health. Having presented startling evidence of a decline in global mental health, she says, 'I believe that the decline in mental health around the world has a lot to do with a decline in the quality of our diet.'[137] Dr Ede points to two dietary patterns that are on the rise: the standard American diet (SAD) – now exported around the world – and the plant-based diet. The SAD gives her cause for concern because it is high in refined/processed carbohydrates and refined/processed fats, both of which are 'very powerful promoters of inflammation and oxidation', to which many mental health disorders are linked. To the extent that the SAD promotes insulin resistance (as previously explained on page 41), she suggests that it could be implicated in the development of Alzheimer's, since fully 80 per cent of Alzheimer's sufferers have insulin resistance or type-2 diabetes.

As for the plant-based diet, Dr Ede has found most studies about its impact on mental health to be epidemiological and the evidence to be weak, mixed and confounded by a failure to control for carbohydrate intake. But, she argues, 'we don't need more studies because we already know so much about what the brain needs'.

One of the things the brain needs is energy. It is, in her words, an 'energy hog'. That energy can come in the form of glucose or ketones. To 'extract energy from these molecules it needs a lot of vitamins and minerals'. Critical among these is DHA (explained on page 80), which research has shown to play an indispensable role in 'the neural signalling essential for higher intelligence'. (In fact, two-thirds of the brain is made up of fat, of which 20 per cent is DHA.) 'Plant foods contain absolutely no DHA whatsoever,' says Ede. They contain ALA, 'but it is widely agreed that it is extremely difficult if not impossible to transform ALA into DHA'. This, she says, helps to explain why vegetarians and vegans have lower levels of both DHA and EPA than omnivores.

Other important nutrients for the brain are folate, vitamins B12, A, C, D, E, K1 and K2, a 'full complement of amino acids' and iron, zinc and iodine. 'All of these nutrients can be found in animal foods and in the most bioavailable form,' Dr Ede says, but 'plant foods are lacking some key nutrients and some of the forms they contain are harder for us to use.' Moreover, and as discussed earlier, plants contain anti-nutrients (Ede lists oxalates, tannins, the goitrogens found in soya, and phytates), which 'reduce our ability to utilise not just the nutrients in plant foods, but the nutrients in the foods we eat alongside them'. These important nutrients don't have to come from red meat, Ede advises. They can be found in other animal foods, such as chicken and chicken livers, pork, duck, salmon, shrimp and oysters. For DHA, seafood, and especially salmon, 'is where it's at'.

'The people that I'm most concerned about, when it comes to a low meat or plant-based diet, in terms of accessing critical brain nutrients, are women,' says Dr Ede. 'Women are more likely to be culturally averse to eating meat and fat – that may help to explain why three-quarters of vegans are women in the United States. They're more likely to prioritise weight and appearance over health. They are more likely to prioritise animal and planet health over their own personal health for compassionate reasons. And this is a problem, not just for the women that we care about in our lives. It is also a problem for future generations because women literally feed the brains – build the brains – of the next generation through their food choices.'[138]

Other researchers are aligned with Dr Ede's proposition that the plant-based diet is suboptimal for brain health. 'To build and maintain a more complex brain,' writes Sujata Gupta, 'our ancestors used ingredients found primarily in meat, including iron, zinc, vitamin B12 and fatty acids. Although plants contain many of the same nutrients, they occur in lower quantities and often in a form that humans cannot readily use.'[139]

DiNicolantonio and Land explain the importance of certain minerals for brain health and function. Magnesium, iron and copper create dopamine (a hormone and neurotransmitter that regulates mood, motivation, well-being and the feeling of reward) and norepinephrine (a stress hormone and neuro-transmitter) in the brain; magnesium, calcium, iron, copper, cobalt and zinc facilitate the making of serotonin (which regulates cognition, mood and sleep in the central nervous system).[140] As we've seen, pure plant-based diets cannot pro-vide the full complement of these minerals as well as a diet that includes animal-sourced foods.

Certain lesser-known nutrients, such as taurine and cho-line, are also important for brain function. The main dietary sources of both these nutrients are eggs, meat and seafood. Creatine, too, helps to optimise brain function and has been shown to improve memory and reduce mental fatigue. Vegans and vegetarians have significantly lower levels of creatine in their bodies because plants and fungi don't contain any.[141]

The consequences of not getting enough of the right nutrients are significant. A 2014 study found iron deficiency to be associated with anxiety, depression, social problems and behavioural abnormalities.[142] An earlier study (2007) highlighted the impact of iron deficiency on intellectual performance, finding that giving young women iron supplements led to significant intellectual gains. (The performance of those whose blood levels of iron increased improved their performance on a cognitive test by five- to seven-fold.)[143] Another study highlighted the importance of B12 to brain function, particularly late in life, finding that the brains of those with lower levels of B12 were found to be more likely to be shrinking.[144]

A more recent study found that vegetarians and vegans had significantly higher rates of depression, anxiety and self-harm.[145] As with all observational studies, this one could show association but not prove causation. Nevertheless, the findings were concerning enough for Dr Aseem Malhotra to comment, 'If you want to avoid increased risk of depression, anxiety and self-harm behaviour, then do eat meat. If you're vegan or vegetarian, then invest in strategies to protect your mental health.'[146] Dr Natasha Campbell-McBride, who holds postgraduate degrees in both neurology and human nutrition, and has direct clinical experience in treating young people who have chosen a plant-based lifestyle, also believes that a plant-based diet poses risks to mental health:

The best building materials to feed your brain come from animal foods. In the clinical practice we see degeneration of the brain function in people on purely plant-based diets ... the sharpness of the mind goes, memory and learning ability suffer, depression sets in and other mental problems follow. These are signs of a starving brain.[147]

Like Campbell-McBride, three experts interviewed for a BBC Futures article stressed how challenging it is to get enough brain food from a vegan diet.[148] One of them, Nathan Cofnas, was unequivocal in his view: 'Without question, veganism can cause B12 and iron deficiencies, and without question, they affect your intelligence.'

Sidestepping the hard questions

Given how poorly plant foods deliver on many of the nutrients required for optimal brain and bodily health, it would be safe to assert that optimal nutrition comes from a diet that includes animal foods. The facts about B12 and DHA alone are a challenge to the plant-based-is-best incantation. Given that B12 is essential to human health, and that it cannot be found in *any* plant foods, shouldn't we question the notion that we can all survive and thrive on a plant-based diet? Given that DHA is essential for a healthy brain, doesn't it make sense to eat the foods that provide it? By eliminating the foods that provide us with these critical nutrients – those foods that humans have been eating for millions of years – would we not be engaged in some sort of fanciful re-engineering project designed to raise two fingers to our evolutionary history?

Plant-based advocates invariably sidestep these questions. Regarding B12, it is often asserted that it is easily obtained from supplements. For many operating in the health and nutrition space, this is an inadequate answer. Relying on supplements for B12, or any of the other vitamins and minerals that are in short supply in a plant-based diet, is not a foolproof solution. Stephan van Vliet explains that 'simply ingesting these nutrients outside of their natural food matrices may not be an optimal solution for promoting health'.[149] Studies have shown that fortification of a low-meat diet with zinc and other minerals found in meat does not result in similar zinc status as when these minerals are provided in the diet as part of the natural matrix of meat.[150] Similarly, omega-3 from supplements does not provide the same benefit as omega-3 from food, failing to lower the risk of disease or mortality.[151] Moreover, it has been shown that adequate intakes of zinc, copper and vitamins A and D were associated with a decreased risk of cardiovascular disease and all-cause mortality when obtained from foods, but not from supplements.[152] Some studies have shown that vitamin A supplements do not decrease the risk of cancer or cardiovascular disease and might even *raise* the risk for some populations; and supplemental calcium has been shown to increase cardiovascular disease risk whereas this is not the case with calcium obtained from food. Similar observations have been made about vitamin C and selenium supplements.[153]

Stephan van Vliet warns against an overly simplistic, supplemental approach that fails to account for the way nutrients from food work: 'When you get vitamins from foods it's always in the presence of other vitamins and phytochemicals. A reductionist approach, where we think we can throw a few artificial vitamins together and replicate the food source? That's not how it works.'[154]

A reductionist approach to vitamin intake also fails to take into account the complexity of the microbiome, says genetic epidemiologist Tim Spector. The microbiome 'consists of a mix of up to 100 trillion bacteria, fungi, parasites and 500 trillion mini viruses, outnumbering the number of cells in our body'. These thousands of different microbe species interact with thousands of different food chemicals to 'produce over 50,000 chemicals that affect most aspects of our body'.[155]

That is how it works.

Diplomacy from dietary advisors

Experts who are asked to comment about meat-free diets in the media almost always opt to tread carefully. But the essential message is written between the lines. In an article in *The Times* titled 'What to eat when you join the no red-meat club', Peta Bee expressed no value judgement as to whether cutting out red meat is a good or bad idea. Instead, she listed the many nutrients found in meat that will have to be sought elsewhere. (This, in itself, would appear to undermine the claim that red meat is bad for us.) In an article written for *The Times* in January 2019, Dr Mark Porter didn't advise against going vegan but he did warn people about the pitfalls of a vegan diet, which included potential deficiencies in calcium, vitamin D, essential fats and, of course, B12. He said that while he is generally opposed to supplements because most are a waste of time 'vegans are an important exception'.[156] A more accurate title for his article would have been 'Vegans can be healthy *despite* their diet provided they take great care and lots of supplements'.

You might have witnessed Dr Hilary Jones dancing on a pinhead on ITV's *Lorraine* in January 2020.[157] He had been asked to comment on Veganuary: was it a good thing for people to do? 'People want to eat less meat to be healthier. I understand that,' he said. In the next breath, he said that if a person was going to adopt a vegan diet, they would need to be 'very careful' about nutrients, implying, but not saying, that vegan diets were not altogether optimal for health. Perhaps he had been asked to remain neutral so as not to offend vegan viewers. Whatever the case, what the viewer got was a soft-shoe, not-altogether-clear statement about the merits of doing Veganuary.

More soft-shoeing was in evidence in a segment of *This Morning* in November 2020. Presenter Phillip Schofield asked the resident doctor what advice he would give to vegans in light of a new study showing that vegans were more than twice as likely to suffer from hip fractures. Tellingly, the doctor's advice was mostly about supplements rather than food. When pressed, he said that vegans could get calcium from foods such as broccoli and insisted that vegans were pretty clued up about these things. He didn't tell the viewer that you would need to eat a mountain of broccoli to get enough calcium, or point out the lower levels of bioavailability of vitamins from plant foods and supplements. Neither did he address the risks associated with calcium supplements. Most glaring, however, was that no explanation was offered as to why, if vegans are so 'clued up', some are so deficient in nutrients that they suffer hip fractures at 2.3 times the rate of omnivores.

In a *Times* article, 'Help! My child has gone meat free', children's nutrition expert Lucinda Miller did not obfuscate. Asked to comment on how a parent could ensure that a vegan child got all the nutrients they needed, she made it clear that obtaining the appropriate nutrients from a vegan diet is a challenging matter. She said that 'to replace what you lose by giving up meat, you really have to pile your plate high'.[158] (Think back to the 1.1 kilos of quinoa you'd have to eat to meet your protein requirements.) She also pointed out that 'many nutrients can easily slip when switching to a vegetarian or vegan diet. These include protein, iron, calcium, zinc, iodine, omega-3, and vitamins A, B and B12.'[159] She went on to list the various supplements that would also be required, and to highlight the bioavailability issues with nutrients such as iron from plant sources. She warned, again, that the plate would need to be stacked high with kidney beans (1 tin), kale (1kg) and beetroot (2kg) to deliver the RDA of iron for a teenage girl.

In an interview with me, Miller said she believes that it is possible to be healthy on a vegan diet, but adds a few provisos:

'When people go vegan for moral reasons, they are often willing to compromise on their health for the sake of the planet. Some say they don't mind feeling low and slow because they think it's all for a good cause. If you value your health and want to eat a vegan diet, you can probably feel well for quite some time provided you really work hard on it. And you will have to supplement and make every mouthful count to get all the nutrients in.'[160]

In 2003, biologist Colin Tudge wrote that 'to thrive on a vegetarian and especially a vegan diet, you have to be astute and conscientious, or to be lucky'.[161] Advice like Lucinda Miller's serves as a guide to the conscientious. But did anyone reading her advice say to themselves: *Hang on a minute, if plant-based eating is supposed to be so healthy, why does it require the consumption of impossibly large mountains of beans and kale, and a cupboard full of expensive supplements?* And reading what Dr Porter had to say, did anyone who was contemplating trying Veganuary stop and think: *If a vegan diet lacks such an essential vitamin as B12, and if the consequences of a B12 deficiency can be felt throughout the nervous system, maybe this plant-based diet isn't all it's cracked up to be?*

Those behind our national and global dietary guidelines have done some very adept sidestepping of these important questions about human health. These guidelines are all variations on a theme, and that theme is one that promotes plant foods at the expense of animal foods.

Eatwell, My Plate, EAT-Lancet: variations on a plant-based theme

The Eatwell Guide – what Dr Harcombe likes to call the Eatbadly Guide – and its US version, My Plate, both evolved from the Food Pyramid (the US federal nutrition guide issued in 1974) and the 1977 McGovern Dietary Goals Report. Neither the Food Pyramid nor the Dietary Goals were based on solid science, says Dr Robert Lustig.[162] Registered nutritionist Maria Cross asserts that the same is true of the UK's Eatwell Guide, revised by Public Health England in 2016.[163] We've previously seen that the recommended amounts of fruit and vegetables – which later became the five-a-day mantra – had no basis in science. Neither did the suggested amounts of grains and cereals, or the fat guidelines. We now know that the evidence against saturated fat and in favour of a low-fat, high-carbohydrate diet was always woefully lacking, yet these guidelines look like Ancel Keys' unfounded theories on a plate.

If the Eatwell Guide is not backed up by science, it *is* backed by industry: the group appointed by Public Health England included significant representation from the food and drink industry.[164] The ramifications of this industry involvement will be discussed in Chapter 12 but, for now, we might at least consider the possibility that the guidelines might have been influenced by factors other than the science of human nutrition.

In 2020 a paper was published claiming that eating according to the Eatwell Guide would reduce your risk of dying early. Dr Harcombe found that the evidence didn't justify the claim, and that the paper should have concluded that 'data from over half a million people found virtually no evidence to support the UK "Eatwell Guide"'.[165]

In fact, much evidence points to the fact that following the Eatwell Guide leads to extremely poor health outcomes. Research by the Public Health Collaboration shows that actual eating patterns in the UK mirror the guidelines closely, with almost 50 per cent of calories coming from carbohydrates. The PHC maintains that this way of eating has resulted in the high rates of obesity, pre-diabetes and diabetes that now cost the NHS around sixteen billion pounds a year.[166]

In September 2019, a new, more extreme version of Eatwell – the Planetary Health Diet – was introduced to the world by EAT-Lancet.[167] Like its predecessors, it stipulated that a plate should be half full of fruit and vegetables, with most of the rest taken up by whole grains and starchy vegetables. There are tiny allowances for animal proteins and dairy. Animal fats are discouraged, but industrially produced seed oils and added sugars are not. The creators of the diet note that the allowances for animal foods are entirely 'optional'. In other words, this is a near-vegan diet that wishes it were a vegan diet. And the entire world is supposed to eat it.

Dr Harcombe found the diet to be high in carbohydrates (51 per cent) and seriously deficient in vitamin B12, retinol (the form in which the body needs vitamin A), vitamin D (and in particular D3, which is the body's preferred form), vitamin K, sodium (salt), potassium, calcium, iron and omega-3.[168] Dr Ede also analysed the diet and the report of which it was a part, concluding that the Commission's arguments are 'vague, inconsistent, unscientific, and downplay the serious risks to life and health posed by vegan diets'.[169] The evidence base for the entire report was judged to be extremely weak by researchers Frédéric Leroy and Nathan Cofnas. 'The case propagated by the EAT-Lancet Commission ... has essentially been based on observational studies with RRs [relative risks] much below 2,' wrote the authors, stressing that it is poor practice to infer a causal connection to meat-eating from such 'weak and confounded data'.[170]

A reliance on weak data is not the report's only failing, however. Adam Drewnowski concluded that 'the EAT-Lancet diet was not actually affordable by many of the world's poor'.[171] Will Masters, a food economist at Tufts University, also accused the EAT-Lancet Commission of overlooking the economics of their diet. He and his research team found that up to half the population of sub-Saharan Africa and more than a third of the population of South Asia wouldn't be able to pay for the EAT diet.[172] The WHO, which had earlier produced a report highlighting that more than one in three low- and middle-income countries face both extremes of malnutrition and obesity, pulled out of sponsoring a launch event for EAT after Italy's ambassador to the United Nations questioned the health and economic implications of its recommendations.[173]

Researchers Francisco Zagmutt, Jane Pouzou and Solenne Costard of EpiX Analytics (a risk analysis and statistical consultancy) criticised the EAT diet on several counts.[174] They calculated that if a person was to eat the maximum recommended intake for each element of the EAT diet, the caloric intake would be a whopping 3,852kcal (kilocalories) daily, something that would not do much for the global obesity and diabetes epidemics. They also pointed out that the EAT authors had overestimated the positive health impacts of their diet on the back of a series of faulty assumptions and spurious associations such as those between red meat consumption, type-2 diabetes and mortality.

The Zagmutt team was also critical of the tiny allowances for animal protein and dairy within the EAT diet, given that backyard animal husbandry is an important source of nutrition in developing countries. 'Reduction of animal production could make these foods less available to children and pregnant or breast-feeding mothers,' said the authors, but the EAT report had not even considered the health impacts on children. The authors conclude that: '[while] issues of obesity have increased in developing countries, the question remains as to whether the reference [EAT] diet proposed by the authors is the best alternative to address all of these issues'.[175]

These concerns were echoed in a 2020 study by the American Society for Nutrition, whose authors maintained that 'a transition to more plant-based diets ... is unlikely to affect obesity [that is, reduce it], and may also have adverse health effects if this change is made without careful consideration of the nutritional needs of the individual relative to the adequacy of the dietary intake.'[176]

The plant-based myth lives on

The EAT-Lancet near-vegan diet has been shown to be inadequate on many levels. It is neither healthful nor economic nor sustainable. And yet, large numbers of people persist in promulgating the essential message underlying the diet, which is that we should all go plant based. We can't blame ordinary people for failing to read the fine print of reports published by organisations such as EAT-Lancet, but we should surely expect more of our politicians and policy makers. Did London's mayor Sadiq Khan do any research before signing London's citizens up to the EAT-Lancet diet? Did he look any further than the latest headline about the environmental consequences of meat consumption? Did the head of a UK school who introduced vegetarian-only group meals to her school in 2020 consult a nutritionist before doing so? It wasn't apparent to me that she had. In response to my letter expressing concern, she sent me a press statement in which she referenced the fact that a vegetarian menu is 'attractive to schools because it allows them to serve better meals for the same money', will generate 'environmental benefits' and allows all children and staff to eat together regardless of their culture or religion. She cited three articles to justify the vegetarian policy, but conspicuously absent from her list of sources was any nutritional research or any opinion pieces by medical practitioners or nutritionists who might claim to have a handle on the research.

She concluded by saying that: 'we are by no means the first school to do this and I believe that if we fast-forward ten years, then many, many more schools will be serving vegetarian meals'.[177] Given the plant-based dogma to which we are all subjected on a daily basis, she may well be right, and school menus might become not just vegetarian but vegan. And we should be worried about that, because if an extreme plant-based diet would put many of us at risk of nutritional deficiencies, it is particularly dangerous for the young, as we'll see in the next chapter.

3

When the Plant-based Diet Goes Badly Wrong

In 2019, an Australian couple who had put their baby daughter on a strict vegan diet were sentenced to an eighteen-month jail term, to be served as a community order. The child was found to be malnourished, underweight and undersized, without teeth and developmentally delayed, having been fed a diet of oats, potatoes, toast, rice and other vegan foods. The judge stated that it 'is the responsibility of every parent to ensure the diet they choose to provide their children ... is one that is balanced and contains sufficient essential nutrients for optimal growth'.[1]

In 2020, a Florida couple were charged with murder and aggravated manslaughter due to neglect and child abuse. They were accused of starving their eighteen-month-old son to death and feeding his three siblings, aged three, five and eleven, a raw fruit and vegetable diet. The older children were found malnourished and with pale, yellowish skin.[2]

Other cases of malnutrition inflicted on children include the 2001 case of a British couple who caused the death of their nine-month-old daughter by feeding her a raw vegan diet, and the 2007 case of an Australian couple who were sentenced to life in prison for the death of their malnourished six-week-old baby boy, who had been fed soy milk and apple juice.[3]

A plant-based diet is not for the young

These are stories of extreme parental ignorance and neglect. But they also beg the important question of whether a vegan diet is safe and appropriate for babies and young children. The official answer to this question is hard to pin down, and it very much depends on which body you consult. The British Dietetic Association, the American Academy of Nutrition and Dietetics, Australia's peak health body, the National Health and Medical Research Council (NHMRC), and Dieticians of Canada take the view that the vegan diet is safe for all life stages, including babies and children.[4] Many European bodies disagree. The Germans, Swiss, French, Spanish, Danish and Belgians all advise against vegan diets for young children.[5] The French Paediatric Hepatology, Gastroenterology and Nutrition Group declared that vegan diets expose children to nutritional deficiencies that can have serious consequences, 'especially when this diet is introduced at an early age, a period of significant growth and neurological development'.[6] While acknowledging that a vegetarian or a vegan diet can be safe if carefully designed, the Spanish Paediatric Association advises that infants and young children follow an omnivorous diet, or at least an ovo-lacto-vegetarian diet (that is, inclusive of some animal foods such as eggs and dairy).[7]

The Vegan Society, on the other hand, states that 'a totally plant-based diet can meet everyone's nutritional needs, including those who are pregnant and breastfeeding'.[8] Their website features guidance for all pre-adulthood life stages, starting with pregnancy and early infant life and ending with eighteen-year-olds.

How are we to know who to believe? We might consult a review of the medical literature on the subject, such as that conducted by researchers Frédéric Leroy and Nathan Cofnas, who found that the risks of nutritional deficiency from meat avoidance are 'documented by an extensive list of clinical case reports in the medical literature', with serious and sometimes irreversible pathological symptoms being reported in infants, adolescents and adults. Those pathological symptoms have included failure to thrive, hyperparathyroidism, macrocytic anaemia, optic and other neuropathies, lethargy, degeneration of the spinal cord, and cerebral atrophy.[9]

A close reading of the Vegan Society's dietary advice should also make us question the position taken by official bodies who support vegan diets for children. For pregnant and breastfeeding women, under-fives, five- to ten-year-olds, and eleven- to eighteen-year-olds, much of the advice consists of lists of the supplements (in the form of pills or artificially fortified foods) that are required to make a vegan diet safe and sufficiently nutritious. By definition, any diet that requires such extensive supplementation is deficient in a range of nutrients, meaning that the diet cannot be considered complete and safe. This is to say nothing about the problem of vitamin and mineral bioavailability from plant-based foods, which is not mentioned by the Vegan Society.

The risk of nutrient deficiencies among children eating vegan diets prompted French professor of paediatric gastroenterology and nutrition Dr Patrick Tounian to speak out in 2019. Claiming that paediatricians are seeing increasing numbers of infants suffering with severe deficiencies as a result of replacing dairy milk with plant milks, he warned of the consequences – some of them irreversible – for their lifelong health, particularly for brain development. He blamed, not parents, but the experts and profit-driven corporations who incite them. Older children and millennials are also at risk, according to Dr Tounian, as more and more succumb to the lure of plant-based diets, risking deficiencies in calcium, iron and B12.[10]

Like Dr Tounian, New York-based associate professor of paediatrics Dr Keith Ayoob highlighted the dangers of feeding plant-based milk to children. 'Infants and toddlers are NOT little adults,' he warned. 'I cringe when parents give kids oat "milk" instead of REAL milk ... dairy ALTERNATIVES are NOT dairy EQUIVALENTS.'[11]

Naturopath and functional medicine practitioner Lucinda Miller spoke to me about the suitability of plant-based milks for both children and adults: 'People don't realise that there is no like for like substitute for real milk. Some of the plant milks are supercharged with calcium, but it's calcium carbonate, which is basically chalk. If they're on reflux medication or they have low stomach acid, they can't absorb this form of calcium. The manufacturers also put in vitamin D2 instead of D3, which is harder to uptake, and there's little to no protein or fat. It's all playing to the marketing angle, not nutrition. There's nothing to fill you up. So, parents who are being health conscious might be giving their kids gluten-free cornflakes with almond milk, and then they go off to school on a half tank and of course they're starving and can't concentrate as the breakfast has not filled them up. I wish there was a better solution as many kids do need to be dairy free for other reasons.'[12]

Despite the expression of such concerns, the Vegan Society continues to insist that plant-based diets are safe for all life stages, while simultaneously alerting us to deficiencies in the diet that must be addressed by supplements. The EAT-Lancet commission takes a similar having-it-both-ways stance, asserting both that its Planetary Health Diet is best for global health, while admitting, a few pages later, that it is not appropriate for pregnant women, babies, young children, pre-teens, teens or the elderly, and requires extensive supplementation.

The Plantrician Project (whose mission is to 'educate, equip and empower our physicians, healthcare practitioners and other health influencers with knowledge about the *indisputable benefits* of whole food, plant-based nutrition'[13] – italics mine) also insists that a vegan diet is healthful for all life stages. The authors of its 'Quick-start guide to paediatric plant-based nutrition' state that: 'A plant-based diet with a wide variety of wholesome plant foods contains *everything* needed to nourish us at any life stage [and that] animal products like meat, fish, poultry, dairy and eggs are not necessary for healthy growth and development' (italics mine).[14] But, since plant foods do not contain B12, which is essential for healthy growth and development, a plant-based diet cannot be said to contain *everything* that is needed. As we saw in Chapter 2, plant-based diets are deficient in a number of important nutrients, including vitamins A, D and B12, and several minerals. Commenting on vitamin D, the guide says that it is 'unrelated to diet' and that it 'only exists in animal foods (mainly dairy products) because it is artificially added'.[15] True, the primary source of vitamin D is the sun. But it's also true that the foods containing the most vitamin D, and in the form that the body wants it, are animal foods. The notion of bioavailability, for vitamin D or any other nutrient, is never mentioned.

In addition to glossing over the nutritional deficiencies in plant-based diets, the Plantrician Project's guide makes questionable claims about the links between meat-inclusive diets and disease. The guide opens with a list of seven frightening claims about disease, including the assertions that hardening of the arteries begins in childhood and obese children are likely to become obese adults. The implication is that meat-eating is responsible for all of these conditions, and that the plant-based diet is a cure-all. But, where evidence is provided, it turns out to have been cherry-picked, and relies on the kind of weak epidemiology discussed in Chapter 1. Theories about saturated fat and high LDL causing heart disease and meat causing cancer are positioned as incontrovertible facts, when we know that they are open to question and believed by many to be entirely incorrect.

The facts about nutrition covered in Chapter 2 belie the claims made by the Plantrician Project, the Vegan Society and some dietitians' organisations. If we take a closer look at some of the nutrients required at each stage of a child's life, we'll see just how far off the mark these claims are.

The plant-based diet and pregnancy

'Without sex hormones there can be no menstruation or any other functioning of the reproductive system.'[16] It follows that the ability to conceive is dependent on healthy hormones, which means healthy cholesterol levels. The body can and does make cholesterol, but this process does not work efficiently in people who are nutrient deficient, as is often the case with vegans. A study by Dr Jorge Chavarro, of the Harvard School of Public Health, led him to claim that 'women wanting to conceive should examine their diet. They should consider changing low-fat dairy foods for high-fat dairy foods, for instance.'[17] The Weston A. Price Foundation also advises women who want to conceive to eat diets rich in healthy fats (such as those in olive oil, avocados and animal-sourced foods) and other nutrients.

Regan Lucas Bailey, a nutrition science professor at Purdue University, has expressed worries not only about the health effect of poor diet on girls themselves but also on the health of any children they might have in the future. 'Going into reproductive age at nutrition risk can cause intergenerational effects,' she has said.[18]

Nutrient-dense foods are equally important during pregnancy. Certain nutrients that are found in animal foods are required for placental function, foetal growth and development of the heart, eyes, limbs and immune system, and a diet that is deficient in one or more can have serious consequences.[19] Lily Nichols, a registered dietitian with expertise in prenatal nutrition and the author of *Real Food for Pregnancy*, writes about the difficulty in obtaining these nutrients if you follow a vegetarian or vegan diet:

> In short, the following nutrients are challenging to obtain in a vegetarian diet: vitamin B12, choline, glycine, preformed vitamin A (retinol), vitamin K2, DHA, iron, and zinc. If you follow a strictly vegan diet, meaning you consume absolutely *no* animal foods – no meat, poultry, fish, dairy or eggs – some of these nutrients may be impossible to obtain from your diet.[20]

Nichols goes on to explain precisely why each of these nutrients is important during pregnancy. (Details can be found in Chapter 3 of her book – essential reading if you're pregnant.)

Nichols has acknowledged that her approach to nutrition was influenced by the work of Dr Weston A. Price (1870–1948), who we first met in Chapter 2.[21] Price was a Cleveland dentist who set out to understand the factors responsible for fine teeth among the people who had them: isolated, non-industrialised people. He studied many isolated human groups, including sequestered villages in Switzerland, Gaelic communities in the Outer Hebrides, Inuit and Indians of North America, Melanesian and Polynesian Islanders and African tribes. (Price used the word Eskimo, but since this term has faded from use I'll use the word Inuit here.) 'Wherever he went, he found that beautiful, straight teeth, freedom from decay, stalwart bodies, resistance to disease and fine characters were typical of native people on their traditional diets, rich in essential food factors.'[22] Price also found that every one of these cultures had a nutrient-rich diet that included animal foods, and that certain of these foods were fed in abundance both to couples trying to conceive and pregnant women. For the Swiss the sacred food was butter made from grass-fed animals; for the Gaelic people it was a fish head stuffed with oats; for the Inuit it was salmon roe. All these peoples seemed to know instinctively that nutrition was particularly crucial for conception and during pregnancy.

In modern, Western cultures many of us have lost our instinct for nutrition. How many pregnant women would be aware of the full range of nutrients that are required for a healthy pregnancy and a healthy baby? I recall having been given very little by way of diet advice during my three pregnancies; nothing much beyond the need to avoid raw eggs, soft cheeses and alcohol, and to take a folic acid supplement. Certainly, no one mentioned DHA, choline or iodine. But because I was eating a whole-food diet that included a wide variety of animal foods, perhaps I ended up with sufficient stores of these nutrients to have healthy pregnancies. A whole-food, omnivore diet could be seen as a kind of insurance policy against nutrient deficiencies during pregnancy and at all stages of life. Leroy and Cofnas use the term 'nutritional robustness' to describe an omnivore diet.[23] Dr David Klurfeld, the programme leader for human nutrition for the USDA, whom we met in Chapter 1, captured a similar idea when he said, 'You have to think less about your diet when you eat a wide variety of foods,' which is why he would like to see an omnivorous diet being recommended as the best diet for health.[24]

The plant-based diet and babies

The Vegan Society says that breast is best and that a child should ideally be breastfed until they are two years old.[25] Breastfeeding vegan mothers are encouraged to take supplements of B12, iodine, vitamin D and omega-3, and to increase their calcium intake (requirements are 80 per cent higher than for other adults) by eating calcium-rich foods such as calcium-fortified foods and calcium-set tofu.[26] At the risk of belabouring the point, the fact that supplements are advised is evidence in and of itself that a vegan diet is not appropriate for breastfeeding mothers.

As to the question of what to do if breastfeeding is not an option, the Vegan Society states that a 'soya-based infant formula can be fed to vegan infants, but *please speak to your health visitor or doctor before using it*'[27] (italics mine). This plea for women to speak to medical professionals strikes me as an attempt to protect the Society's interests in the event that any woman comes to realise that a soya-based formula is not, in fact, appropriate for babies. Which it isn't.

Even Nestlé, manufacturer of several infant formulas, admits that 'soya and rice compositions are not ideal for infants due to the allergen concerns of soya and the amino acid profile of rice-based products'.[28]

Allergen concerns are just one of the problems with soya-based formulas, however. A 2018 study looked at 410 infants born in the Philadelphia area and compared signs of oestrogen impact on infants who were breastfed, cow-milk-formula fed or soya-formula fed. It found that the tissue and organs of the infants who had been fed soya formula showed signs of significant exposure to oestrogen.[29] This was caused by exposure to the oestrogenic isoflavones (which are sometimes referred to as phytoestrogens or plant oestrogens) in soya, which are well-known endocrine disruptors. (Essentially, this means that they disrupt hormonal signalling and can fool the body by mimicking oestrogen.) Another study indicated that a high intake of isoflavones was associated with reduced fertility in animals, and that soya-based formula could be associated with premature sexual maturation and disruptions to thyroid function in humans.[30]

The Weston A. Price Foundation has also expressed concern about the impact of the endocrine disruption caused by soya. 'Soya infant feeding – which floods the bloodstream with female hormones that inhibit testosterone – cannot be ignored as a possible cause of disrupted development patterns in boys, including learning disabilities and attention deficit disorder.' Premature development of girls has also been linked to the use of soya formula.[31]

Recently, researchers in Denmark concluded that 'it was not possible to rule out the potential for health risk if meat and dairy products are replaced with soya-based alternatives in children's diets.'[32] They pointed to the isoflavones in soya which are 'suspected of disrupting endocrine effects in kids', and proposed a safe limit of the most common plant oestrogen found in soya (genistein) of 0.07mg per 1kg of bodyweight for children aged under ten, and 0.09mg per 1kg of bodyweight for pregnant women.[33] A single 200ml serving of soya milk would exceed the recommended daily amount of genistein for a five-year-old by almost three times.[34] No wonder the Vegan Society wants us to check with a doctor before feeding a baby soya-based formula.

Even the baby breastfed for a long period might not thrive if the mother is vegan. Among the sad cases of severe deficiencies in babies breastfed by vegan mothers, with B12 deficiency a common theme, is the case of a ten-month-old boy who suffered ill health across the board: he was failing to thrive, had megaloblastic anaemia and delayed psychomotor development, deficiencies in vitamins B12, K and D, hematocytopenia and developmental disorders. His mother had the same deficiencies.[35]

Vitamin B12 deficiency is a risk for babies being breastfed by a vegan mother, but so is a lack of fatty acids. The omega-3 fatty acid DHA is essential for optimal cognitive development and brain function in both the developing foetus and the newborn baby. If a breastfeeding mother does not consume enough DHA, there will not be enough in her breast milk.[36] DHA is available only from animal-source foods, with fish and seafood being the main source, and levels of plasma DHA have been shown to be significantly lower in vegetarians and vegans.[37] As registered nutritionist Maria Cross has pointed out, a baby that is breastfed by a vegan mother or given non-dairy milk and animal-free baby foods is therefore being short-changed of its essential supply of brain food.[38]

Beyond milk: when babies need solid foods

Whether a baby is breastfed or fed a formula, at the age of about six months they will need some solid food. Should that food be plant based? A US committee overseeing the 2020 dietary guidelines for children under twenty-four months doesn't think so. The committee recommended that 'babies and toddlers eat meat as well as poultry, seafood and eggs to meet the needs for critical nutrients for growth and development, particularly iron, zinc and choline'. Kathryn Dewey, professor emerita in the Department of Nutrition at the University of California, Davis, who chaired the committee, said that the committee's goal was to lay the foundation for a lifetime of healthy eating. Committee member Sharon Donovan, professor of nutrition and health at the University of Illinois, said, 'If we can establish those healthier patterns right away, it will get them used to eating these types of foods.' Both comments suggest that nutrient-dense animal foods should be part of the diet throughout all stages of childhood and on into adulthood.[39]

The committee notes that 75 per cent of breast-fed children between six and twelve months don't consume enough iron or zinc, and that both red meat and chicken livers are a good source of these nutrients. The Weston A. Price Foundation supports this view that puréed chicken liver is a good first food, and emphasises the need for babies to be fed adequate amounts of foods containing cholesterol, animal fats, calcium, phosphorus, vitamins B6, B12, A, D and K2, with red meat, egg yolks and chicken liver the best sources of these nutrients.[40]

Plant-based advocates were unhappy with the US committee's recommendations. The Physicians Committee for Responsible Medicine (PCRM), a non-profit plant-based advocacy group (of which we'll hear more in Chapter 12) insisted that there was no scientific evidence to suggest that infants would be better off eating meat. A representative for the group, Susan Levin, said that infants and toddlers could get iron from fortified cereals, spinach and lentils, but acknowledged neither the problem of poor iron absorption from these foods, nor the fact that a healthy diet made up of nutrient-dense foods should not require artificial fortification.

Other scientists twisted themselves in knots to try to explain why, if animal foods were considered essential for babies and toddlers, the dietary recommendations for adults limit the intake of these foods. Familiar claims were articulated – that diets high in red meat had been linked to cardiovascular disease, cancer and diabetes – followed by an assertion that we need to eat differently at each stage in life.[41] (But, as we saw in chapters 1 and 2, the link between red meat and disease has been based almost entirely on observational studies with weak associations.)

The plant-based diet for children and teens

Even if a vegan mother manages to breastfeed her child for two years, she'll then be faced with the question of what type of milk to feed her toddler. And, as we saw earlier in the chapter, doctors have expressed concerns about the risk to health from substituting plant milks for dairy milk. Rice milk is out due to traces of arsenic[42] and, given the concerns about the effect of isoflavones on endocrine and immune systems, soya milk is no better an option for a two-year-old than it is for a baby. Oat and nut milks can't even begin to match the calcium content of dairy milk and some contain no calcium at all unless it is artificially added.[43] Almond milk has been found to be high in oxalates, which has been associated with kidney stones in children.[44] (I'll cover the problems with oxalates in Chapter 4.)

What about the other nutrients that older children and teens need? The requirements of growing bodies and brains make a nutrient-dense diet even more important in these stages of life, and, as we saw in Chapter 2, a vegan diet can fall down on the job of providing many nutrients. A 2021 study of Finnish children with a median age of three-and-a-half found vitamin A insufficiency and borderline sufficient vitamin D in all the vegan children. Cholesterol, essential amino acid and DHA levels were also markedly low. The researchers commented that the combination of low vitamin A and DHA status in vegan children raised significant concerns for their visual health. They also warned against making dietary recommendations for children based on adult vegan studies.[45]

Clinical practice has led Lucinda Miller to conclude that many key nutrients – including protein, iron, calcium, zinc, iodine, omega-3 and vitamins A and B12 – can easily dip when switching to a vegetarian or vegan diet.[46] In addition to piling plates high with beans, lentils, nuts and whole grains at every meal to ensure adequate intake of these nutrients, supplements for zinc, omega-3 and B12 are recommended. And unless you can get your child to eat seaweed snacks, they should probably take an iodine supplement, too.

Portuguese doctor Mariette Abrahams has also warned that 'following a vegan dietary pattern is not without nutritional risks for adults but even more so for growing children'. She expressed a concern that not all parents who opt to raise their children as vegans will have the information and nutritional understanding needed to provide balanced diets. Alex White, nutrition scientist at the British Nutrition Foundation, echoes these warnings. 'There are some nutrients that may be more difficult to get from a vegan diet in young children such as vitamin B12, vitamin D, iron, iodine and calcium ... the more restrictive a vegan diet, the greater the risk for nutrient deficiencies.'[47] And early in 2022, Ian Givens, director of the Institute for Food, Nutrition and Health at Reading University, said that the health of young women was being compromised by a lack of key nutrients in their diet because they consumed no red meat or dairy products. He said that half of those aged eleven to eighteen were consuming below the minimum recommended level of iron and magnesium, and that a quarter consumed too little iodine, calcium and zinc.[48]

Iron is a particular concern. Although the iron from meat and fish is easily absorbed, the same cannot be said about the iron from plants, so a child needs to eat much more of it. It takes an entire tin of kidney beans, or 1kg kale or 2kg beetroot to deliver the RDA of iron for a teenage girl, and even this might not be enough because iron intake is not the same as iron absorption. Drinking large quantities of iron-rich kale and spinach smoothies might seem like a solution but they can actually cause anaemia, because the oxalates in these vegetables interfere with the absorption of iron as well as other nutrients.

Iron deficiencies can have serious consequences. The WHO notes that there is a 'growing body of evidence indicating that iron deficiency anaemia in early childhood reduces intelligence in mid-childhood', and in its most severe form, can 'cause mild mental retardation'.[49] In May 2020, the *Wall Street Journal* reported that adolescent girls have inadequate intakes of iron, as well as a host of other important vitamins and minerals, including folate, vitamin D and calcium, and that about 20 per cent of girls are anaemic, a condition that can affect both cognitive function and mood.[50] Miller says that 'it is well established that low iron levels are associated with psychiatric disorders', and that, in her clinic, she has found several cases 'where teenage girls have their first psychiatric episode a few months after becoming vegan or vegetarian'.[51]

Omega-3 deficiencies can also impact mental health. Remember, this nutrient is essential for brain development and health. Rampant nutritional deficiencies in omega-3, along with zinc, magnesium, vitamin D and the B vitamins, have been shown to be associated with poor health and mental illness.[52] As we've seen, plants can provide ALA, but conversion to EPA and DHA, which the body needs, is poor. And conversion of omega-3 into EPA and DHA is impaired by omega-6, which is found in high quantities in grains and vegetable oils.

Poor conversion rates between the nutrient forms found in plants to the forms required by the body mean that even if parents follow Miller's advice to pile plates high with vegetables, beans, pulses, seaweed and every variety of seed imaginable, they might not be able to ensure that their child is getting sufficient amounts of the nutrients they need. This is to say nothing of the problem of actually persuading children to eat the way we'd like them to, which is challenging at the best of times. Most children have strong and seemingly irrational likes and dislikes, and some children are very picky indeed. They must be coaxed away from their aversions by parents who are both persistent and savvy about which nutrients their child needs to thrive, and where these nutrients can be found. This situation can only get more complicated if nutrient-dense animal foods are declared completely off limits, effectively removing the 'insurance policy' against malnutrition that they provide.

Can we really afford to remove this insurance policy against malnutrition when children's health in many countries is already at risk? UNICEF reports that over 20 per cent of children in the world aged under five suffer from stunting (impaired growth and development), 6 per cent suffer from wasting, and 7 per cent suffer from being overweight.[53] Almost all adolescents in India are malnourished and suffering deficiencies in one or more micronutrients such as iron, folate, zinc, vitamin A, vitamin B12 and vitamin D, and over 50 per cent of adolescents are too short, thin, overweight or obese.[54] On the other side of the world, in the US, where over 60 per cent of calories come from processed foods, childhood obesity is rocketing, with some states reporting that over 50 per cent of children are obese. Ten per cent of US children have fatty liver disease,[55] and one in four US teenagers is diabetic or prediabetic.[56]

A 2021 study concluded that animal-sourced foods, rich in amino acids, are important for linear growth and development of young children in low- and middle-income countries.[57] On the other hand, the widespread uptake of EAT-Lancet's or any other near-vegan or vegan diet would only exacerbate developmental problems. A study of 187 healthy five- to ten-year-olds in Poland published in the *American Journal of Clinical Nutrition* in June 2021, provides some indication as to how much worse. It found that children on vegan diets (of which there were fifty-two) were negatively affected in terms of growth, bone mineral content and micronutrient status.[58] Vegan children were, on average, 1.2 inches shorter, had 4–6 per cent lower bone mineral content, and were three times more likely to be deficient in vitamin B12 than omnivores.[59]

Meat is more than just protein; it contains essential nutrients, too. Given the evidence that critical nutrients in some vegetables and fruits have fallen in the past fifty years, the consumption of red meat may be more important than ever. Professor Alice Stanton argued as much ahead of her speech at the Oxford Farming Conference in 2020, saying that the drop in vitamins and key electrolytes in plant-based foods, caused by genetic selection for large volume and uniformity of shape and appearance, meant that the nutrients in red meat were essential, particularly for children in the first three years of life.[60]

Kids under pressure

'A little bit of everything will do you good' and 'home-made is best' were my mother's food mantras, repeated regularly when I was growing up. These days, young people are on the receiving end of an entirely different set of messages. Some of those messages are represented by the 'clean food' movement. Lucinda Miller claims to have seen a massive rise in the number of young girls going vegan on the back of this movement, and this sparked a rise in eating disorders and a 'very poor relationship with food'. It also instigated a trend of valuing food for its aesthetics rather than its nutritional content: 'Those bowls of vegan food with all the colours of the rainbow look so pretty and appealing on Instagram,' says Miller. 'You can't make a roast dinner look that good. But often that kind of food is completely devoid of the right nutrition needed for a growing teenager and would likely not be filling enough. This can lead to increased snacking on things like crisps and biscuits instead, which we all intuitively know is not good for us.'[61]

If food must now be clean, pretty and Instagram-ready, it is also politics on a plate. Greta Thunberg and Extinction Rebellion (XR) have established a hold over the imaginations of the young, and their message that avoiding meat and dairy is necessary if we're to avert climate catastrophe is hitting home. Giving up meat and dairy likely gives young people a feeling of empowerment in a situation in which they feel totally out of control – never mind the negative environmental and nutritional consequences of their decisions, which are rarely mentioned.

A British university student (who prefers not to be named), working on a dissertation about how those in her generation (aged eighteen to twenty-three) perceive veganism, says she believes people her age to be reluctant to challenge the dominant message of the day, which is that veganism is required to fix climate change:

> It doesn't help that social media is so powerful, and the message on social media is definitely biased towards the 'meat is bad, veganism is best' message. But there's also the fact that people my age are reluctant to stand out or speak out against the dominant message. People call us snowflakes, and I think we are that. It's easier and safer to fall into line rather than risk causing controversy. Even if someone bothered to do their own research and found facts that contradicted the dominant message, they probably wouldn't be brave enough to speak out about that.[62]

Lessons in veganism: education or propaganda?

The 'dominant message' – that meat-eating is entirely bad and veganism is wholly good – is being propagated not just by actors and activists but via the formal education system. In Coimbatore, India, the effects of one such incident came to light when a twelve-year-old girl, who was anaemic and had been advised to include more iron-rich foods such as liver and eggs in her diet, suddenly began behaving strangely and stopped eating food at home. It was discovered that the girl had been influenced by an animal-rights activist who'd been invited to the school to present videos of mass animal slaughtering as part of a campaign to persuade children not to eat animal foods. The same activist had been presenting unscientific data to promote a vegan agenda in many private, government and corporation schools.[63]

Vegan propaganda slipped into schools under the radar in Coimbatore, but it is being officially endorsed elsewhere. The parent of a child attending a US elementary school was shocked when her child came home with a colourful multi-page booklet he had been given, the contents of which aimed to persuade children that eating animal foods was harmful to their health and to the environment. New Zealand schools have introduced a climate change resource that suggests children eat less meat and dairy, even though teachers cannot know how much meat and dairy any child in their care has eaten.[64] One mother took to Twitter to protest the fact that her son had been 'red carded' at a Scouts meeting simply for saying that eating meat was good for health. Her son had been encouraged to go vegan one day per week to save the planet. 'Our kids are being fed this misinformation daily. No consent,' she said.[65]

In late 2020, one UK school took a stand against the ascendance of the vegan message.[66] Cheltenham Ladies College revealed that while students were at liberty to choose a vegan lifestyle, the school did not actively encourage it because it could be a path to eating disorders. Where students opted to be vegan, they would be offered regular blood tests and support to ensure that their health did not suffer. Commenting on the college's decision not to encourage veganism, psychologist

Nihara Krause, who works with schools and teens with eating disorders, said that it is harder to get a balanced diet as a vegan, and that both vegetarianism and veganism are much higher in girls and women who have anorexia nervosa.

Interviewed in connection with Cheltenham Ladies College's decision, the Vegan Society dismissed these concerns. A spokesperson denied that veganism was linked to eating disorders and said that all schools should let teenagers follow their beliefs. The society has launched a teen hub to encourage more youngsters to stop eating meat and dairy foods and is campaigning for all schools to offer vegan menus.

Plant-based diets for children 'as seen on TV'

The pro plant-based messages that are directed at children by the Vegan Society and some schools are also coming from television. The BBC's *Blue Peter*, for example, offered green badges to any children who could demonstrate that they were 'climate heroes' by making a pledge to 'go meat free', switch off lights or stop using plastic bottles. The 'go meat free' element of the programme drew a furious response from farmers, including Gareth Wyn Jones, who said that it 'overlooked the lower environmental impact of grass-fed British beef and lamb'. The BBC later amended the qualification criteria for a green badge, the new wording saying that children should 'choose a couple of vegetarian meal options during your two weeks as part of a healthy diet'.[67]

A year previously, the UK-based retailer Tesco had communicated an anti-meat message to children via an advertisement called 'Carl's all change casserole', in which a little girl called Chloe says that she doesn't want to eat animals any more. Because 'nothing is more important than his daughter's happiness' the father serves her a casserole of meatless sausages, which Chloe declares 'even better' than the old version. The ad seemed to be aimed at children, while ostensibly communicating to parents. The message was clear: if your child comes home and says they don't want to eat animal foods any more, your job as a parent is to sympathise and head straight to the supermarket to stock up on meat-free meals for the whole family. Caring about a child's happiness is thus deftly conflated with giving in to their desires, however fleeting and ill-informed they might be.

Investigative food writer Joanna Blythman was incensed. 'It's a parent's job to safeguard their children's long-term welfare, not to cave in to modish, ill-informed, potentially dangerous demands from young minds bombarded with propaganda,' she said.[68] Blythman had a go at rewriting the script for the Tesco ad. Her version had the father explaining to his daughter that meat contained important nutrients and that well-raised, well-cared-for animals played a vital role in feeding the soil and maintaining a biodiverse landscape.

Perhaps we shouldn't be surprised by Tesco's ad. The corporation has an eye on the growing and highly profitable vegan food market. In late 2020, former Tesco chief executive Dave Lewis committed to boosting sales of meat alternatives by 300 per cent within five years as part of a wider package of sustainability measures.[69]

The marketing of vegan foods to children is also unsurprising given Big Food's history of deliberately targeting children, documented at length by Mark Hyman in his book, *The Food Fix*. Some 70 per cent of elementary and middle-school students in America see ads for fast food, sweets and soft drinks in their schools, the implicit message being that teachers and schools endorse these products.[70] And the message is reinforced outside school, on TV, hoardings, advertising and via stealth marketing. In the UK, the problem has led the government to announce a ban on junk food advertising online and before 9pm on TV from 2023.[71]

Seeing his son being bombarded with messages from commercial organisations in the UK was, for journalist Jonathan Kent, like 'watching the consumerist equivalent of crack take hold'.[72] Research suggests that this emerging cradle-to-grave consumerism is contributing to growing rates of low self-esteem, depression and other forms of mental illness.[73] Layer a one-sided message about climate catastrophe and the need to stop eating meat on top of all this and you have the perfect recipe for engendering mental illness in children.

The Million Dollar Vegan video: a master class in manipulation

As if young people aren't already being bombarded with enough pro plant-based messages via schools and television, environmental scientists and pressure groups are circumventing formal educational platforms to speak directly to children, disguising personal opinion as irrefutable science. There is no more shocking example of this than Oxford-based environmental scientist Joseph Poore (of whom we will hear more in chapters 7 and 8) talking to a young girl in a short film about diet and the environment. The film was produced and promoted as part of a 'Go Vegan for Lent' campaign organised by a pressure group called Million Dollar Vegan.[74]

The child in the film is Genesis Butler, a twelve-year-old girl from Long Beach, California, who has been vegan since the age of six.[75] Her original motivation for having become a vegan may have been concerns about animal welfare, but the discussion in this film is focused on the effect of meat-eating on the environment. Genesis is interviewing Poore, but given the involvement of the Million Dollar Vegan organisation and the almost twenty-strong production team behind the film, it would be safe to assume that this is no home-grown project initiated by the twelve-year-old. The questions she asks appear to have been scripted – as one might have expected with an experienced presenter – and to have been designed to tee Poore up to deliver a slew of anti-livestock messages. Genesis doesn't challenge any of the claims made by Poore, many of which are entirely spurious, and, in any case, the staging of a genuine question-and-answer session does not appear to be the aim here. The film looks more like propaganda than education.

Genesis begins by asking whether it's better to eat free-range eggs and meat than the factory-farmed versions. 'Not really,' says Poore, who goes on to claim that all kinds of farmland reduce biodiversity. (We'll see just how misleading this is in chapters 8 and 10.) If Genesis has access to the facts about sustainable and regenerative farming that would allow her to challenge this statement (of which there are many), she doesn't use them. Poore moves on to his second point, which is that 'even the grass-fed cows are the equivalent of burning coal to create energy'. This is pure bunkum, as we'll see in Chapter 7, but Genesis accepts everything he says without question.

Next up from our young activist: 'Is reducing meat consumption, like, a good thing for helping the planet?' 'Yes, without a doubt,' says Poore, who proceeds to pop up a chart based on data from one of his own studies, claiming that it demonstrates that even the lowest-impact animal foods have a greater environmental footprint than the highest-impact plant foods. What Poore doesn't mention is that his study fails to account for the different effects of methane and carbon dioxide (CO_2), green water versus blue water use, the soil erosion caused by monocrop agriculture, the regenerative power of properly managed livestock, or the fact that much of the land used for raising livestock cannot, in any case, be used to grow crops. All these points will be discussed at length in chapters 7, 8 and 10.

Poore also talks about how much better soya milk is for the environment, oblivious to the health concerns associated with soya. Then he insists that we need to 'stop this transformation of the environment and treatment of other species' which is 'driven by taste preference for animal products'. Taste preferences? What about the documented nutrient deficiencies of plant-based diets? What about how evolutionary history predisposed us to eat omnivore diets? Poore doesn't explore either of these important points. It appears that he wants his audience to believe that eating animal foods is a selfish habit driven merely by 'taste'.

Poore's *pièce de résistance* is to claim that if we don't do something, current levels of emissions from agriculture are likely to go from 25 per cent of total emissions to a whopping 59 or 60 per cent. Firstly, emissions from livestock farming, which is, after all, the aspect of agriculture that Poore would like to eliminate, are not even close to 25 per cent currently. Secondly, livestock's share of emissions cannot leap to 60 per cent unless emissions from all other sources are so radically reduced that the size of the emissions pie shrinks by three times. This is scaremongering of the highest order.

Genesis's final question is, 'So what would you say to people who want to protect the planet?' Poore replies, entirely predictably, 'Start with the thing in your life that is easy to change: your diet.' Boom – key message delivered, loud and clear. Never mind the risks to child nutrition and health, or to a young woman's ability to conceive and deliver a healthy child. Never mind the facts, full stop. Let's just get the kids to *go vegan for Lent*.

When Vegan for Lent becomes vegan for life

If veganism isn't a diet for the young, neither is it a diet for most adults over the long term. There's an expression used by some nutritionists and physicians to encapsulate what can happen when people spend many years on a vegan diet: ESV, or end-stage veganism. The expression captures a range of health problems, from skin and gastrointestinal conditions to neurological disorders and muscle wasting.

Registered dietitian and author Diana Rodgers collates stories about the vegan experience via her Instagram account: @sustainabledish. Scanning through these stories gives you some idea of the range of ways that health can be impacted by a totally plant-based diet. There are reports of eczema and asthma flare-ups, heart palpitations, stomach pains, bloating, hair loss, anxiety and depression. Similar case studies can also be found at a website for ex-vegans called r/exvegan.[76] One individual messaged the community forum to describe how five years of eating a vegan diet had left him deficient in B12, vitamin D and calcium and caused 'a whole host of horrible neurological symptoms and pain such as facial spasms (similar to Bell's Palsy), ear twitches and nausea' that doctors eventually diagnosed as intercranial hypertension. Another ex-vegan, Daren Gaudry, posted this testimonial on the website:

'Go vegan' they said, 'It's healthy', they said. This was my 2017 result from a strict one-year HCLF [high-carb, low-fat] vegan lifestyle ... I was eating so many so called 'healthy carbs' that I blew up like a balloon ... The vegans I was being coached by said: 'The weight gain is just your body's [*sic*] refeeding and adjusting.' What BS ... It took 2 years to recover. NEVER AGAIN![77]

Elsewhere, ex-vegans have written about the health problems they suffered as a result of the diet. Singer Miley Cyrus said she quit veganism and started eating fish and meat because her brain wasn't functioning properly and she was suffering from hip pain and generally felt as though she was 'running on empty'.[78] Ema Hegberg wrote that after three years of being a stringently 'clean' plant-based eater, she 'started to have severe chest and stomach pain' and suffered from depression. Vitamin B12 supplements helped with the stomach pains, and when she started to eat meat again her depression 'began to fade'.[79] Another woman, Yanar Alkayat, wrote about how a vegan diet ruined her gut health. Symptoms included extreme flatulence and bloating. She was found to have prominent yeast overgrowth and a deficiency in the bacteria that are found in dairy and meat. She learned that a vegan diet – full of grains, dried fruits and sugar-based foods – can feed the harmful bacteria and yeast in the gut, driving issues such as bloating, bowel irregularities and fungal overgrowth in the intestines.[80]

In her ground-breaking book, *The Vegetarian Myth*, former vegan Lierre Keith documented a wide variety of conditions suffered by long-term vegetarians and vegans. These include gastrointestinal disorders of the type suffered by Alkayat, in addition to neurological disorders and autoimmune diseases such as Crohn's disease, rheumatoid arthritis, lupus and diabetes. She writes:

> I'm writing this book as a cautionary tale. A vegetarian diet – especially a low-fat version, and most especially a vegan one – is not sufficient nutrition for the long-term maintenance and repair of the human body. To put it bluntly, it will damage you. I know. Two years into my vegan-hood, my health failed. And it failed me catastrophically. I developed a degenerative joint disease that I will have for the rest of my life ... It took fifteen years to get a diagnosis ... My spine looks like a sky-diving accident. Nutritionally, that's about what happened.[81]

Keith also suffered from flaky skin, gastroparesis (partial paralysis of the stomach), exhaustion, depression and anxiety.

She stopped menstruating and was always cold. Having left veganism behind some two decades ago, Keith still suffers from the damage to her spinal cord and several autoimmune conditions for which she takes medication. About herself and the former vegans who write to her about having similar conditions, she says, 'we will just live with pain for the rest of our lives'.[82]

Lierre Keith urges others to learn from her mistakes. A woman living in the UK, Natasha, wrote to me about her own mistake: a 'disastrous brush with veganism' which severely impacted her own and her son's health.[83] When her children were young she had followed 'the same dietary advice that is still current in the NHS and governments worldwide, that of low fat, wholegrain food'. But from the age of seven, her son steadily gained weight. She tried every way imaginable of eating, but none of them worked for Jacob. Eventually, the whole family went vegan, convinced that it would help them find their ideal weight and make them stronger and fitter than ever. Natasha bought all the books and followed the vegan diet to the letter. The family's carbohydrate intake was very high due to the need to bulk out their meals. Jacob's weight didn't budge, and they were all hungry and constantly eating.

Eight weeks into the diet, out of the blue, Natasha had a mental breakdown. She went from feeling on top of everything to 'feeling as though everything was on top of me'. She was also deficient in vitamins B12 and D3. The only change she had made was becoming vegan. She believes that her body instinctively knew that she was craving animal protein. Adding back eggs, fish and meat put her on an even keel, and she's never looked back.

This experience caused Natasha to question whether the vegan diet really was good for her family's health. She switched her focus from cutting out animal foods to trying not to swamp their bodies with insulin 24/7 from all the carbs they'd been eating. A low-carb diet, combined with intermittent fasting, achieved what a vegan diet never could, which was to help Jacob feel satisfied and in control of what he was eating. He lost all the excess weight and became a 'calm and more positive version of himself', his before-and-after pictures attesting to this transformation.

The vegan honeymoon

Natasha and Jacob never experienced any dramatic benefits from eating a plant-based diet, but this isn't always the case. Ex vegans, doctors and nutritionists talk about the 'vegan honeymoon', which can last for months or even years, convincing converts to veganism that they have made a good decision for their health by giving up animal foods. Cardiologist Dr Aseem Malhotra says, 'I've seen a lot of patients who were initially helped by going vegan but after a few years started to become sick.'[84] The vegan honeymoon phenomenon exists, in part, because people often transition from a very poor diet to one that is better in *relative* terms, and because the health problems arising from the nutritional deficiencies in the new diet can take time to establish. 'The signs of insufficient nutrient intake can take time to set in,' says Stephan van Vliet. 'And it might take five years or more for B12 and fat-soluble vitamins to deplete to a level where deficiency symptoms arise.' This means that positive testimonials from people who have only been on the diet for one or two years need to be taken with a pinch of salt. I came across one such testimonial titled 'I stopped eating meat over a year ago, here's what I learned'. The author said that giving up meat was easy, and that 'vegan food is delicious'. He wrote with enthusiasm about the delicious foods he had tried, but there was nothing in the article to suggest that he had done any research into the nutrients that he might be missing out on; neither was there any acknowledgement of the fact that a year might not be long enough for the effects of a diet to be fully known.[85]

What works for some may not work for others

The vegan diet does not want for high-profile advocates, and many come from the entertainment world. Why does the diet seem to work for these people and not others? How is it that people like Lierre Keith suffer serious adverse health effects from years eating a vegan diet while others, including celebrities Thandie Newton, Zac Effron and Serena Williams, claim to thrive on the diet?[86] The amount of effort and money that is invested into minimising nutrient deficiencies via assiduous food combining and supplementation may have something to do with it, as do genetics. 'Some people appear genetically better adapted to veganism,' says Stephan van Vliet. 'At the same time, differences in nutrient metabolism may preclude others from thriving on vegan diets no matter how well the diet is designed.'[87]

Some who appear to be thriving will be in the midst of the vegan honeymoon and may yet discover that the diet is unsustainable for them. Others who profess to be eating a plant-based diet might actually mean vegetarian or pescatarian and are therefore benefiting from the nutritional value of eggs, fish and dairy. Confusion around the term plant-based certainly appears to be widespread, as was evidenced in the 2021 study referenced in the introduction (I'll talk more about this study in Chapter 13.)[88]

Then there's what Vinnie Tortorich calls the 'chegan' phenomenon – vegans who cheat.[89] In a recent interview, Tortorich and Lierre Keith exchanged stories about the vegans known to them who actually eat meat on a regular basis while continuing to claim to be vegan. Cheating is what keeps them healthy. Keith says she never cheated, which is why her health ended up in such a parlous state.[90]

Keith maintains that, in her experience, many people who try the vegan diet last about three months. (This is borne out by research showing that a third of lapsed vegans reverted to eating animal foods within three months.)[91] Certainly, available statistics point to a high level of recidivism overall – it has been estimated that 84 per cent of those who try veganism end up reverting to eating animal foods in some capacity.[92] Two separate studies found that over 80 per cent of current vegans might have been following the eating pattern for fewer than five years,[93] with just 7 per cent of vegans staying committed to the diet for more than ten years, and 3 per cent for more than twenty years.[94]

For vegans who stay the course for years, transitioning back to an omnivorous way of eating is rarely easy. Diana Rodgers asked her vegan followers what they had found most difficult about returning to eating animal foods. Some respondents talked about being worried about the ethics of eating meat and not being able to find meat that met high animal-welfare standards. Others highlighted the fear of 'judgement from other vegans' and the 'fear of breaking up with the label' to which they had attached themselves.

The fear of breaking up with the label means that many vegans last longer on the diet than they should, ignoring or explaining away the symptoms they experience. When Lierre Keith stopped menstruating, she accepted the explanation given to her by fellow vegans who said that the vegan diet 'is so pure that we don't need to menstruate'.[95] Keith explains that the nature of veganism renders it largely impervious to evidence: '[Veganism] is a kind of all-encompassing ideology, and it becomes your sense of self. There's no way into that kind of fundamentalist mindset. You're not going to reach them until their health collapses, like mine did. Then there's no pretending any more.'[96]

That veganism is often impervious to evidence is illustrated by a story told to me by my son, who recently spent the summer working in a small delicatessen in central London. A young woman came in every day and ordered a coconut milk latte. One day this woman announced, a propos of nothing, that she had been vegan and that she had absolutely loved it. 'It was the best diet,' she said. 'I felt so great on it.' My son asked her why she was no longer vegan. 'Oh, well my hair and nails started to fall out, so I had to stop,' she said. He asked her whether this might be an indication that the diet wasn't all that healthy after all. Her reply? 'Oh no. It's a really, really, healthy diet. I felt incredible.' And with that she headed into the streets of Pimlico, coconut milk latte in hand, a staunch advocate for a diet so lacking in essential nutrients that it can cause hair and nails to fall out.

4

The Bad Guys Lurking in
Your Plant-based Diet

Chapter 3 was largely a story about the effects of deficiency (that is, nutrient deficiency); this chapter tells the tale of abundance. Some things are found in great quantities in the vegan diet, and they are far from benign.

The term 'plant-based' itself, suddenly ubiquitous, sounds not just benign but positively pleasing. Mary McCartney, daughter of Paul and Linda, isn't alone in thinking that plant-based 'sounds more beautiful and natural' than vegan. A survey found that 75 per cent of global consumers found plant-based claims appealing, compared to 42 per cent for meat-free and 39 per cent for vegan.[1] It's hard to object to a term that contains the word 'plants'. After all, plants are gloriously colourful, mostly delicious and replete with those phytochemicals we looked at in Chapter 2. The photographs of all those vegetables, fruits and loaves of wholegrain bread that accompany most healthy eating guides look so attractive. And although we have all these niggling doubts about meat, plants, we've been led to believe, can do no harm.

The truth is that plants can do harm. Eating too many of

the wrong plants at one time, or on a daily basis, can cause severe health problems. Some people cannot tolerate plants in their diet at all. This is because, as Dr Steven Gundry explains, 'leaves, fruits, grains and other vegetable foods aren't just sitting there accepting their fate as part of your dinner. They have their own sophisticated ways of defending themselves from plant predators like you, including the use of toxic chemicals.'[2] Oxalates, phytic acid and lectins are just three of the powerful defences that plants use to stop us from eating them. They can prevent us from accessing plant nutrients and even make some people very sick. Dr Paul Saladino likens their potential effects on those who have an intolerance to them to the effects of a mismatch between a computer program and an operating system. 'They are Android and we are Mac: the programs are not very compatible . . . Plants have evolved these molecules for their own personal biochemistry and metabolism, not ours!'[3]

Oxalates

Oxalates – also known as oxalic acid – are naturally occurring compounds in plants. The oxalate problem made the news in April 2020 when actor Liam Hemsworth had to rethink his vegan diet after an overload of oxalates gave him painful kidney stones that required surgery. Hemsworth's morning smoothie – which included almond milk, plant protein and five handfuls of spinach, in addition to the large quantities of vegetables he was eating on a daily basis – almost certainly caused the build-up of calcium oxalate that causes 80 per cent of all kidney stones. Since getting one kidney stone gives you a much higher chance of getting another if you continue eating in the same way,[4] Hemsworth had little option but to change his diet.

Functional medicine specialist Chris Kresser has warned about the 'dark side' of the type of green smoothie that

Hemsworth was consuming. The cruciferous vegetables from which they are made contain large amounts of oxalates and much else besides, including high levels of thallium (a toxic metal), and goitrogens (a chemical that inhibits the uptake of iodine by the thyroid gland).[5]

Oxalates bind to calcium as they leave the body, which increases the risk of kidney stones.[6] Oxalates have also been implicated in increased inflammation, mitochondrial and gut dysfunction, mineral imbalance, connective tissue problems, urinary tract issues, fibromyalgia and autoimmune diseases such as rheumatoid arthritis and lupus.[7] By binding to minerals such as calcium, oxalates also contribute to the problem of nutrient bioavailability from plants as discussed in Chapter 2. When we eat spinach and other foods containing oxalates, calcium binds to the oxalates, which means that we only absorb about 5 per cent of the calcium.[8]

The oxalate problem has long been known to us. From the early 1850s to the early 1900s, oxalate poisoning was a recognised phenomenon, being referred to as oxalic acid diathesis. It was known to be a seasonal problem that was worse in the spring and summer, when fresh greens were available and oxalate consumption would rise.[9] Today, year-round access to high-oxalate plants like nuts and seeds, spinach, beets, blackberries, quinoa, beans and whole grains means that exposure to oxalates is higher than ever. Most people get between 200 and 300 milligrams of oxalates daily. If you are at risk of kidney stones, you should probably be consuming under 100mg daily, and doctors recommend an intake of less than 50mg per day for some people.[10] A slice of wholewheat bread, a serving of multibran cereal and a serving of okra will put you over the 100mg limit. A daily serving of a normal portion of an oxalate-rich food such as spinach could lead to an intake in excess of 1,000mg per day.[11]

Monique Attinger, a nutritionist who calls herself the Low

Ox Coach, initially became aware of the harm that high oxalate exposure can do when her daughter was diagnosed with an oxalate problem. She decided to join her daughter in following a low oxalate diet, reporting astonishing results. 'Long term issues I'd had (which had been extremely resistant to any treatments I'd done) started to clear up! I'd been dealing with a variety of things: low thyroid; poor sleep; extremely problematic digestion; fat malabsorption; low energy; poor exercise recovery; anxiousness; irritability; low immunity ... all of them started to improve as I started to lower oxalate.'[12]

Of course not everyone will suffer as a result of high levels of oxalate exposure to the same extent as Attinger and her daughter. Many of us are able to excrete the compounds that are formed when oxalate binds to minerals. But those with a genetic predisposition to oxalate sensitivity can experience severe problems.[13] According to Sally Norton, a leading expert on oxalate poisoning, those with damaged gut lining will also absorb more oxalates and suffer more health problems as a result. Unfortunately, thanks to a number of assaulting compounds and chemicals in our food supply and the emulsifiers in processed foods, says Norton, increasing numbers of people have damaged gut lining.[14]

If genetics and gut health play a role in any individual's reaction to oxalates, it's also true that the dose makes the poison, and a plant-based diet is bound to contain a higher dose than a diet that includes animal-sourced foods. As increasing numbers of people adopt strict plant-based diets we might expect to see a rise in oxalate-related health problems.

Phytic acid

Phytic acid (also referred to as phytate) is found in all edible seeds, grains, legumes and nuts. Like oxalates, the phytic acid in foods such as grains impairs absorption of iron, zinc and calcium, and may promote mineral deficiencies.[15] Alarmingly, it prevents not only the absorption of the minerals in the plants being consumed but any other minerals found in the meal. A study on the bioavailablity of zinc (discussed in Chapter 2) showed that eating oysters (which are rich in zinc) with a corn tortilla (rich in phytic acid) completely nullified any absorption of zinc.[16] The anti-nutrient quality of phytic acid is so significant that the requirements for dietary intake of zinc have to be adjusted upwards 'for populations in which animal products – the best sources of zinc – are limited, and in which plant sources of zinc are high in phytates'.[17]

Phytic acid is more than an anti-nutrient, however. It also has alleged and known health benefits. Like other phytochemicals it is believed to have medicinal and chemo-preventative (anti-cancer) effects.[18] The study of these effects represents an emerging field, and it is too soon to say, definitively, that this or that phytochemical reduces the risk of cancer. But we cannot afford to ignore the potentially beneficial effects of these chemicals.

What does this mean in practical terms? Should you or shouldn't you consume foods containing phytic acid? How should you balance the anti-nutrient effects with the potential medicinal effects? Nutrition scientist Stephan van Vliet suggests that there are 'important nuances regarding phytochemicals (type, dose, source),' and that 'in the case of phytochemicals like phytic acid, perhaps some amounts may be beneficial, whereas high doses may be detrimental'.[19] The recommended intake of phytic acid is likely context dependent; the context being a person's nutritional state (particularly with regard to mineral deficiencies), tolerance levels and overall diet. If you are obtaining a sufficient amount of zinc and iron from foods that do not contain phytic acid, you are likely to be able to tolerate, and even benefit from, the phytic acid and other nutrients in the nuts, seeds and legumes that you consume in addition. Researchers DiNicolantonio and Land advise, however, that 'high phytate foods should not make up the majority of the diet'.[20] If you are eating a vegan diet that is based almost exclusively around foods containing high amounts of phytic acid, and excludes the foods that are rich in minerals, you could be setting yourself up for nutritional deficiency. Vegetarians and vegans are already at higher risk of zinc and iron deficiencies than meat eaters; the recommendation that we all embrace the plant-based diet and consume dramatically more of the plants containing phytic acid can only exacerbate this problem.[21]

Lectins

The last of our troublesome threesome, lectins, are large proteins that serve as a crucial weapon in the arsenal of strategies that plants use to defend themselves. The lectins in the seeds, grains, skins, rinds and leaves of most plants bind to carbohydrates in our bodies as we consume the plant. They also bind to sialic acid, a sugar molecule found in the gut, in the brain, between nerve endings, in joints and in all bodily fluids. According to Dr Steven Gundry, these sticky proteins can interrupt messaging between cells and otherwise cause toxic and inflammatory reactions.[22] Brain fog is just one result of lectins interrupting communication between one nerve and another nerve. Gastric distress is another common symptom of lectin overload. Dr Gundry lists a wide range of other health problems – including aching joints, autoimmune diseases, dementia, diabetes, headaches and infertility – that have been resolved in his patients once they eliminated lectins from their diets. Dr Paul Saladino writes that the hypothesis that lectins are implicated in Parkinson's is also gaining credence, with

animal studies showing that 'ingested lectins may be damaging the gut and travelling through the vagus nerve to the brain, where they appear to be toxic to dopaminergic neurons'.[23]

According to research reviewed by Dr Saladino, plant lectins could also contribute to weight gain by mimicking the actions of insulin (thereby signalling fat cells to grow), and by negatively affecting signalling of the satiety hormone known as leptin.[24] Could all those veggies we believe to be so good for weight loss have the opposite effect when consumed in vast quantities?

How prevalent are lectins in our diet? A US study found that the edible parts of twenty-nine of eighty-eight foods tested, including common salad ingredients, fresh fruits, roasted nuts and processed cereals were found to possess significant lectin-like activity. The study's authors concluded that dietary exposure to lectins is widespread.[25]

Kidney beans are touted as a good source of iron for those eating plant-based diets. But kidney beans contain large amounts of a lectin known as PHA, which appears to trigger an inflammatory response known as leaky gut by interfering with the body's ability to produce a healthy mucus layer within the gut epithelium.[26] Another lectin that can cause damage is PNA, found in peanuts. Lectins can also be found in large amounts in vegetables in the nightshade family, such as tomatoes, potatoes, aubergines and peppers. For those who are particularly sensitive, says Dr Saladino, the removal of these vegetables from the diet can result in dramatic improvements in joint pain, arthritis and autoimmune symptoms.[27]

Dr Gundry's programme for patients who wish to alleviate or eradicate the symptoms of these types of conditions comprises lists of acceptable and unacceptable foods. His 'just say no' list of lectin-containing foods includes pasta, rice, bread, flours, cereal, sugar, legumes, chickpeas, soya protein, all beans, all lentils, many seeds, fruit, aubergines and tomatoes. Given that these foods are the mainstay of plant-based diets, it's clear that any vegan wishing to improve an autoimmune condition by eating a lectin-free diet would be hard pressed to find much to eat.[28] And the EAT-Lancet diet, which prescribes the ingestion of large amounts of nuts, seeds, grains, beans and legumes, looks like a recipe for potential lectin overload.

Like phytic acid, however, lectins are complex beasts. In vilifying them, says Tim Spector, we 'ignore the fact that the plants with the most lectin, such as beans, lentils and nuts, contain thousands of other healthy chemicals'.[29] These chemicals might be protective against disease. As with phytic acid, the best approach to lectin consumption would seem to be to eat them in moderation, and to pay close attention to the effect that they have on the body, reducing or eliminating consumption if health problems arise.

Genetics and environmental factors will play a role in determining whether those lectin-related health problems will arise, and to what degree. And the dose likely makes the poison. On a strict plant-based diet, this dose is likely to be very high indeed. This is a particular problem for those with a genetic susceptibility to one or another form of autoimmune disease, whether it be chronic eczema, Hashimoto's disease or rheumatoid arthritis. Those who are not predisposed to any of these illnesses may be able to get away with eating a plant-based diet, but it would be a mistake to suppose that the whole world could do the same.

The potential for an overload of plant toxins isn't the only concerning thing about a plant-based diet. A few other bad guys sneak their way into the diet when animal-sourced foods are removed, each one with potentially deleterious consequences for health when consumed in large quantities. This bad-guy line-up includes soya, vegetable oils, ultra-processed foods and grains.

Soya

Soya is often promoted as a good source of protein for those eating plant-based diets, but many nutritionists and medical practitioners warn that soya is not the health food we are led to think it is. It is a problematic food on many levels.

At the most basic level, soya fails as a complete protein, being low in sulphur-containing amino acids such as methionine. It also interferes with protein digestion, via the effect of its trypsin inhibitors (a form of anti-nutrient), and mineral absorption, thanks to its high phytic acid content. Although phytic acid can be broken down via fermentation, only a few soya-based foods – such as miso, natto, high quality shoyu-style soy sauce and tempeh – are fermented for long enough.[30] (The majority of soya consumed nowadays is processed by modern methods that do not reduce phytic acid levels and comes in the form of foods like protein shakes, veggie burgers, meat substitutes and many other processed foods.)

There are problems with soya beyond its impact on basic nutrient absorption, many of them explored in the extensive literature on the subject. Most worrying is its isoflavone content. You'll recall from Chapter 3 that the isoflavones in soya (of which genistein is one) behave as weak oestrogen mimics, disrupting the body's endocrine system (the collection of glands that produce hormones). One study noted: 'High intakes [of isoflavones] have been associated with reduced fertility in animals and with anti-leuteinizing hormone effects among premenopausal women. Furthermore, concerns have been expressed regarding sexual maturation of infants receiving very high levels of isoflavones in soy-based infant formula. This is of particular importance for baby boys.'[31]

These endocrine-disrupting effects are considered concerning enough for researchers to have set strict limits on the amount of soya that babies, children and pregnant women should ingest (as noted in Chapter 3). But it isn't just babies, children and pregnant women we should be worried about. Adult males and women who are not pregnant are also vulnerable to the endocrine-disrupting effects of isoflavones (that is, phytoestrogens). The authors of a 2010 study concluded that, while these phytoestrogens could have some beneficial effects on health, 'the supporting evidence that consumption of phytoestrogens is beneficial is indirect and inconsistent', and there is sufficient evidence to warrant concern about 'lifetime exposure'.[32]

Dr Jay Wrigley, a specialist in hormonal health, finds the evidence of possible adverse effects of isoflavones compelling enough to warn all women against consuming foods containing soya.[33] The authors of a 2008 study also found evidence of a negative impact on men's health. They noted that high isoflavone intake had previously been shown to be related to decreased fertility in animal studies. The findings of their own study involving ninety-nine male partners of subfertile couples was consistent with these previous findings: a higher intake of soya foods and soya isoflavones was associated with lower sperm concentration.[34]

In 2008, a case of gynecomastia (enlargement of breast tissue – aka man boobs – commonly caused by oestrogen levels that are excessively high or out of balance with testosterone levels) was reported as being caused by the ingestion of soya products.[35] The male patient had been consuming about three litres of soya milk daily. Once he discontinued drinking soya milk, his condition resolved itself.

Genistein (discussed in Chapter 3) can have adverse effects on hormonal processes via its effects on thyroid function.[36] This, says Dr Paul Saladino, can cause 'fatigue, depression, weight gain, cold intolerance, brain fog and many other symptoms'. Saladino also noted that 'soy and the flavonoid

compounds within it also appear to worsen our inflammatory responses to pathogens'.[37]

As with plant toxins, dose is an important consideration. Having reviewed the evidence about the potential hazardous effects of polyphenol consumption, the authors of one study warned that 'it is important to consider the doses at which these effects occur, in relation to the concentrations that naturally occur in the human body'.[38]

So, what's a safe dose of isoflavones, and therefore, a safe level of consumption of soya products? Clearly, three litres of soya milk (containing approximately 300mg of isoflavones) consumed daily by a man is too much and can lead to gynecomastia.[39] Contrary to popular belief, Asian cultures have typically consumed relatively small amounts of soya as a condiment or occasional meat replacement, and often in fermented forms.[40] Isoflavone intake by Japanese populations, which we might take as a guide to generally safe levels, has been estimated at between 23 and 54mg per day.[41] The FDA recommends that adults consume no more than 75mg per day.[42] If you seek to meet your protein needs by eating soya-based foods in place of animal foods, however, you risk exceeding these levels of isoflavone intake. For example, you could obtain 50g of protein by consuming 2 cups of soya milk, a cup of soya beans and 3oz of tofu, but this combination of foods would result in an isoflavone intake of 142mg, almost three times the upper level of Japanese intake.[43]

If isoflavone content should concern us, so should contamination. Some soya samples evaluated by the USDA Pesticide Data Program revealed fourteen total toxin residues, including the herbicide glyphosate.[44] In fact, most soya produced and consumed in the US has been genetically engineered to be resistant to glyphosate (it's often called 'Round-Up Ready', after the biggest-selling glyphosate brand) and contains high residues of glyphosate.[45] In Europe the growing of GM soya is not permitted, but Europeans could still be affected by glyphosate residues via soya products imported into Europe for both human food and animal feed.[46]

Glyphosate reduces the mineral content of vegetables, and also disrupts the microbiome, potentially promoting malabsorption diseases.[47] 'The implications are sobering, given the importance of the gut microbiome in immune function,' writes Fred Provenza. Glyphosate also enhances the damaging effects of foodborne toxic residues and environmental toxins and is considered a pathway to disease. In addition, animal research cited by Provenza has demonstrated worrying effects of glyphosate on liver and kidney function.[48]

Glyphosate contamination, anti-nutrient properties, high isoflavone content – these are reasons enough for us to be circumspect about advising large swathes of the population to increase their intake of soya. Yet this is precisely what plant-based advocates would like to see happen. In early 2021 a self-described vegan advocate tweeted that 'were we to eat *soy rather than meat*, the clearance of natural vegetation required to supply us with the same protein would decline by 94 percent'[49] (italics mine). This assertion fails to account for how most cattle in the world is raised (without soya feed) or for the realities of land use (both of which I'll cover in Part Two). By ignoring the health risks posed by high intakes of soya it also represents nothing short of a proposal for a dangerous experiment with global human health.

That experiment looks even more dangerous in the context of something else we know about soya: it has a high content of omega-6 linoleic acid. Linoleic acid represents over 50 per cent of the fatty acid content of soya beans and tofu.[50] A single 100 gram serving of tofu delivers almost 5mg of linoleic acid. To understand why that's concerning, we need to explore the next foodstuff in our line-up of plant-based bad guys: vegetable oils.

Vegetable oils

If the replacement of meat with plant proteins were to become widespread, consumption of soya would skyrocket. Of course, we already consume a great deal of soya, since it comes into the diet not just as beans, tofu or baby formula, but as bottled oil. Soybean oil is the number one vegetable oil in America, and second only to palm oil in terms of global consumption, with almost sixty million metric tonnes consumed per year.[51]

Soybean oil is made by crushing hard beans, but most vegetable oils are made by crushing the seeds of plants and are thus more accurately described as seed oils. (From this point on, I will refer to them as such.) Other common seed oils include corn, cottonseed, sunflower and rapeseed, also known as canola.[52] The most commonly consumed seed oil in the UK is rapeseed, followed closely by soybean oil.[53] Most oils labelled simply 'vegetable oil' will be a mix of different oils.

Olive oil, coconut oil and palm oil (as opposed to the lesser used variety, palm kernel oil), while often classed as vegetable oils, are different, being made from the fruit, or the 'meat' of the plant. Unlike traditional fats such as butter, duck fat, beef tallow, olive oil and coconut oil, which have been part of the human diet for many thousands of years, seed oils came into the Western diet relatively recently.

All oils are comprised of three different fatty acid types known as SFAs (saturated fatty acids), MUFAs (monounsaturated fatty acids), and PUFAs (polyunsaturated fatty acids). But the amounts of each of these types of fatty acids in the composition of each seed oil varies widely. Soybean oil, for instance, is around 60 per cent PUFA, 21 per cent MUFA and 16 per cent SFA. Corn oil and sunflower oil have similar compositions. Coconut oil, on the other hand, is about 90 per cent SFA, while both olive oil and rapeseed oil are around 70 per cent MUFA.[54] Seed oils like soybean, corn and sunflower are often referred to simply as polyunsaturated oils because of their high PUFA content.

Why have I included seed oils on my list of the 'bad guys' that are likely to sneak their way into a plant-based diet in greater quantities than is good for us? Because these seemingly innocent oils (made from plants, and therefore assumed by many to be good for health) are not so innocent. The biggest problem with seed oils is their linoleic acid content.

Linoleic acid is an omega-6 fatty acid which is found in high concentrations in seed oils. Dietary intake of linoleic acid has risen dramatically over the past fifty years; it now makes up 8–10 per cent of total energy intake in the Western world.[55] The concentration of linoleic acid in human adipose tissue (the connective tissue that stores fat) rose from 9.1 per cent to 21.5 per cent between 1959 and 2008.[56] Why is this a problem? After all, linoleic acid is considered to be an essential nutrient, and small amounts of omega-6, which can be found in chicken, eggs and nuts, can be beneficial. However, the high levels of omega-6 such as that found in seed oils is now recognised as being harmful, driving a range of health problems including inflammation and increased oxidised LDL levels.[57]

The suggestion of a link between excessive linoleic acid intake and ill health emerged from the Minnesota Coronary Study discussed in Chapter 1; the experimental group (the one's consuming the seed oils, which are high in omega-6 linoleic acid) had higher death rates from cancer. They also had twice the rate of gallstones and two to three times more strokes.[58] The PURE study, also referenced in Chapter 1, found that those with the lowest saturated fat intake and the highest levels of PUFA intake had the highest risk of stroke. (It's unclear whether the key factor at work was the low intake of saturated fat or the high intake of PUFAs, but one thing was clear: the findings from this study were no endorsement of the health benefits of PUFAs.) Other research has suggested that oxidised omega-6 (linoleic acid) may be implicated in diseases such as cardiovascular disease, obesity, diabetes, cancer and macular degeneration.[59]

Researchers DiNicolantonio and O'Keefe note that, in Americans, the increased intake of linoleic acid paralleled the increase in the prevalence of diabetes, obesity and asthma. They also note that the amount of linoleic acid in adipose tissue is positively associated with coronary artery disease (CAD) – linoleic acid is found in higher concentrations in individuals with CAD than those without CAD. To explain the link between linoleic acid and CAD, they propose an expansion of what they call the oxLDL theory of heart disease: 'Dietary linoleic acid, especially when consumed from refined omega-6 vegetable oils, gets incorporated into all blood lipoproteins (such as LDL, VLDL and HDL), increasing the susceptibility of all lipoproteins to oxidise and hence increases cardiovascular risk.'[60]

Another consequence of high PUFA intake is the destruction of the all-important balance between omega-6 and omega-3. (Centuries ago, this ratio was estimated to be around 4:1 or less, whereas today it's estimated to be around 15:1.[61]) This is bad news, say DiNicolantonio and O'Keefe, since there is 'compelling evidence that omega-3s protect whereas omega-6 linoleic acid promotes heart disease'.[62] Much of that compelling evidence was amassed by Dr William Lands, one of the world's most respected and published fatty acid scientists, who consistently warned about the risks of excessive intake of omega-6 fats.[63]

A 2013 study by Christopher Ramsden and colleagues (the re-analysis of the Sydney Diet Heart Study discussed in Chapter 1) provided evidence of a link between omega-6 linoleic acid intake and heart disease. The study looked at 220 men with existing heart problems, feeding one group a normal diet containing saturated fats and the other group a diet containing fats and oils high in linoleic acid. Substituting dietary linoleic acid in place of saturated fats 'increased the rates of death from all causes, including heart disease'.[64]

In his book, *Why We Eat (Too Much)*, bariatric surgeon Dr Andrew Jenkinson explains why the imbalance between omega-6 and omega-3s has implications beyond an increased risk of heart disease. Whereas omega-3 functions as a defence against inflammation, promotes insulin sensitivity and provides essential messaging about mood and appetite, omega-6 has the opposite effects, increasing inflammatory responses and blood coagulability (clotting). If the omega-6 to omega-3 ratio goes up dramatically, it could make our immune system hypersensitive. This, in turn, can lead to the development of autoimmune diseases like arthritis and IBS.[65]

Other side effects of a high omega-6 to omega-3 ratio include the reduced ability of cell walls to absorb elements such as calcium, and a decrease in the sensitivity of the cell wall to insulin in muscles and leptin in the brain. Higher insulin levels and leptin resistance increase the risk of obesity.[66] As if this were not bad enough, high levels of omega-6 can prevent the body from converting the omega-3 that we get from plants into the more active omega-3 that we get from fish and animals. 'In other words,' says Dr Jenkinson, 'it doesn't matter how many green vegetables you eat – their conversion into useful omega-3 will be blocked.'[67]

Our understanding of why a dietary imbalance of omega-6 to omega-3 is detrimental to health and why seed oils should be avoided has been enhanced by the work of self-taught researcher Tucker Goodrich (www.yelling-stop.blogspot.com).[68] Goodrich, who has been called a 'PubMed Warrior',[69] has spent the past nine years digging deep into the published medical research about seed oils. Like engineers Dave Feldman and Ivor Cummins, who have contributed so much to our understanding of cholesterol, he has deployed an engineering mindset (focused on data, analysis of root causes and problem resolution) to the study of seed oils, and linoleic acid in particular. (Goodrich's day job is designing and managing complex risk management systems in the financial services industry.)

Goodrich was prompted to embark on this research journey by his personal experience of having seen dramatic improvements to his health simply from eliminating seed oils from his diet. (At thirty-eight, Goodrich suffered from what was initially thought to be a stroke but was later diagnosed as an acute migraine; he had also been suffering from crippling IBS, diverticulosis, 'borderline osteoporosis' and weight gain for years.) By connecting the dots in what he says is a 'vast literature', Goodrich identified a number of mechanisms which could explain the adverse health effects of omega-6 linoleic acid.[70] Animal studies have shown that linoleic acid causes oxidative damage to the mitochondria (the source of energy in all cells) via its oxidation of a specific fatty acid called cardiolipin. This damage can lead to obesity, diabetes and insulin resistance. Linoleic acid is also linked to the oxidation of LDL, which seems to lead to the formation of atherosclerotic plaques. (As noted by DiNicolantonio and O'Keefe on page 153.) Equally alarming is a by-product of oxidised linoleic acid called 4-HNE, which is highly toxic and itself causes damage to an important anti-cancer gene. 'In these animal models, you can't induce cancer and fatty liver disease without linoleic acid,' says Goodrich. 'I can't think of any product that, if you gave it to animals to increase their rate of cancer or fatty liver disease and to cause obesity, it would make it into the [human] food supply, but that's where we are right now.'[71]

The effect of linoleic acid on the body is similar, says Goodrich, to that of smoking, in that it kicks off the oxidative process. And like the damage from smoking, the damage from excess consumption of linoleic acid is cumulative (linoleic acid remains in tissues for many years) and can take many years to materialise. Even when the damage manifests itself in diseases like obesity, diabetes, fatty liver disease or cancer, doctors will likely be slow to connect the dots that lead back to seed oils.

The problems arising from the high linoleic acid content of seed oils are compounded by another of their characteristics. All fats are made up of carbon and hydrogen, but PUFAs have multiple double bonds between carbon molecules. These double bonds create weaknesses in the molecules and make PUFAs less stable and more easily oxidised than SFAs or MUFAs. Oxidation can take place if seed oils are exposed to air (via inappropriate storage) and heat (via cooking), but can also occur when these oils are just sitting on a shelf or in your body. The potential for oxidation, and for damage to health, is exacerbated if seed oils are consumed in a fast-food environment where the oils are repeatedly heated.[72]

Dr Fred Kummerow, a leading researcher on the effects of trans fats and a sceptic of the diet–heart hypothesis, was among the first to raise the alarm bells about the dangers of heated seed oils. He discovered that the high temperatures used in commercial frying caused PUFAs to oxidise, and that soybean oil and corn oils could also oxidise within the body.[73] This oxidisation can lead to oxidised cholesterol, the only form in which cholesterol is dangerous.

Dr Kummerow's early warnings about the oxidising effect of heated PUFAs have been echoed in more recent studies. The authors of one study note that there is considerable evidence that heated cooking oils, especially polyunsaturated oils, can degrade to toxic compounds, posing several health risks to consumers of fried foods and even people working near deep-fat fryers.[74] Other researchers observed that 'acrolein formation is observed even at low temperatures' but that it increases significantly when temperatures are increased from 180 to 240 degrees. (Acrolein is a toxic substance with a strong, unpleasant smell created by the burning of fossil fuels, tobacco smoke and the heating of oils.) They also note that foods fried in oils with a high PUFA content absorb more acrolein than foods fried in oils with a high saturated fat content.[75] The risk to people working with seed oils was highlighted by a study in China, which attributed high rates of lung cancer among non-smoking women to their exposure to toxins while cooking with seed oils at high temperatures in improperly ventilated environments.[76] The oils in fryers can also turn into polymers (like those in paints) that prove almost impossible to remove, as Nina Teicholz discovered while researching *The Big Fat Surprise*. She writes that industry experts considered this to be a 'cleaning problem', when in fact, as she details in her book, it is likely to be much more of a health problem.[77]

The weight of the evidence (epidemiological, mechanistic and clinical) led Tucker Goodrich to the conclusion that excess consumption of linoleic acid is the fundamental problem of modern health. 'Other things play into it,' he says, 'but if you fix this you can get away with a lot else.' Many doctors and researchers agree with him. Among them are the aforementioned Dr Jenkinson and Dr Jason Fung, who has labelled seed oils 'garbage'. [78] Dr Saladino and Ivor Cummins regularly warn against their consumption. Dr Chris Knobbe has asserted that the 'omega-6 apocalypse' resulting from high PUFA intake underlies diseases such as obesity, cancer, Alzheimer's, Parkinson's and macular degeneration.[79] Dr Michael Eades has proposed that rising intake of PUFAs, the vilification of saturated fat and the increased consumption of carbohydrates have created a 'perfect storm' which has resulted in the massive increase in obesity since 1980.[80]

All of these views run counter to the official guidelines, of course. Both the US and UK guidelines advocate the consumption of large amounts of those foods that Dr Eades holds responsible for the 'perfect storm' – carbohydrates and polyunsaturated fats (aka, seed oils) – as does the EAT-Lancet Planetary Health Diet. Moreover, the promoters of these diets would have us eat copious amounts of the foods that are high in linoleic acid, such as grains, nuts and seeds.[81]

We saw how the guidelines for fat intake came into being in Chapter 1. As those in charge of the dietary guidelines lined up against saturated fats, they had no choice but to embrace seed oils. This suited the industrial producers of seed oils just fine, as it provided an ever-expanding consumer market for what had initially been an industrial product. (The original seed oils, mainly cottonseed oil, started life as lubricants for industrial machinery, before Proctor & Gamble had the bright idea of using them in soap, and then as the basis of a lard substitute product called Crisco.) In 1980, the USDA also threw its weight behind seed oils, paving the way for food companies to use them in most processed and restaurant food.

'There's a huge disconnect between what the lab science tells us we should be doing and what our dietary guidelines are telling us,' says Tucker Goodrich. He also points out that the guidelines are founded on an inherent contradiction. 'On the one hand, they want us to eat lots of polyunsaturated fats because they're supposed to be good for us. On the other hand, they want us to avoid fried foods as these are bad for us. But what are fried foods except foods fried in polyunsaturated oils?' Regarding the proponents of the guidelines, Goodrich says, 'you just have to not listen to those people'.[82]

If we can't take our guidance from the guidelines, what should we do? Bring our intake of linoleic acid back in line with that of our ancestors, whose minimal consumption (estimated to be less than 5g a day) was associated with chronic disease rates that were a tiny fraction of those we see today. This means avoiding seed oils and the processed foods in which they are found, as well as pork and chicken meat from grain-fed animals. (The meat from grain-fed monogasts like pigs and chickens contains more linoleic acid than that from animals raised without grain feed. This effect is less marked in meat from ruminants.)[83] If you must consume seed oils, your best bet is to choose a rapeseed oil (canola) with high oleic acid content. Linoelic acid content will be in the region of 18 per cent, double that of olive oil, but significantly less than that in corn and sunflower oil.

A wholesale, planet-wide shift to plant-based eating would likely exacerbate the problem of excess consumption of linoleic acid. Animal fats would be off the menu, and supplies of olive, coconut and palm oil could never be sufficient to satisfy demand from consumers or the manufacturers of the plant-based processed foods on which consumers would find themselves dependent. (This is to say nothing of the environmental destruction that would come from increased production of palm oil.) Consumption of seed oils would inevitably increase.

Seed oils are, of course, highly processed foods (known in the industry as RBD: refined, bleached and deodorised). They are also ubiquitous as ingredients in ultra-processed foods, the next of the 'bad guys' I want to consider.

How ultra-processed foods sabotage your health

Unless you grow or catch all your own food and eat it raw, almost everything you eat will have been processed to a certain extent. A pea may be frozen. Cooking is a process. So is fermentation.[84] But ultra-processed foods – UPFs – are different. The NOVA food classification system groups food into four categories: unprocessed and minimally processed foods (natural and whole, with inedible parts removed); processed culinary ingredients (such as butter and lard); processed foods (such as canned or bottled vegetables and tinned fish); and ultra-processed foods, which are defined as being 'formulations of ingredients, mostly of industrial use, typically created by a series of industrial techniques and processes'. These processes include fractioning, hydrolysis, hydrogenation, extrusion, moulding and pre-frying. 'Colors, flavours, emulsifiers, and other additives are frequently added to make the final product palatable or hyper-palatable.'[85] Common ultra-processed products are carbonated soft drinks, packaged snacks, mass produced packaged breads, buns, cake mixes, margarines and other spreads, cereals, pre-prepared meat, cheese, pasta and pizza dishes, chicken and fish nuggets, instant soups, noodles and desserts.

Plant-protein specialist Paul Hart puts the NOVA classification in simpler terms. Processing, he says, is what goes on in your own kitchen or at the bakers or butchers. Ultra-processing is done on a huge scale in computer-controlled industrial plants running 24/7. Nutrition scientist Stephan van Vliet offers an equally simple distinction: the formulations and ingredients in UPFs are things you can't reasonably put together in your kitchen.

The convenience and attractiveness of UPFs, combined with aggressive marketing, have driven rising consumption. UPFs now account for more than half of the total dietary energy consumed in high-income countries such as the US, Canada, the UK and Australia. Their sales in middle-income countries are growing at a rate of up to 10 per cent a year.[86] Within Europe, the UK has succumbed to the lure of UPFs to a greater extent than some other countries: while 50 per cent of the UK's household food purchases are ultra-processed, this compares to 14 per cent for France and 13 per cent for Italy.[87]

The rising consumption of UPFs is bad news for global

health. In a report on the dietary challenges of the twenty-first century, the FAO asserted that if the direction of current policies remains the same, the number of overweight and obese people will have increased from 1.33 billion in 2005 to 'around a third of the projected global population by 2030'. Specific reference is made to the consumption of UPFs as a reason for this increase in obesity.[88] In the UK, those responsible for crafting the National Food Strategy (2021) asserted that the consumption of UPFs could be a key factor in rising obesity rates, noting that these foods tend to be high in calories and 'interfere with the feedback mechanisms of our appetite'.[89] Researchers from the Francis Crick Institute, a biomedical research centre, suggested that diets high in processed foods could be causing an increase in the number of people developing autoimmune diseases across the world.[90]

There's a growing body of evidence that UPFs are not only obesogenic and bad for the immune system, but addictive. Dr Joan Ifland, food addiction expert and author of several books about processed food addiction, cites thousands of studies which illustrate that processed food addiction is real.[91] Ifland explains how the tobacco industry, which was tragically good at spreading addiction, came into the processed food industry in the 1980s, managing to apply everything they'd learned about how to make products addictive while also suppressing awareness of that addiction. Processed food addiction, like any other addiction, 'impairs learning, decision-making, memory, impulse control, emotional processing and satiation' and has resulted, according to Ifland, in the epidemics we see today in attention deficit, learning difficulty, memory loss and poor impulse control.[92]

Ifland is far from alone in believing processed foods to be addictive and harmful to health. In his book, *The Hacking of the American Mind*, paediatric endocrinologist Dr Robert Lustig details how a bad diet comprised of large amounts of processed foods has contributed to the hacking of our minds and helped to fuel the epidemics of non-communicable diseases such as diabetes, heart disease, cancer and dementia.[93]

Dr Andrew Jenkinson attributes the addictive, mood altering effect of processed foods, in part, to their high omega-6 content. Omega-6 fatty acids act as precursors to endocannabinoids, which are signalling molecules that stimulate the cannabinoid receptors in the brain. (The same receptors that are triggered when cannabis is smoked.) The effect of stimulating the cannabinoid receptors is an elevated, happy mood. Later, there will be a sudden increased appetite combined with food-seeking behaviour.[94] A 2019 controlled trial led by Kevin Hall showed definitively that UPFs do in fact cause people to consume more calories and to gain weight.[95]

Processed foods are also nutritionally inferior to whole foods, being depleted in dietary fibre, protein, various macronutrients and other bioactive compounds.[96] 'The processing of foods typically robs them of nutrients, vitamins especially,' warns Michael Pollan. 'Store food is designed to be stored and transported over long distances, and the surest way to make food more stable and less vulnerable to pests is to remove the nutrients from it.'[97]

What does any of this have to do with the plant-based diet? It's simply this: those following a plant-based regime are likely to ingest high quantities of the ultra-processed foods that are so deleterious to health. To make a vegan cheese, you have to engage in some serious processing. Ditto with a meatless burger or a dairy-free cream. PUFAs, derived proteins, additives, preservatives, stabilisers and emulsifiers are likely to become a regular part of a plant-based diet. The Veganuary Facebook page is testimony to this link between vegan diets and processed foods: every single food they promote is highly processed, such as Pizza Hut pizzas and Morrisons vegan sausage rolls and pasties. I couldn't find an image of a single actual vegetable anywhere on the site. Equally, Tesco's new plant-based range doesn't consist of lush baskets full of fresh broccoli, tomatoes and cauliflower, but of ultra-processed dishes like the Plant Chef BBQ Jackbake, made with over fifty different ingredients including seed oil, sugar, acidity regulators and thickeners.

This is the kind of food that many vegans will end up eating. 'Vegans and vegetarians are not automatically eating heaps of fruit and veg because there are all these products out there that are fully processed, fully refined,' said Dr Megan Lee, a researcher in nutritional psychiatry, who found that a high intake of processed plant foods is a risk factor for increased depression.[98]

Plant-based burgers constitute a significant share of this processed plant food intake. They are chosen by many because they believe them to be better for health[99] but, says Sara Keough, an integrative eco-nutritionist and technical advisor to Understanding Ag (of which more in Chapter 10), 'evaluating the healthfulness of a product based primarily on its caloric and macronutrient content completely disregards the importance we should be placing on the specific food items, additives, or chemicals contained within that product'.[100] The list of 'specific food items, additives and chemicals' found in one top-selling brand of plant-based meat burgers includes soya protein concentrate, yeast extract, sunflower oil, methylcellulose, cultured dextrose, soya leghemoglobin and soy protein isolate. Another top brand contains a similar list of ingredients but replaces soya protein with pea protein and rice protein, and substitutes canola oil for sunflower oil. Keough warns that many of these ingredients are far from healthful. The plant oils are full of PUFAs that are likely to be highly oxidised as a result of intense processing; additives like methylcellulose and cultured dextrose are derived from laboratory manipulation, and ingredients like genetically engineered soya leghemoglobin 'lack adequate safety studies and could also pose potential new health risks for consumers'.[101]

The pea and soya isolates in these plant-based meat replacements are particularly concerning, says Keough. She points to 'over eighty years of research [that] has shown that soy can produce many harmful health effects'[102] (having read the first part of this chapter, you'll be familiar with these effects), and says that soya and pea protein isolates could be particularly damaging, since high heat processing and isolation 'separates proteins from their whole food form and generates compounds that are not naturally occurring in food and may trigger inflammation or immune system reactions'. Soya is already ranked as one of the top eight allergens in the US and there are concerns about the allergenicity of pea protein. Many could develop a 'food sensitivity' that 'may not produce an acute immune system reaction but can still lead to severe and chronic health issues such as autoimmune diseases, obesity, digestive disorders, neurological conditions, skin issues and many other common ailments'. Keough reminds us that consumption of peas and soya products that are 'free of genetic modification and chemical contaminants and in relatively small, infrequent portions as part of a diverse diet' looks strikingly different from consuming the processed versions found in alternative meat products. 'Consuming industrially isolated proteins from chemical-laden, GMO soybeans or peas as a staple food is completely unnatural and poses many health risks,' she concludes.

Not only do plant-based meat replacements contain ingredients we would hope not to find but they cannot be said to be nutritionally equivalent to their meat-based counterparts. 'Attempts to mimic meat with plant-based alternatives – using isolated plant proteins, fats, vitamins and minerals,' say researchers Fred Provenza and colleagues, 'underestimate the nutritional complexity of whole foods, which contain tens of thousands of phytochemicals that promote health nutritionally and pharmacologically.'[103] A metabolomic analysis (a technique that allows for the measurement of large numbers of nutrients and metabolites present in biological samples) conducted by van Vliet, Provenza, Kronberg and colleagues revealed 'a 90 per cent difference in nutrient and metabolic profiles of grass-fed beef and a popular plant-based meat, many of which can have important consumer health implications. This information could not be determined from their Nutrition Facts [food labels], which suggests nutritional similarity.'[104] The authors highlight the absence of creatine, hydroxyproline, anserine, glucosamine, cysteamine and many other nutrients with 'important physiological, anti-inflammatory, and/or immunomodulatory roles' in the plant-based product.[105] Elsewhere, they have pointed out that only a quarter of plant-based meat substitutes are fortified with B12.[106]

Given that plant-based meat substitutes are not a perfect match for meat in nutritional terms, we are storing up problems for the future in populations who think they are a like-for-like alternative, says Dr Shawn Baker: 'My concern is that this will lead to a decline in the number of people who eat meat, leading to a further decline in our population's health ... it will be a matter of how sick people get before they realise that nutrition is the answer'.[107]

Are plant-based fish and chicken any better? Vuna, a plant-based tuna launched by Nestlé, is made up of six ingredients – water, pea protein, wheat gluten, rapeseed oil, salt and a natural flavour blend – most of which are highly processed. Damning the product with faint praise, the company deemed it 'quite comparable to tuna'.[108] As for chicken 'alternatives', most brands are made from ingredients like soya, wheat and other textured vegetable proteins, plus a long list of ingredients required to keep the product fresh and tasty. For example, one variety examined included soya protein isolate, pea protein, 'vital' wheat gluten, canola oil, methylcellulose, yeast extract, potato starch, added colours, salt, sugar, and four types of flour. (At least the flours were organic, though. That's a relief.)

Like fake meats, vegan dairy substitutes are highly processed and stuffed full of unnatural ingredients. Most contain upwards of fifteen ingredients, including coconut oil, seed oils, various starches and acids, acidity regulators and sugar. And, unlike dairy cheese, they are poor sources of protein, most supplying less than 1g of protein per 100g compared to the 25g of protein in the same amount of dairy cheese.[109] Flora Professional Plant, a non-dairy plant-based double cream, is billed as being 'every bit as good as regular dairy cream'. The trouble is, it's full of seed oil, palm fat, sugar, sugar esters, corn starch, various emulsifiers, stabilisers and colourant. It has a shelf life of nine months.[110] No wonder, with all those compounds to bolster its defences against natural processes.

These sorts of additives take their toll on the body. When food writer Bee Wilson tried a Beyond Burger she was pleasantly surprised at how much it tasted like meat, but said it felt nothing like meat to her digestive system. Half an hour after lunch she was gripped by stomach pains and a terrible junk-food aftertaste. When she looked up the ingredients she saw exactly why. She had been lunching on pea protein isolate, expeller-pressed canola oil, refined coconut oil, yeast extract, maltodextrin, natural flavours and gum Arabic.[111] Yum.

The inmates of an Illinois prison were alleged to have suffered much worse adverse effects than stomach pains when they were fed a 'planet-saving' diet devoid of meat but loaded with imitation foods containing soya protein isolate and soya protein concentrate, with naked soya flour added to baked goods, between 2003 and 2009.* The women stopped menstruating after just a few months, so the Department of Corrections had to cut the soya from their diets and give them meat again. The men suffered from digestive problems, nausea, constipation, flatulence, thyroid problems, heart arrythmias, growth of breasts and erectile dysfunction.[112]

There's hardly a plant-based meat, dairy or egg substitute out there that isn't a highly processed blend of artificial ingredients swimming in seed oil. Paul Hart maintains that plant-proteins don't yet have the functionality of animal proteins, and that the packaged products currently being offered 'could be so much better'. There need to be improvements in aspects such as product texture and nutritional profile, sustainability of ingredients (lower food miles and carbon footprint), and level of processing, with a 'rule of five' applying to the number of ingredients. Hart believes that plant proteins are necessary to meet future demand for protein and, in particular, to meet the needs of those who can't or do not wish to eat animal foods. Consumers must have choice, he says, but 'this should not be at the expense of turning over centuries of dietary practice to be subverted by a rather too modern single Plant-Based agenda'.[113]

By increasing intake of ultra-processed food, might that plant-based agenda be adding fuel to the fire that is the obesity epidemic, which began in the 1980s, just as greater and rising quantities of processed foods were introduced into the diet, alongside more vegetable oils and grains?[114] It's reasonable to hypothesise, as Dr Jenkinson does, that excess quantities of these three foods played a role in making many of us fat and sick. We've looked at seed oils and processed foods; it's time to consider the last of our bad guys, grains.

---

* The Weston A. Price Foundation filed a lawsuit on the prisoners' behalf.

Grains

Was there ever a more revered food group than whole grains? They sit front and centre of every eating guide from the food pyramid, the Eatwell Guide and MyPlate guides to the near-vegan Planetary Health Diet brought to us by EAT-Lancet. A belief in the benefits of whole grains has been expressed so often, by so many, that, like the belief that saturated fat is bad for us, it is taken as gospel. There are a head-spinning number of grains to choose from including the commonly known, such as oats, wheat, rye, brown rice, corn and quinoa (a pseudo-grain), to the less familiar including spelt, buckwheat, sorghum, millet, teff and kamut. They are good sources of fibre, which is generally deemed to be good for our health (although some nutritionists and doctors maintain that the recommended daily intake of fibre is not evidence based). But, aside from their fibre content, are these grains as good for our health as they are made out to be?

A study by GAIN (Global Alliance for Improved Nutrition) that I referenced in Chapter 2 compared the nutrient density of different foods by looking at the calories and grams needed to provide an average of one-third of recommended intakes of six nutrients deemed essential for optimal health: vitamin A, folate, vitamin B12, calcium, iron and zinc. With a few exceptions, whole grains were deemed to be of low nutrient density in terms of their delivery of these six nutrients. (The exceptions were teff and quinoa – rated 'moderate' to 'very high' in terms of delivery of iron, zinc and folate; and millet and sorghum – rated 'moderate' for the same three nutrients.) The category labelled simply 'whole grains' was rated 'low' for delivery of everything except zinc. But we know that obtaining zinc from grains is problematic, since the anti-nutrients in the grains inhibit absorption.

If we look at a broader range of nutrients, whole grains do

not fare much better in terms of nutrient density. USDA data for whole wheat, for example, evidences reasonably good levels of magnesium and manganese (when assessed against the RDA for these nutrients) but low levels of phosphorus, potassium, sodium, selenium, thiamine, riboflavin, vitamin D and vitamin K.[115] The data for brown rice, another popular grain, paint a similar picture,[116] namely that grains can be said to provide moderate amounts of nutrition and can make contributions to nutrient needs when eaten in combination with other foods, but nutritional powerhouses they are not. If they are consumed as part of a strict plant-based diet, they cannot be counted on to make up for the nutrient shortfalls resulting from the removal of animal-sourced foods from that diet.

Neither are grains necessarily 'heart healthy'. Three studies published in 2016 made the claim that eating grains, such as wholemeal bread, could slash the risk of dying of heart disease by 25 per cent. But when Dr Harcombe worked her analytical magic on these studies, she found that the evidence behind the claims amounted to a hill of beans:

> It's not causal, the absolute difference is tiny and it's *whole lifestyle* being depicted in these studies – not a *whole grain* ... To prove me wrong, the authors of these studies need to give 3oz of whole grains daily to the smoking, drinking, obese, sedentary, aimless fourth generation unemployed, living on benefits, deprived populations ... and change nothing else. Do you think that will 'slash their risk of dying from heart disease by 25%'?[117]

A 2020 study, which looked at randomised controlled trials (RCTs), further undermined the much-repeated claim that whole grains are heart healthy.[118] The efficacy of using whole grains to manage cardiovascular risks in overweight people had previously been, in the words of the authors, 'inconsistent' and 'not well established'. This study did nothing to establish it, for it found that although whole grain consumption was *associated with* slightly lower body weight and lower C-reactive protein, it made no positive difference to LDL-C, waist circumference, blood pressure or fasting glucose – the last three of which are indicators of insulin resistance.

Grains cannot reliably be said to be heart healthy and they are not nutritional powerhouses. Some doctors believe that they do play a role in powering something else, however: systemic inflammation in the body – including the intestines – which is damaging to the brain.[119] In his book, *Grain Brain*, Dr David Perlmutter provides convincing evidence that brain dysfunction and disorders such as chronic headaches, depression, epilepsy, and even Alzheimer's, begin with our daily bread:

> Modern grains are silently destroying your brain. By 'modern', I'm not just referring to the refined white flours, pastas, and rice that have already been demonised by the anti-obesity folks; I'm referring to all the grains that so many of us have embraced as being healthful – whole wheat, whole grain, multi-grain, live grain, stone ground, and so on. Basically, I am calling what is arguably our most beloved dietary staple a terrorist group that bullies our most precious organ, the brain.[120]

Cardiologist Dr William Davis has also written about the negative effects of grain consumption. In *Wheat Belly* he writes that wheat, 'the world's most popular grain, is also the world's most destructive dietary ingredient':[121]

> Documented peculiar effects of wheat on humans include appetite stimulation, exposure to brain-active *exorphins* ... exaggerated blood sugar surges that trigger cycles of satiety

alternating with heightened appetite, the process of *glyca-tion* that underlies disease and ageing, inflammatory and pH effects that erode cartilage and damage bone, and activation of disordered immune responses. A complex range of diseases results from the consumption of wheat, from coeliac ... to an assortment of neurological disorders, diabetes, heart disease, arthritis, curious rashes and paralysing delusions of schizophrenia.[122]

Part of the problem with wheat, says Davis, is that it is 'genetically and biochemically light years removed from the wheat of just 40 years ago'.[123] In her book, *The Real Food Solution*, Izabella Natrins explains this transformation.[124] Wheat was hybridised in the 1960s, which altered its protein and nutrient content. Protein content went up and nutrient content went down.[125] Using the Chorleywood Bread Process, developed in 1961, manufacturers then added hard fats, extra yeast and chemicals to this deficient wheat and mixed it all at high speed, producing dough that was ready to bake in a fraction of the time it took to bake bread by traditional methods. Now, therefore, our freshly baked loaf is good to go in a mere three hours.

Most of the bread in the UK is produced using the Chorleywood method. Some two-thirds of it also contains traces of at least one pesticide, most commonly glyphosate. Much bread – even the super-seeded wholewheat variety – also contains a host of unnatural ingredients and additives, including vegetable oils, which have no business being there.

The lectins in grains are another reason why they can wreak havoc on the body. And 'the lectin load on humans is higher than ever before, in part because corn, wheat and soya, all packed with lectins, are in most processed foods'.[126] Dr Steven Gundry generally limits whole grains and legumes in diet plans for his patients but finds that if he *removes* all grains and pseudo grains (quinoa, buckwheat and the like), along with all legumes, including tofu, edamame and other soya products, his patients experience even greater improvements.[127]

Direct personal and clinical experience also led registered dietitian Lily Nichols to conclude that 'the argument that you need grains just does not stand up to scrutiny' and that 'of all the food groups you can push to the side and make up the micronutrients elsewhere, grains are the top of the list'.[128] Dr Andreas Eenfeldt, founder of the low-carb website Diet Doctor, has said that just because whole grains are better for you than refined grains that doesn't make them good, it simply makes them less bad.[129]

Grains can have the same effect on the body as other carbohydrates, which is to raise blood sugar levels. Wholewheat bread, for example, can increase blood sugar as much or more than table sugar.[130] Former type-2 diabetic Debra Scott was shocked to learn that her blood sugars spiked to dangerously high levels when she ate brown seeded bread. The oatmeal breakfast, advertised as heart healthy, can also cause massive blood sugar spikes in some people. This excursion into high glucose levels is OK once in a while, but it's become normalised, which goes some way to explaining why so many (25 per cent of people in the UK and 40 per cent of Americans) have metabolic syndrome, and many more (almost 90 per cent of Americans for example) are deemed metabolically unhealthy.[131] (See page 44 for a definition of metabolic syndrome.)

Understanding the effects of grains in the body led Vinnie Tortorich to trademark the term NSNG (no sugar, no grains): four letters that encapsulate his approach to helping clients lose weight and get healthier. It's a simple formula that requires no calorie counting. It's also a formula that has helped him to keep his cancer in remission for more than twelve years. The no-grains part of the formula is really an extension of the no-sugar part, since grains behave like sugar once in the body. But sugar comes in many other forms too, and sugar in all its guises is arguably the most pernicious ingredient in the plant-based diet, the worst of all the bad guys lying in wait to hijack your health. We'll take a close look at why in the next chapter.

5

Sugar: The Biggest of the Bad Guys

In an article about what she eats on a normal day, a vegan woman, whom I'll call Jan, sets out to dispel the myth that vegan food is dull. Detailing her food intake on a typical day (which includes lots of oatmeal, peanut butter, tofu, plant milk, vegetables, beans and cereals), she proclaims that while vegan diets have a bad reputation for being bland and expensive, they can be inexpensive, exciting and good for health.

Inexpensive and exciting, perhaps. Healthful? Less so. The typical day's menu outlined by Jan would contain around 300 grams of carbohydrates. To put that into perspective, that's three to six times the carb intake advocated by most low-carb experts and practitioners and fifteen times what those on a very low-carb (ketogenic) diet would consume, and approximately equivalent to the carb content of the standard American diet (SAD) that has helped to fuel the obesity epidemic in the US and elsewhere.

Let's look at that 300g of carbohydrates in the context of IR (insulin resistance). (As we saw in Chapter 1, IR can lead to type-2 diabetes and other chronic diseases.) IR expert Ben Bikman recommends the following levels of carbohydrate intake for people wanting to reverse or prevent insulin resistance, a condition that could affect almost 90 per cent of adults:[1] If you definitely have IR (which you can ascertain using a simple questionnaire of his design), consume less than 50g of carbohydrates per day; if you show some signs of being insulin resistant, consume less than 75g of carbohydrates per day; if you are not insulin resistant and never want to be, you have more freedom, but would ideally keep carbohydrate intake to under 100g a day.[2] Nowhere in Bikman's protocol for preventing and managing IR is there an allowance for the consumption of 300g of carbohydrates. In fact, Jan's high-carb diet, consumed on a daily basis over the long term, could be said to be a recipe for IR.

Why do plant-based diets tend to be high in carbohydrates? (The exception is the vegan low-carb, high-fat diet, which I'll discuss at the end of this chapter.) When you remove animal proteins and fats from the diet, you have to put something else in, and that something is invariably carbohydrates. Take breakfast, for example. With eggs, bacon and cheese off the menu, a typical vegan breakfast would likely be based on what Ben Bikman has called 'the worst possible foods' for metabolic health (a non-insulin resistant state): juice, cereals, bagels, rice or toast.[3]

The need to replace animal protein is also a driver of carbohydrate intake. Let's look at a protein intake of 45g, which would equate to the RDA for a 56kg (8st 11oz) woman. For an omnivore, this amount of protein could be obtained from two eggs and 120g of tuna, giving a carbohydrate price tag of 1.2g. For a plant-based eater, the same amount of protein could, in theory, be found by combining 100g each of lentils, kidney beans, brown rice, tofu and cashew nuts. But since these plant proteins have lower digestibility scores (see Chapter 2), slightly more of each of these foods would have to be consumed to get the 'delivered' protein up to 45g. Bumping up the amount of ingested plant protein by 9 per cent to account for the lower levels of digestibility would give you a combination of plant foods with a carbohydrate price tag of almost 110g. So that's 1.2g of carbohydrates versus 110g in order to obtain protein that is not even complete (that is, it does not contain all essential amino acids).[4]

Nutritionist Tim Rees maintains that high-carbohydrate intake by those on plant-based diets can drive carb addiction. Clinical psychologist Dr Jen Unwin has also witnessed how plant-based diets can fuel addiction: 'The problem with plant-based diets is that people tend to rely on eating a lot of rice and pasta and processed foods, vegan brownies and that sort of thing. It's all completely devoid of nutrition and primes the system to rely on sugar. Some sugar addiction specialists won't even work with vegans. Bitten Jonsson [an expert in food addiction whose background is detailed at bittensaddiction.com], for instance, says that it's not possible to cure a vegan sugar addict, because there aren't enough alternatives for them to eat.'[5]

Dr Unwin uses the words 'carbohydrate' and 'sugar' interchangeably, and rightly so, since they are more or less the same thing once in the body. Dr Nasha Winters reminds us that 'all types of carbohydrates – including vegetables, fruit, grains, legumes and all sugars – are naturally converted into glucose in the digestive system'.[6] Dr Zoë Harcombe says that 'every time we talk about carbohydrate, we should be mindful of the fact that we're talking about sugar'. In her 'Carbohydrates 101' lecture,[7] Dr Harcombe explains that there are three main types of sugar: single sugars (glucose, fructose and galactose); two-sugars (such as everyday table sugar, or sucrose, which is 50 per cent glucose and 50 per cent fructose); and many sugars or polysaccharides (including digestible forms such as glycogen and starch, and indigestible forms that include fibre).

Carbohydrates are the starchy foods contained in the

'many-sugars' category around which the government guidelines suggest we build our meals and around which many
vegans build their meals: bread, pasta, oats, rice, maize,
beans, couscous, potatoes and sweet potatoes. Starch and
other forms of sugar also constitute the backbone of many
processed foods, plant-based varieties being no exception.

Fructose, and therefore high-fructose corn syrup and the
table sugar often listed as 'added sugars' on packaged food
labels, is now believed to be a particularly damaging form
of sugar. Rick Johnson, Professor of Nephrology at the
University of Colorado, has shown fructose to have profound
metabolic effects, regardless of its source, because it causes
a drop in cellular energy (called ATP). This sets off a chain
reaction that results in the creation of uric acid, which then
leads to the generation of body fat, insulin resistance, fatty
liver and hypertension.[8]

Dr Robert Lustig also warns about the negative effects of
fructose, which drives fatty liver disease and insulin resistance, causes an ageing reaction that is seven times faster
than that caused by glucose, and activates the reward system,
thereby stimulating consumption and addiction.[9] In his book,
The Case Against Sugar, Gary Taubes suggests that it's the
fructose in table sugar (sucrose) that differentiates it from
other carbohydrate-rich foods such as bread and potatoes,
making pure sugar particularly toxic.[10]

Taubes, Johnson and Lustig aren't the first to have written
about the harm that sugar can do. One of the original scientists to bang the drum against sugar was British physician
John Yudkin, author of *Pure, White and Deadly: How Sugar
Is Killing Us and What We Can Do to Stop It*. Yudkin's theories were discounted by Ancel Keys and his supporters, and
any concerns about sugar were obscured by a decades-long
obsession with saturated fat. But now Yudkin is having his
day, with many scientists and doctors acknowledging the

harmful effects of sugar. Sugar, it is now widely acknowl-edged, causes blood sugar to rise, which in turn causes insulin to be produced. When this happens to excess, it leads to insu-lin resistance and metabolic dysfunction, which manifests as many diseases including non-alcoholic fatty liver disease (NAFLD), obesity, diabetes, hypertension, CVD, cancer and dementia.[11]

The precise impact of a given food on the body's metab-olism can be calculated in terms of its glycaemic load – GL. This is a measure that accounts for the food's glycaemic index, or GI – the speed with which it raises blood sugar – as well as the quantity of carbohydrates in that food.[12] Dr David Unwin, an award-winning UK family doctor who has had enormous success helping his patients to reverse type-2 diabetes, came up with a simple way of thinking about gly-caemic load, expressing it in terms of table sugar equivalents. His sugar infographic helps people to identify and avoid high-sugar foods. So, for example, a bowl of Bran Flakes has a GI of 74 and a GL of 13, making it the equivalent of 4.8 teaspoons of sugar.[13] Seeing that a breakfast of Bran Flakes, milk, brown toast and apple juice equates to 16.3 teaspoons of sugar (22 if you add a sliced banana to the cereal) you might want to make your choice bacon, eggs and avocado instead.[14] Different people will react differently to each of the foods shown in the infographic, with some people's blood sugars rising more than others, but the principle remains generally applicable. Carbs equal sugars, which equal a rise in blood glucose levels.

Dr Jamie Seaman conducted an interesting experiment to establish precisely how her own blood sugars responded to different foods. She followed three different diets – a carnivore diet (animal-sourced foods only), a ketogenic diet (very low in carbohydrates), and a whole-food vegan diet – for three days each, while wearing a continuous glucose monitor (CGM), which enabled her to track exactly how each diet affected her blood sugars. The carnivore and ketogenic diets affected them very little, but the whole-food vegan diet caused some significant spikes. The foods included in this diet were those you would find in almost any vegan diet, such as tuberous vegetables, fruit, beans and oats. The worst spike in her blood sugar came from a bowl of oatmeal.[15]

Does this mean you should never eat oatmeal, beans or bananas? Of course not. But should you eat them in great quantities every day? Ideally not. If you are in tip-top metabolic health, you may be able to get away with it. Otherwise, the constant excursion into high blood sugars will do you harm. Eating large amounts of these high-glycaemic carbohydrates, as we would all be doing if plant-based advocates had their way, would do many of us harm, sending our blood sugars through the roof, and with them, rates of obesity, diabetes, heart disease, cancer and other chronic diseases.

Stay with me as I explore these diseases and their connection to excess carbohydrate consumption. It might feel like a diversion but it will provide a better understanding of why carbohydrate-rich, plant-based diets can lead to poor health.

Carbohydrates and obesity

We are in the midst of an obesity epidemic. Today, almost one in three adults in England is clinically obese, and two-thirds are overweight or obese.[16] The National Food Strategy report (2021) notes that 'a significant chunk of the population is now severely obese' (BMI above 40).[17] The picture is dramatically worse in the US,[18] and according to the WHO, worldwide obesity has tripled since 1975, with around 2 billion people now overweight.[19]

The fact that levels of obesity began their dramatic ascent

after the introduction of new dietary guidelines (1977 in the USA and 1983 in the UK) suggests that either people weren't following the guidelines or that the guidelines were inadvertently promoting obesity. Research by the Public Health Collaboration, a UK-based charity dedicated to informing and implementing healthy decisions for better public health, shows that people's diets did largely reflect the guidelines. It follows that some of the blame for the surge in obesity levels must be laid at the door of the guidelines themselves, with their advice to 'base your meals on starchy foods'. (As we saw in Chapter 4, the increased consumption of ultra-processed foods, which themselves tend to be starchy, is also undoubtedly a factor.)

In her book, *The Obesity Epidemic*, Dr Zoë Harcombe offers up an analysis of the laws of thermodynamics to prove that old, widely held beliefs about obesity and how to address it ('eat less, move more', and 'a calorie is a calorie') are incorrect, and that starchy foods are more likely to blame for weight gain:[20] 'Weight gain and weight loss is not a simple matter of energy in and energy out, but a matter of fat storage and fat utilisation. And since carbohydrate facilitates fat storage and debilitates fat utilisation [because it stimulates the production of insulin], dietary advice that leads someone to eat more carbohydrate is, therefore, fundamentally flawed.'[21]

In 2021, the 'energy in, energy out' (sometimes called the Energy Balance Model of obesity, EBM, or the 'calories-in, calories-out' model – CICO) was challenged by a group of leading researchers that included David Ludwig, Gary Taubes, Jeff Volek, Eric Westman and Walter Willett. The authors proposed an alternative model of weight gain and obesity, the carbohydrate–insulin model (CIM), in which fat accumulates in response to the hormonal responses triggered by a high glycaemic-load diet. They called for rigorous research to 'compare the validity of these two models'.[22]

Dr Fatima Cody Stanford, an obesity specialist at Harvard

Medical School had previously made it clear what she thought about the CICO model, stating that it is 'not only antiquated, it's just wrong'.[23] Gary Taubes made a similar assertion in his 2007 book, *Good Calories, Bad Calories* and later in *The Case for Keto*. A calorie is not a calorie. It matters very much *what type* of food the calorie comes from and whether it facilitates fat storage or utilisation. Trying to lose or control weight simply by applying the CICO principle does not work in the long term.

UK physician Dr Andrew Jenkinson, who has spent his entire career helping severely overweight patients, grew frustrated by the gap between what scientists were saying about obesity and what his patients were experiencing. Like Dr Harcombe and Gary Taubes, he stresses that obesity is not simply a matter of too many calories in and too few expended. Instead, appetite and metabolism are controlled by powerful hormones.[24] These hormones are involved in a process called homeostasis, or negative feedback, which is the mechanism the body uses to try to maintain a healthy environment. This negative feedback system leads the body to burn more energy when we take in too much food, and to conserve energy when we take in too little. This is one reason calorie-restrictive diets don't work over the long term. The body simply fights against any long-term deprivation by reducing its metabolic rate.

Dr Jenkinson provides a blueprint for weight loss that recognises the way different types of food impact both our hormones and the negative feedback system within our bodies. To lower insulin and cortisol, he recommends eating only three meals a day (including a low-carb breakfast), cooking your own food, and avoiding all sugar, wheat, corn and fruit juices, as well as all vegetable oils and foods prepared with them. His is a low-carbohydrate route to health.

Toronto-based obesity doctor Jason Fung also maintains that the CICO and 'eat less, move more' mantras are flawed, and that weight gain and weight loss are a much more complex matter. Insulin and cortisol are drivers of weight gain. Therefore, anything that stimulates the secretion of these hormones, as high-carbohydrate foods stimulate insulin secretion via their blood-sugar-spiking effects, will drive or exacerbate weight gain. His protocol for weight loss includes the removal of all added sugars from the diet, reduced consumption of refined grains and increased consumption of natural fats (as opposed to refined seed oils).[25]

Dr Fung's message is getting through to some, even if it isn't getting through to those who design the dietary guidelines. At a PHC workshop for health practitioners that I attended in 2020, when participants were asked to specify what had shifted their perspectives on obesity and diabetes and transformed the way they treated patients, a large number said that it was reading Dr Fung's book, *The Obesity Code*.

Whereas obesity experts such as doctors Harcombe, Jenkinson and Fung offer programmes for obesity management that differ at the margins, they are agreed on one thing: obesity is a hormonally driven disease that is exacerbated by a high carbohydrate intake. A low intake of carbohydrates, on the other hand, assists with weight loss. The most recent meta-analysis confirms that a low-carbohydrate, real-food diet results in better weight loss and better health outcomes such as reductions in triglycerides and increases in HDL.[26] Research conducted by the PHC shows that low-carbohydrate diets have outperformed low-fat diets in fifty-seven of sixty-six randomised controlled trials, and that low-fat diets have *never* significantly outperformed low-carbohydrate diets.[27]

Diets compared

Sam Feltham, founder of the PHC, conducted a personal experiment during which he tested the efficacy of three different diets: low-carb, real-food; low-fat, fake-food; and low-fat vegan.[28] He ate 6,000 calories (essentially overeating by 3,000 calories) per day for three weeks on each of the diets. On the low-carb, real-food diet he gained just 1.3kg, whereas the CICO formula would predict a gain of 6.1kg. On the low-fat, fake-food diet (which included cereals, sandwiches and pasta) he gained a whopping 7.1kg – a full 1kg more than the CICO formula would have predicted. Finally, he tried a low-fat vegan diet, which was almost 70 per cent carbohydrates and included foods such as porridge, potatoes and bananas. Because of the very high fibre content of this diet, his calorie intake fell short of that eaten on the other diets, but he still gained 4.7kg. This experiment demonstrated not only that the calorie-based model of weight gain and loss is incorrect but also that a low-carb, real-food diet is streets ahead of low-fat, high-carbohydrate diets, whether vegan or omnivore, in terms of its ability to help people to control their weight.

For those who 'fatten easily', a carbohydrate-free diet might represent the only means of losing weight and keeping it off. In his book, *The Case for Keto*, Gary Taubes makes a compelling case for keto as a necessity for those with a 'metabolic disorder of fat accumulation': 'It is that simple. Just like smokers who quit cigarettes and drinkers who abstain from alcohol, fixing the condition requires a lifetime of restriction.'[29]

The link between carbohydrates and the accumulation of fat isn't just a concern for those who are obviously overweight or appear to 'fatten easily'. Some 40 per cent of normal-weight people in the US have what is known as TOFI syndrome: thin on the outside, fat on the inside. The 'inside fat' has accumulated in and around their organs, most notably the liver. When someone consumes a high-sugar food, such as a 590ml soda, or even a daily mountain of lentils and beans, there's a tsunami of sugar that the liver can't handle. It sends some of this out as fat, and this creates risk factors for heart disease and obesity. The rest is converted to fat *in* the liver, becoming a risk factor for diabetes and NAFLD.[30] Wherever the extra fat ends up, it's a marker for metabolic syndrome.

If an excess of carbohydrates causes fat to accumulate and inclines people towards metabolic syndrome, what might be the impact of mandating carbohydrate-rich plant-based diets for the world?

Carbohydrates and diabetes

Diabetes is a 'modern-day scourge',[31] responsible for huge suffering, millions of deaths, and billions of dollars in healthcare spend worldwide. Globally, the number of people with diabetes (of which the vast majority will suffer from type-2 diabetes) has quadrupled since 1980 (rising from 108 million in 1980 to 422 million in 2014). The latest UK figures showed that 3.9 million people had been diagnosed with diabetes, but there could be as many as 4.8 million with the condition,[32] the treatment of which accounts for 10 per cent of the NHS budget.

The cause of this type-2 diabetes epidemic, says Dr Tim Noakes, is not hard to uncover. 'It is predicted in at least seven published works by credible medical scientists over the past century.' Those scientists include Dr Thomas Cleave, Professor John Yudkin, Dr Weston Price and Dr Walter Yellowlees, all of whom blame the replacement of traditional foods with refined flour and processed foods.[33]

Type-2 diabetes is characterised by excessive amounts of glucose in the blood. As Dr Verner Wheelock writes, 'it is like having a flood in your home from a burst in the plumbing system'.[34] As long ago as the late 1800s, doctors discovered that diets with a high meat content and low carbohydrate content improved the conditions of diabetes patients. Then came the discovery of insulin, which shifted the focus away from the presence of carbohydrates in the diet and towards treating diabetes with drugs. The carbohydrate content of diets for type-1 patients (type-1 being a condition whereby the pancreas produces little or no insulin) crept upwards, so that by 1940 it had increased to around 172g per day. Diabetologists also began to prescribe higher carbohydrate diets for type-2 patients.[35]

Another step backwards came in 1982, when the British Dietetic Association followed the National Advisory Committee for Nutrition Education (NACNE) in reversing previous advice to diabetics to consume diets high in protein and fat and low in carbohydrate. Since the anti-saturated-fat movement was in full swing by that time, and the prime consideration for all health authorities was to reduce fat within the diet, it was inevitable that recommended levels of carbohydrate intake would rise. This despite the fact that increased consumption of carbohydrates would result in higher levels of glucose in the bloodstream.

Some current official advice is not much better. The NHS site advises those with diabetes to 'base meals on higher fibre starchy foods like potatoes, bread, rice or pasta'.[36] The bulk of the advice on the site is of the generalised 'healthy eating' type, with references to the Eatwell Guide and five-a-day, and does not seem to have been tailored to the needs of people with a blood sugar disorder. (People are encouraged to sprinkle dried fruit on their cereal as a way of obtaining one of their five-a-day, for example, despite the fact that dried fruit is loaded with sugar.) Diabetes.org acknowledges that some starchy foods can raise blood glucose levels quickly, but it does not recommend a low-carb diet as the best way of managing or even reversing diabetes. Instead, it recommends that '*if* you're trying to cut down on carbs, cut down on things like white bread, pasta and rice first' (italics mine), going on to suggest that patients eat multigrain toast, brown rice, pasta, noodles and sweet potatoes.

The dietary advice issued by NICE (the National Institute

for Health and Care Excellence) is equally indefinite. NICE guidelines are difficult to navigate at the best of times, but trying to find clear dietary advice for type-2 diabetes is a needle-in-a-haystack problem in the extreme. After rummaging around for a while, you'll eventually be sent off to the NHS Choices website where you will find yourself in Eatwell hell, encouraged to base meals on starchy foods and sprinkling sugar-laden dried fruit on equally sugar-laden breakfast cereal.[37]

Going back to the Wheelock analogy of the flood in your home, this is like suggesting that you continue to pump more water into the house rather than trying to fix the plumbing system.[38] Many medical practitioners believe this to be counterproductive, which is why they are taking matters into their own hands, prescribing low-carbohydrate diets for their type-2 patients. Dr Gary Fettke, an orthopaedic surgeon in Tasmania, and a well-known proponent of low-carb diets,* started talking to diabetic patients about cutting their sugar intake after having to perform an increasing number of diabetes-related amputations and tiring of 'hearing the sickening sound of limbs dropped into buckets'.[39] (Dr Fettke encountered much resistance to his attempts to reduce sugar intake by diabetic patients, as we'll see in Chapter 11.)

Dr David Unwin, who created the sugar charts referred to earlier in this chapter, has achieved drug-free remission in 46 per cent of his patients with type-2 diabetes, and normal blood sugar levels for 93 per cent of pre-diabetic patients, reducing his surgery's annual bill for diabetes medication by over £50,000.[40] (The PHC estimates that if every surgery in the UK were to do the same, the savings to the NHS would be around £470 million.) David's wife, Dr Jen Unwin, works

---

* Low-carb diets are often referred to as LCHF – low carb, high fat. Some people use the term LCHF to mean lower carb, higher fat.

alongside him to help patients manage the behavioural challenges they face as they try to change their diets.

Dr Unwin has published several papers demonstrating the efficacy of the low-carb method.[41] Other GPs in the UK, many of them aligned with the Public Health Collaboration, are following his example.

In the US, VIRTA Health, founded by Sami Inkinen, Stephen Phinney and Jeff Volek, has shown the low-carbohydrate diet to be highly effective in reversing type-2 diabetes. A recent two-year, non-randomised clinical trial conducted by VIRTA (involving 349 patients) resulted in a high level of resolution of diabetes (reversal 53.5 per cent; remission 17.6 per cent) among those in the CCI group (following the low-carb protocol), but this was not seen among patients in the UC (Usual Care) group.[42] Research by Sarah Hallberg, the medical director of VIRTA, and colleagues has demonstrated that there is significantly more evidence for efficacy in treating diabetes for carbohydrate-restricted diets than for any other eating pattern, including the DASH diet (a flexible and balanced low-fat eating plan that restricts saturated fat intake), the Mediterranean diet, and the plant-based diet.[43] The American Diabetes Association changed its recommendations in line with this evidence, stating, in its 2020 report, 'Standards of Medical Care in Diabetes, 2020', that 'reducing overall carbohydrate intake for individuals with diabetes has demonstrated the most evidence for improving glycemia' and that 'for individuals with type-2 diabetes not meeting glycemic targets or for whom reducing glucose-lowering drugs is a priority, reducing overall carbohydrate intake with a low or very-low carbohydrate eating pattern is a viable option'. This view has also been endorsed by other US bodies, as well as the EASD (European Association for the Study of Diabetes).[44]

Research by Phinney, Volek and colleagues has also shown that the high fat part of the low-carb, high-fat (LCHF) approach is not a cause for concern. Their studies demonstrate that a hypocaloric (very low in calories), carbohydrate-restricted diet can lead to a *reduction* in plasma saturated fatty acids (that is, fatty acids within the blood) and a decrease in inflammation, despite a high intake of dietary saturated fat.[45] Hallberg explains this in a lecture titled, 'You are (not) what you eat'.[46] Just because you eat a higher level of saturated fat does not mean that you will end up with a higher level of saturated fat in your blood.

Individuals taking charge of their own health

The oil tanker that is the traditional dietary advice for diabetes is tough to turn around, even when the likes of Dr Unwin and VIRTA deliver evidence that low carb works. Many continue to cling to the familiar line on diet and diabetes. One patient, who managed to reverse his own diabetes by doing independent research that led to his following a low-carb diet, tried to explain to his GP how he had done it, but she was not interested. Another patient, Mark, tells a similar story. Diagnosed with type-2 diabetes in September 2015, he was initially advised to base meals around 'starchy carbohydrates' and given a prescription for metformin, but he felt so terrible on this programme that he decided to try the low-carb approach that he had found via an online search. Three months later he had reduced his HbA1c level to 45mmol/mol.* The nurse was shocked to learn that he had thrown his metformin pills in the bin and had lowered his blood sugars with diet alone. A year later Mark had reduced his HbA1c to

---

* The HbA1c reading measures how much haemoglobin in the blood has become glycated (bonded with glucose). It can be expressed in terms of mmol/mol or as a percentage. An HbA1c less than 42 mmol/mol (6.0%) is considered normal; 42– 47 (6.0– 6.4%) indicates pre-diabetes; 48 (6.5%) indicates diabetes.

27mmol/mol, but the practice nurse attributed this entirely to his weight loss and warned him against continuing the low-carb regime. 'I tried to explain how I had cut carbs and both controlled blood sugar levels and lost a few pounds. "No, no" was her reply, "carbs are essential, your brain will stop working without them." I must admit the thought going through my mind was yours obviously has but I bet you still eat them. The meeting did not end well.'

In 2017 Mark was called into the surgery for a review, but the practice nurse remained uninterested in how he had achieved such low HbA1c levels (which were then consistently in the 20s). Shortly afterwards, Mark joined his surgery's Patient Participation Group (PPG) in an effort to get the treatment for type-2 diabetics modified but to date he has not had success and he fears that 'this is going to be a long fight'.[47]

Like Mark, many newly diagnosed type-2 diabetics have found the best advice via unofficial online resources. Chris Rooney said that doctors told him his diabetes was a slippery downhill slope and that the best they could do was to try to flatten out the slope. Luckily, one of them referred him to diabetes.co.uk (rather than diabetes.org.uk), where he found a wealth of information about the low-carb approach, and a community of people who were making the approach work. He devised a plan, starting by swapping bread and cereals for eggs, then he gradually removed more carbohydrates. By testing his blood glucose levels he was able to establish which carbohydrates affected him most – brown rice being among them. By 'cutting out the beige', as he describes it, Chris lost 21kg (3st 4lb) in four months and brought his HbA1c score down from 66 to 40 (that is, below the level deemed normal) in eight weeks. He now actively spreads the word about the low-carb approach, speaking out on Twitter and giving talks at his own and others' workplaces.

Debra Scott watched her mother suffer terribly from

advanced diabetes: 'She was blind, had sores on her legs, numbness in her fingers, neuropathy in her feet, high blood pressure, kidney issues and skin problems.' When Debra was diagnosed herself, she was determined to be proactive. She wasn't offered the low-carb option by her doctor, but a quick online search (using the phrase 'reversing type-2 diabetes') led her to diabetes.co.uk. Like Chris Rooney, she banished the beige and swapped high-carb foods for low-carb foods. Courgette spaghetti replaced pasta, full-fat Greek yoghurt or bacon and eggs replaced cereal, and almond flour replaced refined white flour. Debra lost 25.4kg (4st) and took her HbA1c levels down from 62 to 36. She says, 'I felt like I'd discovered some sort of miracle cure. I just felt so much better. And it wasn't hard.'

Debra's GP surgery was supportive. She now runs low-carb groups for their diabetic patients, helping them to put their diabetes into remission and come off medication, which she calls just 'a mop and bucket'. She believes that the low-carb approach to diabetes management is gaining traction and she is determined to be part of the process of spreading the word:

> In the two years since I was diagnosed, Doctor Unwin and many more doctors around the world, like Joanne McCormack and Jason Fung, have been talking about the low-carb approach, and on any forum – Facebook, Twitter, diabetes.co.uk – diabetics are saying that this is the best way to do it. The low-carb voices are getting louder. They can't be ignored much longer.[48]

The low-carb voices are indeed getting louder, and acceptance of the low-carb approach to managing obesity and diabetes is gaining credence. Doing research for his latest book, Gary Taubes interviewed over a hundred physicians who are supportive of the low-carb approach and points out that more than a hundred Canadian physicians had 'cosigned a letter to the *HuffPost* publicly acknowledging that they personally follow LCHF/ketogenic regimens and that this is the eating pattern they now prescribe to their patients'.[49]

The Noakes Foundation, based in South Africa, has provided training in low-carb approaches to over two thousand medical professionals around the world, and reports a high level of enthusiasm for the approach in some African countries.[50] When I spoke to Professor Noakes, he was pleased to report that the *BMJ* had just published a meta-analysis which had concluded that 'patients adhering to an LCD [low-carbohydrate diet] for six months may experience remission of diabetes without adverse consequences'.[51] 'This is astonishing,' he said, 'I didn't think I would read that in my lifetime.'[52]

As the low-carb approach slowly gains acceptance within the medical mainstream, doctors like the Unwins remain focused on the daily work of helping patients. Meanwhile, there are still many who believe that calorie reduction and weight loss is the key to diabetes remission. (The practice nurse at Mark's surgery being one of them.) And, indeed, it is possible to put diabetes into remission with a calorie-restricted diet that results in weight loss. Proponents of LCHF maintain, however, that LCHF is more effective and more sustainable over the long term because it quickly and directly addresses the main problem (high blood sugar levels) and because of the satiating effect of fat (which helps people to stick to the diet). If weight loss is the key, the review carried out by the PHC (referenced earlier in this chapter) suggests that LCHF has the edge, since it has consistently outperformed the low-fat diet (which tends to be low calorie) in clinical trials. And we know from Sarah Hallberg's research that there is more evidence for the efficacy of the low-carbohydrate diet for treating diabetes than for any other eating pattern.

Carbohydrates and heart disease

Heart and circulatory diseases still cause a quarter of all deaths in the UK and cost the NHS approximately £7.4 billion annually. Almost six million people in England live with the daily burden of heart disease.[53] In the US, CVD is responsible for one in four deaths, or 600,000 deaths every year. Given that diabetes patients are at a greater risk of heart disease, any diet that fuels diabetes – namely a high-carbohydrate diet – will also increase the risk of CVD.[54] A 2015 study confirmed this to be the case, finding that 'when saturated fats are replaced with refined carbohydrates, and specifically with added sugars (like sucrose or high fructose corn syrup), the end result is not favourable for heart health'.[55]

Over fifty years ago, John Yudkin identified the role of high triglycerides and low HDL-C levels (both of which are linked to carbohydrate intake) in heart disease and gathered extensive epidemiological and patient-specific data to show that high-carbohydrate consumption increases the risk of heart disease.[56] In his article titled 'It's the insulin resistance stupid, part one', Professor Tim Noakes provides a neat summary of the work of other scientists whose investigations have shown that the real culprit in heart disease is not raised cholesterol but high levels of triglycerides, which is one of the best measures of a person's degree of insulin resistance.[57] Since blood triglyceride concentrations rise in response to carbohydrate ingestion, a high-carbohydrate diet is ill-advised not just for those at risk of heart disease but also for those wishing to minimise their risk.

Having reviewed the research, Patrick Holford and Jerome Burne, authors of *The Hybrid Diet*, assert that 'years of a high carbohydrate diet, which creates regular spikes in blood glucose each and every day, is one of the main drivers of high insulin levels and insulin resistance'. And 'insulin resistance equals increased susceptibility to heart disease'.[58]

A 2018 study corroborates these conclusions.[59] The study looked at the indicators of CVD (such as high blood pressure, CVD mortality and high blood glucose) in 158 different countries and compared these with the mean intake (supply) of sixty different foods. The results identified high carbohydrate consumption (mainly in the form of cereals and wheat) 'as the dietary factor most consistently associated with CVDs'. The authors wrote that their 'results agreed with the changing view of the causes of CVDs and pointed to high-glycaemic carbohydrates as the major CVD trigger'.

Dr Malcolm Kendrick argues that heart disease is caused by a number of factors that create endothelial dysfunction. (The endothelium is the thin, fragile, single-celled layer that lines the arterial wall.) These factors include 'high blood-sugar levels, especially spikes of blood sugar following a meal' and 'high insulin levels'. Smoking is also on his list of risk factors, along with acute mental stress and high levels of the stress response hormone, cortisol.[60] The point here is that a high-carbohydrate diet that causes repeated blood sugar spikes and insulin production could be as much of a risk to heart health as smoking and extreme stress. It follows that a low-carbohydrate diet ameliorates that risk. A recent documentary, *Extra Time*, highlighted the fact that low-carbohydrate diets can even be effective in treating heart disease and lowering the risk of cardiovascular events.[61]

If a high intake of sugar is implicated in heart disease, it follows that the widespread adoption of any diet that includes large amounts of carbohydrates would put more people at risk of heart disease. Unless plant-based eaters watch their sugar intake and eschew the mountains of grains, beans and pulses usually recommended as part of a plant-based diet, they are likely to consume far more carbohydrates than is good for their hearts.

Carbohydrates and cancer

In the UK in 2017, 366,303 cases of cancer were diagnosed, and there were 165,267 cancer deaths. One in two people will be diagnosed with cancer in their lifetimes.[62] Worldwide, in 2018, there were 17 million new cases of cancer and 9.6 million deaths from cancer.[63]

Cancer Research UK puts a positive spin on the cancer story, reporting that 50 per cent of people diagnosed with cancer today will survive the disease for at least ten years, whereas in the 1970s just a quarter would survive this length of time.[64] But, writes Professor Dominic D'Agostino, associate professor in the Department of Molecular Pharmacology and Physiology at the Morsani College of Medicine (University of South Florida), 'on the whole, treatment has remained largely ineffective, especially for advanced metastatic cancer and brain cancer'.[65] Naturopathic physician Dr Nasha Winters describes cancer as 'the most elusive, cunning, adaptable, intelligent and innovative disease in history'. She says that we must take a new approach because 'right now we're not winning the war on cancer – not even close'.[66]

John Bailar of the US National Cancer Institute claimed in 1985 that the US national cancer programme had failed, that there were 'no wonderful cancer cures out there waiting to be found', and that, to prevent cancer 'we will have to change our lives'. He and his colleague Elaine Smith reiterated this point in an article in the *New England Journal of Medicine*, advocating a shift in the research approach to focus more on prevention.[67]

A focus on prevention requires an understanding of what causes cancer. The fascinating story of the search for this understanding is recounted by Travis Christofferson in *Tripping Over the Truth: How the Metabolic Theory of Cancer is Overturning One of Medicine's Most Entrenched*

Paradigms. For a long time, writes Christofferson, the dominant view has been that cancer is a genetic disease. Nobel Laureate Otto Warburg's observation, made in 1924, represented a challenge to this view:

> Warburg's observation was this: cancer cells have a perverted method of generating energy. They truncate the conversion of glucose (sugar) into energy. They depend much less on the efficient process of aerobic respiration, using oxygen to produce energy – instead relying much more on the ancient and highly inefficient pathway known as fermentation.[68]

Later in his career, says Christofferson, Warburg would contend that this was the true origin of cancer, saying, 'Cancer, above all other diseases, has countless secondary causes. But, even for cancer, there is only one prime cause. Summarised in a few words, the prime cause of cancer is the replacement of the respiration of oxygen in normal body cells by a fermentation of sugar.'[69]

By the 1960s Warburg's theory had 'all but faded into oblivion'.[70] However, in the past five to ten years, cancer research has begun to heed Warburg's message and has shifted towards understanding tumour metabolism. Christofferson points to the work of Professor Thomas Seyfried, who provided evidence 'supporting the origin, management, and prevention of cancer with metabolic based approaches' in his book, *Cancer as a Metabolic Disease*.[71]

What does it mean to say that cancer is a metabolic disease? For Christofferson, it means that 'every type of cancer is treatable, because every type of cancer has the same beautiful, metabolic target painted on its back, regardless of the tissue or origin or the type of cancer'.[72] And that metabolic target might be susceptible to treatment with diet. 'A dietary protocol developed by Seyfried has shown promise in slowing the growth of cancer and working synergistically with existing therapies while mitigating side effects,' says Christofferson. 'Although unquestionably in their infancy, metabolic therapies have demonstrated incredible promise.'[73]

Simply put, diets that are low in sugar may slow the growth of cancer. The connection between sugar and cancer makes complete sense, given that there are close links between type-2 diabetes and cancer. Type-2 diabetes is a disease of insulin resistance (IR) caused by high levels of glucose in the blood, and IR is a critical element in the development of many diseases, including heart disease. Insulin also 'stimulates cancer cells to absorb and utilise more glucose, thereby speeding up the fermentation process, resulting in further damage to cells' and driving cancer-cell growth, says Dr Verner Wheelock.[74] Wheelock points to a number of studies that have shown the close connection between blood glucose levels and cancer, including a Korean study of over 1.2 million people which showed that all-cause mortality and cancer death rates increased in line with fasting blood glucose levels.[75]

Although the majority of cancer biologists still believe the origin of cancer to be genetic, others are pursuing metabolic approaches to treating cancer. Christofferson identifies the first documented use of the ketogenic diet (which, as we have seen, is a very low-carbohydrate, high-fat diet) to treat cancer in 1995 by Linda Nebeling, PhD. Then, in 2007, two German scientists began a trial at Wurzburg Hospital to test the ketogenic diet in cancer patients, the results of which confirmed what Nebeling's study had suggested: the ketogenic diet seemed to be affecting the growth of cancer cells. Meanwhile, Seyfried had some success treating cancer by combining fasting with a restricted version of the ketogenic diet alongside standard treatments.[76]

By 2010, writes Christofferson, 'with the results of the

Wurzburg trial, Nebeling's trial, and the Seyfried case study known, restricted, therapeutic ketosis [that state achieved through a ketogenic diet] appeared to be a viable approach against cancer'.[77] Although the ketogenic diet could stand alone as a protocol, its true power was in combination with other treatments, as it seemed to 'prep' up the therapeutic landscape in a spectacular way.

Dr Nasha Winters believes not just in the power of prepping the therapeutic landscape but also the necessity of prepping the original terrain. If the body is the terrain, prepping it to be an inhospitable host to cancer is the equivalent of attending to a garden's soil, ensuring that plants receive adequate sunshine, providing plentiful water supplies and so on. For the body, the most essential thing to care for is the mitochondria, which are the factories of cells in charge of telling the cell when to produce energy, when to reproduce and when to die. Winters says: '90–95 per cent of cancer cases are caused by poor diet and unhealthy lifestyles that also damage mitochondrial function. This is where we absolutely have to start focusing. Cancer is a mitochondrial disease related to a person's physiology, psychology, and ecology.'[78]

Winters' 'Terrain Ten' protocol is described in her book, *The Metabolic Approach to Cancer*.[79] The first step is to follow a ketogenic diet, limiting carbohydrates while increasing the amount of fat consumed and ensuring an adequate intake of vegetables. Winters applied the approach to treating her own cancer some twenty years ago and has been applying it with patients ever since. Under her care, most patients experience better clinical outcomes and a better quality of life living with cancer than patients adhering strictly to the conventional medical model.[80]

Canadian cancer researcher Dr David Harper uses a garden analogy to explain how a high-carbohydrate diet acts like the rain and sun for cancer cells, feeding their glucose addiction and causing them to grow. The ketogenic diet, on the other hand, limits insulin secretion, prevents the growth of cancer cells and upregulates the immune system. A 2020 breast cancer study in which Harper was involved showed that just six weeks on a ketogenic diet (alongside conventional treatment) could result in a remarkable level of regression in cancer patients.[81] Other medical institutions are using the ketogenic diet to try to achieve similar results. Dr Robert Lustig is advisor to two such trials being conducted by two US hospitals, Memorial Sloane Kettering Hospital and MD Anderson.[82]

Harper is at pains to emphasise that 'ketogenic diets are not a cure for cancer. They have not been proven to do anything unless it's adjunct with the standard of care.' And no one would be advised to embark on the ketogenic diet as adjunct treatment without consulting their doctor or a specialist in ketogenic therapies. The precise nature of the ketogenic diet used by cancer patients can vary widely, incorporating different amounts and types of animal proteins for instance, and the diet needs to be adapted to suit each individual patient's needs. Nevertheless, the diet can provide cancer patients with another valuable tool to help them fight the disease, and therein lies hope.

Hope for other illnesses

The ketogenic diet offers great hope for those suffering from cancer, and those who wish to be proactive in tending to their 'terrain' so as to avoid getting cancer, but it is also recognised as a powerful tool in the treatment of many other serious conditions. An article in the *European Journal of Clinical Nutrition* maintains that there is 'strong evidence' for the effectiveness of ketogenic diets in treating epilepsy, diabetes, obesity and cardiovascular risks, and that there is 'emerging evidence' for its effectiveness in treating acne, neurological diseases such as Alzheimer's and Parkinson's, cancer and polycystic ovarian syndrome (PCOS).[83] There is even some early evidence that a ketogenic diet might confer resistance to Covid-19.[84] More research will doubtless follow in this area.

Dr Eric Westman, co-founder of the Duke Keto Medical Clinic at Duke University, 'did some of the earliest clinical trials comparing the kind of low-fat, portion controlled, weight-loss diets advocated by the American Heart Association to the Atkins diet, an LCHF/ketogenic diet'. He reported that 'the Atkins diet allowed his patients to lose weight almost effortlessly and to become healthier in the process'.[85] He has since treated over 6,000 patients (some of them being the 'sickest patients who are still alive') with the ketogenic diet, improving conditions such as obesity, type-2 diabetes, PCOS, IBS, NAFLD, heart failure and post-bariatric surgery weight gain.[86] He's also seen people on plant-based diets who are severely overweight but have never considered that it could be their diet that's the problem, 'because everyone says it's so good for you'. Invariably, the root cause of the weight gain is excess carbohydrate intake.

The fact that some people following very low-carb or ketogenic diets can see their LDL levels rise significantly is alarming to those in the medical establishment, however, but Dave Feldman's model (the triad discussed in Chapter 1) suggests that it need not be. These people – termed 'hyper-responders' – also seem to be in the minority. Dr Westman estimates that only a fraction of people who try very low-carbohydrate diets will be hyper-responders. (In one of his trials, from 2004, just two people out of fifty-nine were forced to drop out because their LDL levels rose.) Westman and others say that the hyper-responder response is found most often in people who are slim and relatively muscular.[87] Another doctor, Vipan Bhardwaj, a family doctor in the UK, saw LDL rise in two out of his thirty-eight patients who began following a low-carb diet to reverse their diabetes. But, says Bhardwaj, these two people had other health markers that were all moving in the right direction (HDL and triglycerides among them), and scans showed that their arteries were free of plaques.[88] This would seem to indicate that high LDL is not a cause for concern in the context of good readings for the other members of Feldman's 'triad': HDL and triglycerides.

The keto diet and epilepsy

The efficacy of the keto diet in the treatment of epilepsy has been known about for some time. Film producer Jim Abrahams stumbled across the diet in an old textbook back in 1993 after conventional medications and approaches had failed to help his epileptic son Charlie. Within a month of following the diet, Charlie was drug- and seizure-free. Abrahams was angry that no one in the medical community told him about keto for epilepsy. He founded the Charlie Foundation to provide information for people with epilepsy, other neurological disorders and selected cancers. The foundation does the work that the medical establishment and industry are reluctant to do: 'the medical industry sells products to address these issues (such as epilepsy), so it has no interest in a sugar-free diet,' says Abrahams.[89]

Another story was recounted to me by Andy, whose youngest son, Toby, was diagnosed with epilepsy at the age of five. Toby was prescribed many medications over the years, but none seemed to work. He also suffered through having countless tests and interventions, during which he was either sedated or fitting. At the age of seven, he told his father he wanted to die. The last straw, when Toby was having over 150 seizures a day, was a drug called Zonisamide, which made his condition even worse. Toby's reaction to the drug led his parents to wean him off all medication and try a ketogenic diet. Within two months of starting keto, Toby's seizure activity was down to forty per day, with no anti-seizure drugs. It continued to improve. Andy found a world of keto people on Twitter who continued to help him and his family. Two years on, the whole family eats a ketogenic diet, and credit it with resolving their previous ailments (IBS, psoriatic arthritis, psoriasis and headaches). They've all lost weight, too. Andy said, 'I can honestly say keto saved our family. Toby just has a few twitches in the morning now, which he manages really well. It doesn't stop him doing anything. He is our hero.'[90]

Are very low-carb diets compatible with plant-based diets?

The keto diet might work wonders for people like Toby, but is it compatible with veganism? A tweet by VegNews suggests not: 'The high fat #keto diet is based heavily on red meat, fish, nuts, cream, eggs, cheese, oil and non-starchy vegetables and mostly avoids fruit, starchy vegetables, whole grains, beans, and lentils. No thanks! #notveganfriendly.'[91] Although keto experts are reluctant to discourage plant-based eaters from trying keto, most acknowledge that it can be challenging to try to eliminate carbohydrates from the diet when animal fats and foods are off limits. An online guide to the vegan ketogenic diet highlights why.[92] The list of permitted foods that meet both low-carbohydrate and plant-food criteria is vanishingly small. There are few sustaining foods on the list, meaning that the vegan keto dieter will likely be ravenous most of the time. Quality protein is also in extremely short supply. Tofu, for example, provides just 8g of protein per 100g, and, as discussed previously, this is protein that is much less complete and digestible than animal protein. The consumption of large amounts of nuts and seeds might also drive omega-6 levels up to unsafe levels.

Combining ketogenic principles with plant-based eating is difficult, but some are doing it. I found a dozen Facebook groups operating in the plant-based/LCHF/keto space, with followers numbering anywhere between a few hundred and several thousand.[93] The biggest of these, Vegan Keto Made Simple, boasts 58,000 members. This group is private, so it's impossible to know what foods members are eating, the challenges they face in combining keto with veganism or how many of its members have found the keto vegan diet sustainable and stayed the course for the three years that the page has been in existence.

From the other Facebook groups it is possible to glean that keto vegetarians have more choice and therefore an easier time of it than keto vegans. The allowance for eggs and dairy in their diet gives them a much broader range of satisfying recipes from which to choose.

It remains to be seen whether keto veganism is a movement that can attract and retain more than a small community of dogged enthusiasts. Of all the diets available to us, it strikes me as the most restrictive and the least sustainable in terms of adherence. (It's interesting to note that one of the doctors interviewed by Gary Taubes for his book, *The Case for Keto*, professes to following a vegan keto eating pattern because it works for her but recommends to her patients that they eat meat if they have no ethical issues doing so.)[94]

If veganism has a high rate of recidivism, keto veganism must surely have a higher one. In a mandated plant-based future, such as that envisioned by the most vociferous of plant-based advocates, it's likely that many would find the challenge of combining plant-based and ketogenic dietary principles too difficult and would therefore be denied the benefits of the healing powers of the ketogenic diet. Although plant-based advocates promote the potential of their chosen diet to generate widespread improvements in human health, the reality could be very different.

Why the architects of the global diet are missing a big trick

The evidence that a very low carbohydrate (ketogenic) diet aids weight loss and can have therapeutic effects is accumulating. That doesn't mean that everyone needs to eat a keto diet. Many will be able to garner the health benefits of a low-carbohydrate diet simply by cutting down on refined carbohydrates while continuing to eat starchy vegetables like potatoes and sweet potatoes. Remember, Dr Bikman suggests different levels of carbohydrate intake depending on the circumstance, and some people will be able to get away with eating more than his top level of 100g per day.

But those within organisations like the WHO and EAT-Lancet who advocate the roll out of a plant-based diet across the planet seem to have missed the lower-carbohydrate message altogether. They don't appear to have considered either the power of low-carb diets to prevent and cure disease, or the fact that animal foods are an important part of a nutrient-rich, low-carb approach. Neither do their public statements recognise any of the downsides of eating too many plant foods, which were discussed in Chapter 4. Environmental scientists rarely factor these things into their models, which are often based on flawed assumptions about how food impacts health. Their reports and public proclamations are replete with statements about how the plant-based diet could be one of the healthiest diets but generally fail to consider all the ways that this diet – deficient in nutrients, high in plant toxins and stuffed full of carbohydrates and industrial seed oils – could actually increase the burden of chronic disease around the globe and deprive people of a powerful dietary means of treating and curing these diseases.

We need to send these architects of the global diet back to the drawing board. In the meantime, let's take a look at how a diet based solely on animal foods – often called the ultimate ketogenic diet – can lead to dramatic improvements in health for some people. Follow me to the next chapter, where we'll learn about how animal-sourced foods can heal.

6

The Healing Power of Animal-sourced Foods

In the opening pages of *The Big Fat Surprise*, Nina Teicholz recounts the story of Vilhjalmur Stefansson, the son of Icelandic immigrants to America and a Harvard-trained anthropologist, who, in 1906, went to live with the Inuit in the Canadian Arctic.[1] Like his hosts, he lived exclusively on meat and fish for the entire year. Almost 80 per cent of his calories would probably have come from animal fat. He observed that if a healthy diet required carbohydrates and vegetables, then the Inuit should have been in a wretched state, but, to the contrary, they seemed to him the healthiest people he had ever lived with.[2] He witnessed neither obesity nor disease.

Following his return home in 1928, Stefansson devised an experiment. He and a colleague checked themselves into a hospital in New York City and vowed to eat nothing but meat and water for an entire year. After three weeks in the hospital the men were sent home but kept under close supervision. They continued to eat nothing but meat. Stefansson fell ill just once, when his team encouraged him to eat lean meat without the fat. His symptoms were quickly cured by a meal of sirloin steak and brains fried in bacon fat. Stefansson followed this carnivore diet for the entire year and for much of his life. He remained healthy and died at the age of 82.[3]

A few years after Stefansson conducted his year-long hospital experiment, Canadian dentist Dr Weston A. Price (discussed in chapters 2 and 3) started travelling the world with his wife, Florence. The couple visited fourteen countries on five continents, travelling Indiana Jones-style on prop planes, steamships, canoes, automobiles and on foot.[4] Troubled by the massive increase in dental problems among his patients, Price wanted to see what could be learned from indigenous groups. He observed that those who ate traditional diets rich in animal foods enjoyed superior health. In Africa, for example, he compared the Maasai, who eat an almost entirely animal food-based diet, to the neighbouring Kikuyu tribe, who consumed mainly sweet potatoes, corn, beans, bananas and millet. Price noted that the Maasai were taller and more rugged, and had far superior dental and all-round physical health. Like Stefansson, he also found that the Inuit (whom he referred to as Eskimos) thrived on an animal-food diet.

Fast forward to 12 February 2020. A young man posted exciting news via the Twitter account of P.D. Mangan, a microbiologist and keto–carnivore activist: '[In July] I was completely anemic, had horrible Crohn's disease and arthritis at the age of 19. Now, here I am after 6+ months of eating 90% beef, chicken, eggs and some dairy and I'm completely healed from Chrons [*sic*] and Arthritis and for the first time ever since I was nine years old I'm on ZERO prescription drugs ... I've tried going vegan, fruit-based diets and almost every other diet in the book and this is what finally worked for me.'[5]

This young man's story is not unique. Social media abounds in testimonials of individuals who have healed themselves of Crohn's, epilepsy, autoimmune diseases, arthritis, depression and bipolar disorder by following a carnivore diet. Like Vilhjalmur Stefansson and some of the indigenous populations studied by Weston Price, these individuals thrive by eating almost nothing but animal foods. These are modern-day carnivores. They are among that section of the population who have an intolerance of plants and whose bodies simply work better without them. Using Dr Paul Saladino's analogy, you might say that their operating system is completely antithetical to that of plants.

What, exactly, is a carnivore diet?

Like the plant-based diet, the carnivore diet can mean different things to different people. To some it means eating only meat, whereas for others it means eating eggs, dairy and fish in addition, but a key characteristic of the diet is that it comprises mostly animal foods and largely excludes plant foods. (I say 'largely' because carnivores are not averse to consuming small amounts of certain fruits and vegetables if they can be tolerated.) It sometimes represents the first stage of an elimination diet embarked upon to determine the cause of an allergy or other medical condition. It is also the ultimate low-carbohydrate diet.

For Professor Tim Noakes, who describes himself as 'essentially carnivore', a very low intake of carbohydrates is essential. When diagnosed with type-2 diabetes more than a decade ago, Professor Noakes started out on a low-carbohydrate diet, but the carb count was still too high for him:

> Starting out low carb I couldn't get my fasting glucose down to normal. I had to take medication. Now I eat eggs, bacon, steak, fish, dairy, nuts and very few vegetables, so my carb intake is close to zero and my diabetes is under

control. But my diabetic control is right on the edge. If I take in any carbs my glucose goes haywire. I'm motivated to stick to the [essentially carnivore] diet because I believe that if I eat carbs I'll kill myself. My father died ten years after his [type-2 diabetes] diagnosis and I'm ten years in and I'm asymptomatic. I'm healthy, when I should have lost a leg or had a heart attack by now.[6]

Professor Noakes is one among a carnivore community that is sizeable and growing. A Twitter search for carnivores will turn up thousands of results. Carnivore advocates such as Dr Shawn Baker (@SBakerMD, otherwise known as the Carnivore King), Dr Paul Saladino (@CarnivoreMD), and Carnivore Aurelius (@ketoaurelius) number their Twitter followers in the many tens of thousands. A Facebook group called Women Carnivore Tribe has almost 24,000 members. Travis Statham's website, carniway.nyc, which is 'dedicated to the science and history of a carnivorous way of eating', attracts new members every day, many of whom submit their stories of health regained via the diet.

The value of N=1*

Stories and anecdotes are not clinical trials, but neither should they be discounted. History is replete with examples of medical treatments that began as personal experiments or observations which, when tested, proved to have general significance. It's worth remembering that germ theory began as one doctor's personal observations, which were initially dismissed

---

* N=1 is shorthand for a science experiment with a sample of one. It is often used to refer to the evidence derived from the recounted experience of individuals.

as being the ravings of a madman. Hungarian obstetrician Ignaz Semmelweis (1818–1865) observed that mortality rates from infection were much higher in wards staffed by doctors than in those staffed by midwives. He realised that this difference was due to the habit of doctors performing autopsies and then examining women in the maternity wards without disinfecting their hands, a practice that caused infection.[7] Semmelweis instructed doctors to wash their hands in a chlorine solution in between attending patients. This resulted in a dramatic drop in mortality rates in the wards staffed by doctors. But, despite this clear evidence, Semmelweis was not able to convince his peers that hand washing was an effective and essential practice. 'His stubbornly pursued hand-washing suggestions were rejected by his contemporaries who even mocked and stigmatised the "weird man", and some doctors refused to accept his idea "on the grounds that a gentleman's hands could not transmit disease".'[8] It was not until Louis Pasteur arrived on the scene and germ theory became widely accepted that Semmelweis would be vindicated. Semmelweis's story inspired the concept called the 'Semmelweis effect': the automatic rejection of new knowledge that contradicts established norms, beliefs and paradigms. Journalist Monika Baár calls it 'the arrogance of mainstream hierarchy vis-à-vis fresh insight coming from the margins'.[9]

Dr Shawn Baker aims to bring the carnivore dietary approach in from the margins. He initially became a carnivore advocate after noticing how the diet improved his own health. His joint pain and tendinitis disappeared, the quality of his sleep improved, and he no longer experienced bloating, cramping or other digestive problems.[10] He also gained muscle, had more energy and saw his athletic performance improve. His personal experience initially led him to document case studies of people who had also transformed their health with the carnivore diet. He went on to form an online community called Meat Heals, which later became MeatRX, of which he is now CEO. Through this community he has amassed survey data on more than 12,000 people. 'This is self-reported data,' he says. 'But it's incredibly compelling. And while one individual data point [N=1] does not make a scientific study, many N=1s taken together generate a powerful case for the potential health benefits of a carnivore diet.'[11] (Or, as Nobel Prize winner George Stigler famously asserted, 'the plural of anecdote is data'.)

Dr Baker holds daily meetings with people in his community, which enables him to continue to gather data. He is also raising funds for a controlled interventional trial and has been involved in a trial being carried out at Harvard University.

Can the carnivore diet deliver on nutrition?

Both Dr Baker and Dr Paul Saladino have written books (*The Carnivore Diet* and *The Carnivore Code,* respectively) in which they explore the science behind a diet based on animal foods. Leading carnivore L. Amber O'Hearn[12] has also done extensive research into the power of an animal-food diet to resolve many health conditions. But can the diet deliver complete nutrition? According to Dr Harcombe, the answer is yes, provided careful attention is paid to the specific foods eaten. She mocked up a 2,000-calorie-a-day diet that included chicken liver (100g), steak (300g), sardines (500g) and eggs (300g). This provided sufficient amounts of most vitamins (both water and fat soluble), minerals, amino acids and fatty acids, but there were deficiencies in manganese and vitamin C. The manganese deficiency could be resolved by varying the intake of seafood. To reach the minimum required levels of vitamin C (65mg for an adult), you would have to increase the amount of liver eaten to around 360g.[13]

Dr Harcombe hypothesises that vitamin C deficiency might

be less of an issue for carnivores because they don't eat carbohydrates. (The glucose in carbohydrates competes with vitamin C for uptake in cells.) L. Amber O'Hearn's research suggests an alternative explanation for why carnivores do not suffer from scurvy (a condition long believed to result from a simple vitamin C deficiency): 'Many of the symptoms of scurvy are due to lack of carnitine, which can be derived endogenously using vitamin C, but can also be absorbed in large quantities from the meat in the diet ... given that meat is an excellent source of carnitine, it may be that carnitine spares vitamin C that would otherwise be needed for synthesis, while the small amounts of vitamin C it [meat] provides are enough for the remaining functions.'[14]

Manganese is another nutrient for which the requirement is lower in the absence of carbohydrates.[15] And the absence of plant anti-nutrients in the carnivore diet means that the required levels of vital minerals such as iron, zinc and magnesium will be more easily achieved and maintained.[16] The requirement for fibre is also greatly reduced. (One of the roles of dietary fibre is to help process carbohydrates and control blood sugar levels.)

Although nutrient deficiencies need not be a concern with a well-planned carnivore diet, a surplus of certain nutrients might be. 'The carnivore diet provides an abundance of complete protein; some would argue too much,'[17] says Dr Harcombe. Levels of zinc, B12 and iron might also be high.[18] Does an excess of certain nutrients 'mean overdose, or super health?' Dr Harcombe asks.

Dr Baker's trial, when completed, may well answer this question and others about the carnivore diet. In the meantime, says Dr Baker, it would be unwise to dismiss the diet simply because trials have not yet been done: 'There are few controlled studies showing the outcomes of any diet. There are only observations in populations [epidemiology] and these are widely confounded by lifestyle variations. And when people say the carnivore diet will give you scurvy, or kill your microbiome – well, none of these things are happening to people who eat this way. You can dismiss this based on observation alone.'[19]

When medicine fails us

Individuals with experience of the diet deserve a fair hearing. Their stories can teach us something, even if we have no intention of becoming carnivores ourselves. Mikhaila Peterson's story is one of the most well-known. The daughter of the Canadian psychologist Jordan Peterson, Mikhaila adopted a meat-only diet after years of ill health. She was diagnosed with severe juvenile rheumatoid arthritis (JRA) when she was two, and a series of chronic health issues during her teens (including chronic fatigue, severe body itching, depression, ulcers, rashes and blisters).[20] The medical community had no answers for her, so she started experimenting with her diet, trying Paleo and then a dairy-free ketogenic diet of meat and greens. Every time she tried to reintroduce foods to the diet, her symptoms would return. Over time it became apparent that there were just very few foods that she could eat, and that for her the only safe foods were ruminant meats. Within a few weeks on an all-ruminant diet, her depression lifted and her other symptoms began to improve. Following a strict carnivore diet, she regained control over her health.

A woman named Neisha suffered for years with Hashimoto's disease (an autoimmune disorder whereby the body's immune system attacks the thyroid). At age twenty-eight, she suffered from extreme fatigue, depression, weight gain, cold intolerance, dry skin, muscle cramps, decreased concentration, problems with fertility and a lack of libido. Her symptoms improved on a ketogenic diet, but after doing more research she decided to follow a carnivore diet that included beef, butter, eggs, bacon and fat-based ice cream. She felt even better on this diet. Latterly, after having a baby, she began doing what she calls 'cyclic carnivore', meaning five days carnivore and two days ketogenic. Writing about her extreme intolerance of carbohydrates, she said: 'I was floored by the fact that carbs had ruined my health. Not just bad carbs. All of them. After all, I had been eating "healthy". I ate whole wheat, and sweet potatoes and Ezekiel bread. I ate freakin' quinoa … I even tried cutting out gluten. All this time, I was just trading poison for poison. Those carbs were killing me.'[21]

A website called Ketogenic Endurance, which is managed by an athlete whose conversion to a carnivore diet in 2017 led to his experiencing fewer colds, improved digestive function, better energy and mental focus, and the resolution of the arthritis in his ankles,[22] showcases the stories of other individuals who have resolved a range of health issues by swapping to a carnivore diet.[23] Rich, one of the success stories, lost 31.75kg (5st) and saw his IBS, gas, bloating and lower abdominal pain resolved; another, Rosie, found that the diet alleviated her anxiety, depression and insomnia and made her feel 'like a normal, functioning human again'; Cory experienced the end to his chronic bloating and noticed a big boost in energy and muscle growth; Yuval went from a 'vegetarian carbivore' weighing 120kg (18st 12lb) and with 32 per cent body fat, to a carnivore weighing 77kg (12st 2lb) with 13.7 per cent body fat. He reports having more energy and resolving the bloating, which was something he had dealt with constantly as a vegetarian.

Preventative interventional cardiologist Dr Christian Assad has seen carnivore success stories in his own practice. In November 2019 he tweeted that one of his patients, a vegan of fifteen years, saw massive improvements in his psoriasis within four weeks of eliminating all plants from his diet. This was the third individual he had seen whose condition had been improved by the carnivore diet. He urged us not to dismiss this direct evidence simply because it is of the N=1 type.

More N=1 stories were recounted directly to me while I was doing research for this book. One man claimed to have reversed an autoimmune disease, eradicated IBS, improved gum and teeth health and built a stronger body.[24] Another former long-term vegetarian claimed to have reversed a twenty-year-long loss of taste and smell with a carnivore diet. A number of people reported increased sun tolerance: carnivores seem to be able to stay out in the sun for longer without burning. One explanation for this could be that carnivores don't consume as much omega-6 (found in vegetable oils and processed food) as others. Omega-6 oils are easily oxidised, so the less you have in your skin cells, the less you might experience of the oxidation that leads to burning.[25]

Dr Paul Saladino is, himself, testament to the healing potential of a carnivore diet. He originally investigated an animal-foods-only diet after suffering from incurable eczema throughout his time at medical school and as a physician assistant. He recalls hearing Jordan Peterson talking about how the carnivore diet had transformed his daughter's, and subsequently his own, health. There followed a light-bulb moment: *what if my own autoimmune issues and so many of the inflammatory problems we see manifested as chronic disease today could be triggered by the plants we are eating?*[26] After months of studying the literature and considering the ideas behind the carnivore diet, he decided to give it a try. Within three days he began to feel more emotionally calm and positive, a change he attributes to the gradual resolution of the low-level inflammation in his body that began in his gut and was translated to his brain. His eczema resolved itself, and he felt healthier in every way. What's more, tests consistently showed that he was healthier, and he remains so, his inflammatory markers almost undetectable and his blood sugars in the ideal range at all times.[27] Dr Saladino's experience led him to explore how other people had been helped by the diet and to investigate the science behind it:

> My story is not unique. There are thousands of people with experiences similar to mine demonstrating improvement and resolution in a variety of diseases such as ulcerative colitis, Crohn's, lupus, thyroid disease, psoriasis, multiple sclerosis, rheumatoid arthritis, and psychiatric illnesses like depression, bipolar, and anxiety. This is in addition to those who have used the carnivore diet to lose weight, reverse diabetes and insulin resistance, or to improve libido and performance. Many of their incredible stories are catalogued at the website MeatHeals.com, which is indexed by condition.[28]

Like Saladino, L. Amber O'Hearn became a carnivore and a carnivore advocate after the diet helped her to resolve serious health issues. Her online 'book in progress', titled *Eat Meat. Not Too Little. Mostly Fat*, describes her journey from mostly vegetarian and then vegan beginnings to her carnivorous lifestyle: 'In an unexpected turn of events, a whimsical foray into eating meat eliminated not just my excess weight but all symptoms of my then-progressing bipolar disorder. Faced with this perplexing result, I turned my study from mathematics, linguistics, and cognitive psychology to the subjects of nutrition, physiology, biochemistry, and anthropology.'[29]

Both her own experience and her extensive study led O'Hearn to reach many conclusions that fly in the face of conventional thinking and dietary advice: 'Recommendations to eat a large and varied amount of fruits and vegetables are based on inconclusive and questionable science; heavy reliance on animal-sourced foods, including animal fat, was critical to the evolution of our brains; ketosis is not only natural but is normally involved in human brain development before and after birth; evolutionary forces shaping plants have resulted in some less than savoury health effects; removing plants from the diet altogether may improve your health.'[30]

That a carnivore diet helped O'Hearn to eradicate her bipolar disorder makes sense in the context of what we know about how diet affects the brain and mental health. As we saw in Chapter 2, meat and other animal foods provide essential nutrients for the brain. And the connection between meat abstention and poor mental health has been documented in research, with a review of eighteen studies concluding that those who avoided meat consumption had higher rates, or risk, of depression, anxiety and/or self-harm behaviours.[31] It follows that a diet rich in meat and other animal foods would be beneficial to brain function and mental health.

For most people, it isn't necessary to become a carnivore to reap these kinds of benefits. Simply adding some meat and animal-sourced foods back into the diet can improve mental health and brain function. Dr Jen Unwin, now a low-carb advocate, was vegetarian for eight years when she was young. She says her mental health 'really suffered', and she noticed immediate improvements when she started eating meat.[32] The Ethical Butcher, Glen Burrows, and his wife were vegetarians for 25 years. His wife went back to eating meat as part of a Paleo diet after experiencing hormonal problems and severe adrenal fatigue. Seeing her health 'transforming before his eyes', Glen started adding quality animal foods back into his diet. Cutting out the grains and pulses on which his diet had been based led to an immediate alleviation of digestion issues and brain fog. 'I'd got to the point where I couldn't think straight half the time, but everything changed when I left the vegetarian diet behind,' he says.[33]

A carnivore diet is certainly not for everyone and might not even suit many people. But it's important to recognise that, for some, the diet has proved to be the best route to both mental and overall health. And it is all about health, says Dr Baker. Carnivores are not simply 'reverse vegans', trying to convert everyone else to their worldview: 'There's no ideology attached. We're not out to save the broccoli. This is a diet for the sole purpose of improving health. There's no other agenda ... we [carnivores] are not extreme about it. If you eat a few blueberries or an avocado, who cares? Whatever works for your health.'[34]

When something works, news spreads. Anecdotal evidence about the carnivore diet – found on Facebook, Twitter and websites such as MeatRX – represents an invaluable resource for people who have health problems that have not been resolved by mainstream medical and dietary advice. For the rest of us, the carnivore story is an antidote to the plant-based-is-best dogma that threatens to engulf us; a useful reminder that animal foods abound in important nutrients, that plant foods are not always benign, and that there is no such thing as a one-size-fits-all diet.

Part Two

Will a Plant-based Diet Save the Planet?

'What is sold as sustainable, ethical, and healthy is a food system without animals, or at least one that involves substantially less meat than our current levels of consumption. These notions are accepted largely as fact. But the evidence – although it is difficult to unpack – is clearly not consistent with these ideas.'

DIANA RODGERS, RD, and ROBB WOLF,
former research biochemist, authors of
Sacred Cow: The Case For (Better) Meat

'There is nothing "saving the planet" in choosing a vegetarian lifestyle, just the opposite: you become an activist for the destruction of the planet.'

NATASHA CAMPBELL-MCBRIDE, MD,
Vegetarianism Explained

'There are very few ecosystems that have functioned in the absence of animals and the cycling of nutrients through animals; there's no way to exclude animals from a truly sustainable agricultural system.'

PETE HUFF, the Pasture Project, an initiative of
the Wallace Center at Winrock International

Part Two

Will a Plant-based Diet Save the Planet?

7

Emissions Stories: The Truth About CO2, Methane and All Those Cow Burps

Early in 2020, UK broadcaster Jeremy Vine hosted a discussion about veganism on Radio 2. His guests were a farmer and the author of a book about sustainable living.[1] Vine raised a few questions about the health and environmental impacts of vegan versus omnivore diets, giving each of his guests a chance to respond. All of this went pretty smoothly, with the discussion favouring neither one side nor the other. Then Vine closed the programme by giving the author the final say, and she said this: 'A study by Oxford University shows that if you go vegan you can reduce your carbon footprint by 73 per cent.' This looked like a home run for her, because if what she said is true, wouldn't we all consider eschewing animal foods? Certainly, these last words will have given listeners pause for thought and a big reason to feel guilty about the ham sandwich they might have been eating while listening to the programme.

The trouble is, the author was wrong, and she was wrong in a big way. In the study on which her claim was based it had been asserted that, for the US, where per capita meat consumption is three times the global average, dietary change (moving to a diet that excludes animal products) has the potential to reduce food's different emissions by 61–73 per cent.[2]

Setting aside, for a moment, the question of whether this study by Poore and Nemecek is entirely robust, or whether any results achieved in the US could be replicated in countries as diverse as, say, the UK and India, let's consider the key words in this claim. These words are *food's different emissions*. The authors are not claiming, as Vine's guest did, that an individual's entire carbon footprint could be reduced by 73 per cent if they adopted a vegan diet. They are claiming that the footprints of *different foods* could be reduced by 61–73 per cent. Given that an individual's food footprint in much of the world is, at most, around 16 per cent of their *total* footprint[3] one might say that converting to a vegan diet has the potential to reduce a person's entire footprint by between 61 and 73 per cent *of* 16 per cent, or a *maximum* of 10 per cent. Of course, 10 per cent is nowhere near as impactful a number as 73 per cent. And given the questions surrounding the economic and health impacts of a wholesale switch to a vegan diet, many might regard a 10 per cent payoff as insufficient.

The 73 per cent number is out there now, with millions of Radio 2 listeners possibly persuaded that it is true. It will undoubtedly stick in many people's minds, as will a claim in *The Economist* that 'die-hard leaf eaters can claim to have knocked off 85 per cent of their carbon footprint'.[4] What *The Economist* should have said was that vegans could claim to have knocked 85 per cent off their *food* footprint, which equates to a maximum of 14 per cent of their total footprint. That's if the study being cited is definitive, which it isn't, as we'll see later in the chapter.

This kind of coverage is causing untold damage to our

understanding of the true causes of the climate crisis and to our ability to address it. As Frank Mitloehner (the professor and air quality extension specialist at UC Davis whom we met in earlier chapters) points out: 'This kind of reporting, and the studies on which it is based, is immensely misleading because it makes people believe that changing what we eat will have a major impact on our climate, when that is not the case.'[5]

In addition to conflating reductions in individuals' food emissions with reductions in total emissions, plant-based advocates and the media that gives them a voice contribute to a misrepresentation of the emissions story in five important ways: exaggerating total emissions from animal foods; neglecting to account for the carbon sequestration effect of livestock farming; misrepresenting the difference between methane and CO2; disregarding nutritional considerations; and treating the outcomes of some studies as though they were definitive and incontrovertible. We'll take a look at each of these shortcomings in turn to see just how skewed a picture is being painted for us.

Emissions from animal agriculture: the real story versus the usual story

It has been claimed that animal agriculture accounts for 51 per cent of all greenhouse gas emissions. The makers of the documentary *Cowspiracy* made this assertion to great and long-lasting effect in 2015. (Although they were later forced to retract it, as we'll see in Chapter 13.) Popular publications took to throwing the 51 per cent number around without questioning it.

The fantastical 51 per cent number came from a 2009 non-peer-reviewed article by Goodland and Anhang, published in *World Watch Magazine*, a Worldwatch Institute publication.[6] The number stood in stark contradiction to existing data from the Food and Agriculture Organisation (FAO) of the UN, showing that animal agriculture generates 14.5 per cent of global emissions. Defending the numbers used in his documentary, co-director Keegan Kuhn said that 'regardless of whether animal agriculture is responsible for 14.5 per cent of GHGs or 51 per cent it is still a primary driver of climate change',[7] seemingly untroubled by the fact that his film had exaggerated the then-accepted facts by 3.5 times.

Like the saturated fat-clogs-arteries myth, the notion that animal agriculture causes more than half of all emissions doesn't seem to want to die. Running alongside it in popular discourse is another claim, which is that animal agriculture generates more emissions than *all of transport*. As discussed in the introduction, this accusation is based on a 2006 report by the FAO, 'Livestock's Long Shadow: Environmental Issues and Options' Report', which claimed that animal agriculture was responsible for 18 per cent of emissions.[8] Although the FAO revised this number down to 14.5 per cent, the idea that eating meat generates more emissions than transport has stuck. Vegan activists, director James Cameron and his wife Suzy, used the transport comparison in a *Guardian* op-ed piece in support of their claim that 'animal agriculture is choking the earth'.[9]

Even the lower FAO estimate overstates the case. This is because, while the number for livestock includes life-cycle emissions (emissions from rumen digestion and forages, crops grown for feed, processing and transportation) the number for transport includes only direct (tailpipe) emissions. Life-cycle emissions for transport would be at least 1.5 times the operational ones, according to Henning Steinfeld, head of livestock sector analysis at the FAO. Steinfeld explains that were we to compare livestock and transport on an apples-with-apples basis, the global emissions from livestock would be just 5 per cent of total emissions, as compared to transport at 14 per cent.[10] An accurate newspaper headline – the likes of which I've not yet seen – might therefore be 'transport generates almost three times the emissions of livestock'.

The other problem with the global number for emissions from livestock is just this: it's global. And as Richard Young of the Sustainable Food Trust noted, 'looking at global averages and drawing conclusions from them isn't actually very helpful'.[11] The global percentage disguises the enormous differences between countries around the world. In Paraguay and Africa, for example, livestock represents 50 per cent and 90 per cent of emissions respectively. These percentages reflect different levels of industrialisation, the importance of agriculture within these countries relative to other sectors, and different approaches to, and levels of, efficiency in livestock farming. The global numbers don't mean very much in places such as the US, the UK or Ireland, and they don't help us to understand the relative trade-offs between animal agriculture and other sectors in terms of addressing the emissions problem.

Mitloehner explains how this distorts the picture for consumers:

> The global [lifecycle] number is 14.5 per cent, but in the UK it is in the order of 4 per cent. They use the global number because it sounds big. They haven't lied, but they haven't told the British consumer what matters to them when they choose between a British burger or a Beyond Burger. The honest way would be to use numbers as they apply in the market where the products are sold and the decisions are being made.[12]

Looking at the GHG numbers country by country tells us far more about the significance of agricultural emissions. In the US, where the per capita consumption of meat is the highest in the world, agriculture as a whole generates 9 per cent of emissions, whereas transportation generates 29 per cent, and industry 22 per cent.[13] Within the number for agriculture, there lies an even more interesting story. Emissions from animal agriculture are around 4 per cent of the total for agriculture, whereas those from non-animal agriculture are 5 per cent. Even if you account for the fact that a percentage of crops grown are fed to animals (I'll discuss this in Chapter 8), you end up with emissions numbers for animal agriculture that are on a par with those for crops grown for human consumption. The other interesting thing to note is that the US emissions number is even smaller for beef cattle, at around 2.2 per cent.[14] The maligning of beef is completely out of proportion to its actual contribution to emissions and climate change.

The case for UK-produced meat

UK-produced meat is among the most sustainable in the world. Taking into account grassland sequestration (the process by which grassland draws carbon out of the atmosphere and stores it in the soil, of which more in a moment), cattle and sheep account for 3.7 per cent of UK emissions. Even excluding sequestration, cattle and sheep account for just 5.7 per cent of emissions. Very little meat consumed in the UK comes from systems that deplete rainforests and generate large amounts of emissions. UK beef imports from Brazil, for example, make up just 1 per cent of beef imports.[15]

The emissions picture varies widely between continents. Latin America and the Caribbean generate 35 per cent of global cattle-related emissions but just 20 per cent of protein. North America demonstrates an inverse ratio, generating just

10 per cent of global emissions while delivering 17 per cent of the protein. (The US also produces 18 per cent of the world's beef with just 6 per cent of the world's beef cattle.) Western Europe has a similar protein-to-emissions ratio, delivering 19 per cent of the world's protein while generating 8 per cent of global cattle-related emissions. Clearly, the region from which we get our protein – and the systems deployed in that region – matter immensely.[16] Regional differences are due to a wide range of factors, including variations in feed digestibility, slaughter age and weight, climate conditions, management practices, and the economic, cultural and religious context in which management is practised.[17]

If the high-level, global numbers for emissions are misleading, so are the various claims about the carbon cost per kilo of beef. Frank Mitloehner explains this using a car analogy:

> If I asked you about the emissions generated by a car, you would have to ask: what car are we talking about? A Fiat or an S-class Mercedes or an electric car? Is it diesel or gas? How old is it, and who's driving it? All these questions and more. It's the same with cows. What breed is she? Where is she? What is she fed? Is there a veterinary system to treat her diseases? There are so many issues to consider. So, when you try to produce a global estimate and apply it to a specific region or farm, you are almost certainly going to be wrong, perhaps by 10, 15 or 20 times.[18]

The problem identified by Mitloehner goes some way towards explaining why estimates for the carbon costs per kilo of meat vary so widely. Sources I consulted gave estimates ranging from minus 4 kilos to plus 400 kilos of CO_2 per kilo of meat (the latter being a real outlier). The research organisation Our World in Data (OWiD), for example, has published two different estimates: 100 kilos and 60 kilos. The per kilo CO_2 cost of beef in sub-Saharan Africa is estimated at 40–50 kilos CO_2e, versus 5–10 kilos in Europe.[19] A report by the NFU (National Farmers Union) estimates the carbon cost of British beef at 17.2 kilos (as compared to 46 kilos for the rest of the world).[20] The claims in a BBC *Horizon* programme which aired in early 2021 were (according to the online material provided by the scientist who provided the data for the programme) based on yet another emissions-per-kilo-of-beef number – 25 kilos of CO_2e.[21]

Clearly, where and how the beef is produced, and what factors are accounted for in the calculations, makes a difference, but it remains a fact that emissions in places such as the UK and the US are dramatically lower than is regularly claimed, and represent a very small part of the emissions pie. Yet the cumulative effect of the arguments put forward by plant-based advocates is to condition people into thinking that swapping all animal foods for plant foods will make a significant difference in our quest to reduce emissions and fight climate change.

A 2017 study by Robin White and Mary Beth Hall concluded that the impact of eliminating all meat consumption would be very small indeed. Modelling a US food system without animals, they found that total US emissions would be reduced by just 2.6 per cent, and this at some considerable cost to nutritional adequacy.[22] Two point six per cent is not nothing, but it is not even close to the kinds of numbers that are regularly bandied around. Environmental economist Bjørn Lomborg concurs with White and Hall, asserting that 'eating carrots instead of steak means you effectively cut your emissions by about 2 per cent'. Lomborg, a vegetarian for ethical reasons, says 'there are many good reasons to eat less meat. Sadly, making a huge difference to the climate isn't one of them.'[23]

Professor Frédéric Leroy confirms that the impact on the climate of adopting a vegan diet is very small and becomes even smaller if one also factors in such contextual factors as natural carbon cycles, carbon sequestration and *actual* nutritional value. Whatever the exact number is, he says, 'it's not big. It's something, but not much, and what the data from White and Hall also suggest is that there is likely going to be a cost in terms of nutrition.'[24]

White and Hall's findings have been replicated at the level of the individual. An individual's annual carbon footprint is around 12 tonnes of CO_2 and their food footprint is estimated to be around 16 per cent of this, or 2 tonnes of CO_2 (although this number varies greatly by country).[25] The estimated reduction in emissions generated by a switch to a vegan diet is 0.8 of a tonne, representing a 6 per cent reduction in the total per-capita footprint. When you compare this to the reduction in emissions resulting from one fewer return transatlantic flight (3 to 3.2 tonnes)[26] or living car-free (between 1 and 5.3 tonnes), the benefit of switching to a plant-based diet looks relatively inconsequential, particularly when the negative impact on nutrition and health are factored in.[27] Once any unintended consequences – sometimes referred to as rebound effects[28] – are accounted for, the benefit of switching to a vegan diet looks more inconsequential still.

These hard truths about the carbon savings made possible by different individual actions makes a nonsense out of the frequently heard claim that eating a plant-based diet is 'the most important contribution every individual can make to reversing global warming'.[29] For someone who regularly flies, forgoing just one transatlantic flight that they would otherwise have taken would make a far bigger contribution. (The data in Sarah Bridle's *Food and Climate Change: Without the Hot Air* makes this abundantly clear: the emissions from a single transatlantic flight are 50 per cent more than those from an entire year's worth of food consumed by the average individual.)[30] For someone who drives a car, ditching the car or driving it less often also constitutes an important contribution. Do both of these things and you could wipe 6.9 tonnes of carbon off your total footprint.[31]

The comparison between the amount of CO2 saved by forgoing all animal foods as compared to that saved by forgoing a single flight makes a mockery of publicity stunts such as that of Richard Branson, CEO of Virgin Airlines, who declared that beef would no longer be served on Virgin flights. Let's look at the carbon costs of a serving of beef (say, 112g). Even if we take one of the higher estimates, 11 kilos of CO2 per 112g,[32] the CO2 cost of a serving of beef is utterly dwarfed by the per-person CO2 cost of the flight (1.6 tonnes, or 1,600kg, for a one-way flight). Equally specious is the concept of the Hollywood elite demonstrating their commitment to combating climate change by taking meat off the menu at the Golden Globes while travelling to the awards ceremony by private jet.

Putting emissions from meat into perspective

Equating the environmental impact of meat to that generated by air travel is problematic, and not just because the carbon cost of an individual flight so clearly outstrips that of any meat consumed on the flight. Looking at the bigger picture, it's clear that flying has a bigger impact than is captured by Environmental Protection Agency (EPA) estimates, which put emissions from aviation at 2 per cent of the total. This percentage accounts only for direct emissions of CO2 as planes travel through the atmosphere. It ignores the other greenhouse gas emissions that come in the form of nitrous gases, water vapour, soot, particles and sulphates, and (as with other forms of transport) fails to consider life-cycle elements such as the manufacture of materials for aeroplane parts, the transportation of materials and parts to factories, wear and tear on roads and runways, and many other factors.[33]

Looking at the real emissions from single flights, and from aviation as a whole, puts the emissions from animal farming into perspective. Still greater perspective is gained by looking at the emissions generated by other sectors. As previously noted, the emissions from global transportation, as currently calculated, amount to 14 per cent of the total, and could be as much as 1.5 times as much if a life-cycle calculation is used.[34] Global information and communications technology (ICT), including smart phones, also generates close to 14 per cent of all emissions.[35] A single steel factory in Flanders produces more greenhouse gasses (9 million tonnes) than all agriculture combined for that region, and almost twice as much as animal agriculture (5 million tonnes). And with a quarter of all food produced globally going to waste, whatever gains could be achieved by a global conversion to veganism are outstripped by the emissions-reduction potential of curbing food waste.[36] There are plenty of ways to view the numbers, but whichever way you choose to view them, it's clear that there are emissions culprits that we need to be looking at before and beyond animal agriculture.

The individual versus the collective

Of course, the emissions numbers look different depending on whether you are viewing them from the perspective of the individual or the collective. As currently calculated (and setting aside the enormous distortions created by applying life-cycle principles to livestock but not to aviation) collective global emissions from livestock, at 14.5 per cent, outstrip collective global emissions from aviation, estimated at 2 per cent. But looked at from the perspective of the individual, the emissions from a single transatlantic flight (1,600kg CO_2) outstrip those from, say, eating a 4oz serving of red meat twice a week for a year (1,144kg CO2), even if one uses one of the higher of the available estimates for beef. The discrepancy arises because so few people in the world fly on an annual basis (an estimated 5–10 per cent) whereas everyone in the world eats.

How are we to make sense of all these numbers and use them as a guide for action? Collectively, we could ban flying, and save 2 per cent in direct emissions (more if lifecycle emissions are accounted for). Or we could eliminate livestock and mandate a vegan diet, resulting in a similar reduction in total emissions – around 2.6 per cent if we take White and Hall's estimate for the US as a guide. We wouldn't lose the full amount of emissions now attributed to livestock because, at the risk of stating the obvious, humans still need to eat, and a large part of the emissions saved would be recreated by the production of replacement food sources. The total elimination of both of these activities would thus result in fairly negligible reductions in overall emissions. So where lies the biggest potential for reducing emissions?

Identifying the gorilla in the room

The common thread linking emissions from the aviation, transport, cement, steel and electricity industries is fossil fuels – what Dr Mitloehner calls the gorilla in the room. They account for a whopping 37 billion tonnes, or 75 per cent, of all global emissions.[37] According to analysis done by the Climate Accountability Institute, twenty fossil-fuel companies can be directly linked to more than a third of all greenhouse gas emissions in the modern era.[38] And emissions from fossil fuels are rising: they increased by 60 per cent between 1990 and 2019, while agricultural emissions rose by just 16 per cent.[39] But 'Big oil distracts from their carbon footprint by tricking you into focusing on yours,[40] writes Frank Mitloehner, who regularly calls for a more realistic appraisal of the contribution of fossil fuel use to climate change.

Among those echoing Mitloehner's view is Professor Michael Mann, co-author of *Dire Predictions: Understanding Climate Change*, who points out that meat-eating is a modest slice of the carbon emissions pie.[41] Identifying actions that individuals can take to help address climate change in *Dire Predictions*, Mann and co-author Lee Kump focus on energy usage and transportation choices. They don't even mention diet. The authors of a 2020 study also stress that although we are talking about diet and flying, we should be talking about the massive impact of fossil fuel use and, in particular, road transport.[42]

These bare facts of fossil fuel use and comparisons between the emissions generated by different sectors should make us think twice before we accuse animal agriculture of choking the earth. It's also important to recognise that the numbers being used overstate the impact of animal agriculture in the first place because they neglect to account for the carbon-storing effect of ruminants on pasture.

Ruminants on pasture: carbon culprits or carbon heroes?

Carbon sequestration – the process by which carbon is removed from the atmosphere and stored in soil – is the holy grail of climate-change mitigation. But how does sequestration work? Plants take in carbon dioxide from the air and combine it with water to form simple sugars. These sugars are transformed into a range of other compounds that are then used by plants for growth, but a significant amount are transferred to the root tips and leaked into the soil as liquid carbon and stored there, feeding soil microbes.[43] The entire process is often referred to as the 'liquid carbon pathway', and, when it's working, environments can store more carbon than they create, thus becoming what's known as carbon sinks.

Agriculture is already a significant carbon sink. An IPCC report[44] noted that the sequestration effect means that the 'net flux' of CO_2 from agriculture is approximately balanced at a global level.* The soil already holds 2,700 gigatonnes of carbon, or 80 per cent of the total held by the earth.[45] In the US, agriculture and forestry together are a greater sink than a source of GHGs.[46] In the UK, 10 million hectares of grassland (land used for grazing animals) store approximately 600 million tonnes of carbon, absorbing another 2.4 tonnes annually. This is enough to offset all the methane emissions of UK beef cattle and about half those of dairy cattle.[47] Farmer Joe Stanley has pointed out that 'this makes agriculture unique among British industry in that it can act as a sink, and not just a source, for greenhouse gases – it is part of the climate change solution'.[48]

Listening to those who are keen to see the reduction or even the elimination of animal agriculture, however, you might think that the only way to sequester carbon is to convert land currently used for grazing into forest. But the IPCC has recognised that grasslands, including those used for livestock grazing, can store as much or more carbon as some types of forest, and more carbon than either wetland or cropland.[49] And calculations of the carbon-capturing potential of rewilded and reforested land often underestimate the carbon that would be lost during the planting process, thereby overblowing the benefits.

---

* This means that most of agriculture's own emissions are reabsorbed into the soil. It does not mean that agriculture as a sink counteracts the emissions from other sectors, such as fossil fuel production and use.

Mongabay, the non-profit organisation dedicated to providing reader-supported news and inspiration from nature's front line, recently reported on the downside of the current tree planting frenzy. Planting trees can seem like the easiest way to battle climate change and the collapse of biodiversity and 'this narrative is what many are relying on', they say, highlighting the example of the trillion tree initiative from the World Economic Forum (WEF), launched in January 2021. They cite experts who say that 'many tree planting campaigns are based on flawed science: planting in grasslands and other non-forest areas, and prioritising invasive trees over native ones'.[50] And forested areas don't always trump non-forested areas such as grasslands and meadows. A study published in *Nature* in 2021 suggests that they can, in fact, be less effective at storing carbon. The researchers found that forest soils did not store any more carbon at all, whereas grasslands experienced an 8 per cent growth in soil carbon.[51]

Farmers are discovering this for themselves. UK farmer Rob Halliday, who describes himself as being 'in the very early days of a long journey', is discovering the benefits of converting an arable farm back into a mixed farm that includes livestock on grassland. He discovered that his grassland is sequestering almost twice the amount of carbon per hectare as his woodland. 'Woodland is a great resource,' he says, 'but let's see it as a part of a mosaic landscape, not some environmental panacea.'[52] Farmer James Rebanks found something similar. He hypothesised that 'in ungrazed woodland, grasses can ossify on the surface and lose photosynthetic performance', whereas when cattle are brought in to pull off old grass periodically, the soil improves rapidly.[53]

A study by the University of California, Davis, showed that the carbon-storing potential of grasslands could be particularly important in semi-arid environments, which cover about 40 per cent of the planet. In California (where decades of fire suppression, warming temperatures and drought have increased wildfire risks, turning forests from carbon sinks into carbon sources), grasslands and rangelands are more resilient carbon sinks than forests. Lead author, Pawlok Dass, explains: 'Looking ahead, our model simulations show that grasslands store more carbon than forests because they are impacted less by droughts and wildfires ... this doesn't even include the potential benefits of good land management to help boost soil health and increase carbon stocks in rangelands.'[54]

The reason grasslands are more reliable sinks is that they sequester most of their carbon underground, while forests store it mostly in woody biomass and leaves. When wildfires set trees alight, the carbon they formerly stored is released back to the atmosphere. When fire burns grasslands, on the other hand, the carbon fixed underground tends to stay in the roots and the soil.

Another study found that carbon sequestration from well-managed grazing at finishing stage might help to mitigate climate change.[55] (Finishing stage is the period during which a cow gains its final weight before slaughter.) The study looked at two different beef-finishing systems in the USA: AMP (adaptive, multi-paddock grazing) and FL (feedlot, or confined feed yard). Data showed a positive four-year sequestration for the AMP pastures in addition to a lowering of finishing emissions.

How exactly do animals on grassland work this sequestration magic? Dr Christine Jones explains that animal grazing keeps plants in a vegetative state, which means that the carbon produced by photosynthesis will stay below ground longer. Without grazing, the plant would recall carbon for use in seed production and growth. Grazing also stimulates exudate production (carbon secretion) through the roots, because a bite from an animal is like a wound that requires healing (via a process that is much like scab formation in humans). The plant uses nutrients from the soil to heal and sets about collecting these nutrients by releasing more root exudates, thus feeding more carbon-hungry microbes. This level of stress is good for plants, which otherwise tend to be lazy. Plants, much like humans, need stress – but not too much – to reach peak performance.[56]

In providing this much-needed stress for plants, managed grazing imitates what herds of herbivores do on wildlands: cluster, eat, disturb the soil, nourish the soil with urine and faeces, then move on. French biochemist and farmer André Voisin first put forward the theory in 1957 that managed grazing could generate the same benefits as wild herbivores. He realised that *how* cows grazed on grass was the main determinant of a pasture's health and productivity. Grasses should neither be overgrazed nor undergrazed. Improved grazing 'typically sequesters a few hundred pounds of carbon per acre, but in some cases as much as three tons per acre'.[57]

According to Seth Itzkan, co-founder, with Karl Thidemann, of Soil4Climate (a charitable organisation dedicated to the mitigation of climate change via improved soil health and land restoration), the sequestration possibilities could be even greater. His research has shown that up to 60 tonnes of carbon per hectare (or 24 tonnes per acre) per year may be sequestered on semi-arid grasslands and savannas, and that the total global potential for capturing soil organic carbon in grasslands is around 88–210 gigatons. This, he says, 'is enough to significantly mitigate global warming'.[58] (Soil4Climate has prepared a comprehensive list of peer-reviewed publications showing that well-managed grazing can be a means of improving rangeland ecology, building soil carbon and mitigating global warming: 'Hope Below Our Feet', available at www.soil4climate.org.)[59]

Managed grazing is one of three important agricultural practices involving animals that is proven to increase carbon sequestration rates, the other two being regenerative agriculture and silvopasture. (There's considerable overlap between the three practices, and they are sometimes referred to, collectively, as regenerative agriculture.) **Regenerative agricultural practices** restore degraded land. These practices include no tillage (no ploughing), the use of diverse cover crops, minimal use of pesticides and synthetic fertilisers, and multiple crop rotations, all of which can be augmented by managed grazing.[60] **Silvopasture** is a farming practice that integrates trees and pasture into a single system for raising livestock.[61]

The impact of these practices can be hard to measure, and will vary by farm, but results seen to date are impressive, as noted by the authors of *Drawdown: The Most Comprehensive Plan Ever Proposed to Reverse Global Warming.* Regarding regenerative agriculture, they say that 'Farms are seeing organic matter levels rise from a baseline of 1 to 2 per cent up to 5 to 8 per cent over ten or more years. Every per cent of carbon in the soil represents 8.5 tons per acre. That growth adds up to 25 to 60 tons of carbon per acre.'[62] Research suggests that silvopasture may even outpace the pure grassland technique in terms of rates of carbon sequestration, since 'silvopastoral systems sequester carbon in both the biomass above ground and the soil below'.[63] The *Drawdown* authors estimate that if silvopasture were expanded from current levels (351 million acres globally) to 554 million acres, carbon dioxide emissions could be reduced by 31.2 billion tons by 2050. (To put this into context, this equates to a 3 per cent reduction in annual global carbon emissions.)[64] Taken together, the three agricultural practices – managed grazing, regenerative farming and silvopasture – are powerful tools in the fight against climate change. Of eighty ways to alleviate climate change, they jointly rank number one as ways to sequester GHG emissions.[65]

The full potential of regenerative practices has been

demonstrated at White Oak Pastures, a diversified family farm in the south-eastern United States (characterised as an MSPR – multispecies pasture rotation – enterprise). A study led by Jason Rowntree (with analysis carried out by Quantis, a leading environmental sustainability consultancy) showed that regenerative practices applied over a twenty-year period led to dramatic improvements in carbon sequestration rates, reducing the net GHG emissions of the farm by 80 per cent.[66] This means that White Oak pasture-raised beef sequesters more carbon than it emits, leading to 1.6 kilos of CO2e sequestered for every 450 grams of beef. This compares with net emissions of 15 kilos of CO2e for the same amount of conventional US beef, and around 1.8 kilos for the same amount of the plant-based burgers, Beyond Burger and Impossible Burger.

Rowntree and colleagues acknowledge that MSPRs like White Oak Pastures require considerably greater land areas than input-intensive commodity systems, suggesting that efforts to reduce emissions may come with land-use trade-offs. However, the greater land area needed could be partially mitigated by the implementation of MSPR on marginal lands, including degraded cropland, which could free up more productive land for production of higher value and more nutrient dense crops.[67] (The land-use question – and the difference between marginal and arable land – will be considered in greater detail in Chapter 8.)

Dr Allen Williams and his colleagues at Understanding Ag have been working with farms across the US to increase the adoption of regenerative practices, achieving similar results to those achieved at White Oak Pastures. Williams estimates that if just 40–50 per cent of arable farmland and grassland acres in the US were converted to regenerative agriculture, 'the emissions issue would disappear. The agricultural component would be taken care of and we'd also be countering much of the emissions from other sources.'[68]

Globally, increasing the uptake of advanced regenerative practices has huge potential to mitigate against emissions. Diversified farms (as opposed to intensive, feedlot-style operations on the one hand, and extensive pastoralism on the other) currently supply 60 and 75 per cent of the world's meat and dairy, respectively.[69] But a small percentage of the farms supplying these products are truly regenerative operations (an estimated 5 per cent of farms in the US and the UK, for example).[70] The White Oak authors assert that expanding the use of diversified farming methods for animal production 'can lead to improved environmental outcomes and beneficial ecosystem services in addition to food production'.[71] Expanding the use of *regenerative* diversified farming practices would surely lead to even better environmental outcomes.

If Bill Gates has considered the potential benefits of regenerative agriculture, there is little evidence of it. In a chapter on food and farming in his new book, *How To Avoid A Climate Disaster*, he briefly touches on the chemical compounds that have been found to reduce methane emissions, and the possibility of introducing better veterinary practices, improved breeds and best practices, but fails to mention the regenerative agriculture methods that have the potential to reduce net farming emissions by up to 80 per cent, and indeed are already doing so on some farms. Instead, he praises plant-based meat companies (in which he is invested[72]), and waxes lyrical about the miracle of chemical fertilisers, of which he would like the developing world to use more.[73] (I'll talk about how fertiliser use has adversely impacted soil health and biodiversity in Chapter 8.)

Though Gates' book gives short shrift to the work being done by regenerative farmers, I aim to give it due respect in Chapter 10. In the meantime, I'd like to look at another aspect of the emissions story that's been distorted: the depiction of the methane problem.

Methane: the most egregious of greenhouse gases?

The data from White Oak Pastures is based on CO2e and therefore takes into account the production of methane by livestock. But most of the time, methane gets singled out as the bad boy of emissions from livestock, so it warrants closer inspection.

Methane (CH4) is one of three main greenhouse gases, the others being carbon dioxide (CO2) and nitrous oxide (N2O). Carbon dioxide is by far the biggest contributor to emissions overload, making up 81 per cent of all US emissions, for example. This compares to 10 per cent for methane and 7 per cent for nitrous oxide. (The remainder is made up of fluorinated gases.)[74]

Any discussion about livestock's contribution to methane emissions needs to be placed within an accurate picture of just how significant these emissions are. Around 737 million tonnes of methane are emitted globally every year.[75] What few people realise is that methane sinks in the atmosphere and soils *remove* almost 625 million tonnes (or 85 per cent). 'The media have mostly failed to grasp or report this message,' says Frank Mitloehner.[76]

Another fact that is rarely reported is that, although 44 per cent of livestock emissions are in the form of methane,[77] livestock isn't the only or even the biggest source of methane. Of the estimated 737 million tonnes of methane emitted globally every year[78] approximately 50 per cent comes from natural sources (including wildfires, wetlands, termites, oceans and volcanoes). Seventeen per cent comes from fossil fuel production and use, 9 per cent from landfills and waste, and 4 per cent each from rice and biomass and biofuel burning. Just 15 per cent of methane is derived from enteric fermentation and manure, i.e., cattle.[79] Moreover, it has been found that methane emissions attributable to leaks from oil and gas fields, abandoned uncapped gas wells, and landfills are likely much higher than has been reported.[80] And yet most of the hysteria around this greenhouse gas is directed at the livestock industry. The focus on methane from livestock could have perverse, unintended consequences. If rewilding plans were to involve replacing grassland (where cattle graze) with wetland (the source of at least 20 per cent of methane emissions), for example, it would exacerbate the methane problem.

A report by the UK Soil Association highlighted other possible perverse, unintended consequences of focusing too much on reducing methane from livestock:

> Advocates of a shift from red meat to grain-fed white meat to reduce methane emissions could therefore find that this has the perverse effect of exchanging methane emissions for carbon emissions from soils and the destruction of tropical habitats (to produce soya feed), as well as having a far-reaching impact on our countryside, wildlife and animal welfare.[81]

The authors of the UK FIRES report, *Absolute Zero* (published in January 2021) appear to have fallen into the trap described by the Soil Association – that of failing to factor in unintended consequences.[82] The stated reason for their call to eliminate all beef and lamb from our diets by 2050 is the fact that 'ruminants release methane as they digest grass'. The preoccupation with the methane from ruminants leads the authors down a path mined with contradictions. For example, in addition to eliminating beef and lamb from the diet, they also want to see total energy required to cook or transport food reduced by 60 per cent, and a dramatic reduction in the consumption of frozen ready meals. But they have not accounted for the fact that if you eliminate a highly nutritious (and local) whole food source like red meat from the diet, you'll likely see increased, not decreased, consumption of imported frozen processed foods (mostly of the plant-based variety), fillers like rice (itself a source of methane), and chicken (much of which is currently fed on grains grown at a cost to the rainforest).

Not all methane is created equal

While failing to connect the dots between the goal of eliminating red meat consumption and the goal of reducing processed food consumption and food miles, the UK FIRES report also neglected to recognise the difference between methane from cows and methane from industrial sources, a common failing that underlies the scapegoating of meat and livestock. Methane is a potent greenhouse gas with an estimated warming potential twenty-eight times that of CO_2. But biogenic methane (produced by living organisms), a short-lived 'flow gas' (staying in the atmosphere for around twelve years), is very different from CO_2, a 'stock gas' (meaning that it persists in the atmosphere for hundreds of thousands of years, creating a cumulative effect). Moreover, methane is derived from atmospheric carbon; it is part of the biogenic carbon cycle and eventually returns to the atmosphere as CO_2, making it recycled carbon. Methane from fossil fuels, on the other hand, acts more like CO_2 because it isn't derived from atmospheric carbon but is pulled from the earth (where it has been stored for millions of years) and is therefore new to the atmosphere. Mitloehner has described it as a 'one direction carbon highway'.[83]

The features of biogenic methane have important implications. Because methane is a flow gas with a short life span, it is always being destroyed as well as emitted. Its warming impact isn't determined by how much is being emitted (since it is destroyed relatively quickly) but by how much more or less methane is emitted over a period of time. If livestock herds are stable, the methane emitted equals the methane destroyed, and thus the warming impact is neutral.[84]

Additionally, biogenic methane is derived from atmospheric carbon. Unlike a fossil-fuel gas like CO_2, methane from sources such as cattle begins as CO_2 that's already in the atmosphere and is pulled down via the biogenic carbon cycle. This is the process through which plants absorb carbon dioxide and, via photosynthesis, harness the energy of the sun to produce carbohydrates such as cellulose (as described earlier by Christine Jones). Indigestible by humans, cellulose is a key feed ingredient for cattle and other ruminants. As they break it down, they emit methane. After 12 years, this methane is converted to carbon dioxide – the same carbon that was in the air prior to being consumed by the animal. It is recycled carbon.

The current standard for determining how greenhouse gases warm the planet, GWP100,* does a good job of representing CO_2, but it overstates the impact of methane. (GWP100 applies a multiplier of twenty-eight for methane, based on the rationale that emitting 1 kilo of methane will have twenty-eight times the warming impact of 1 kilo of CO_2 over one hundred years.)[85] Researchers from the LEAP (Livestock, Environment and People) project based at the Oxford Martin School, have proposed a new measure, denoted GWP*, which provides a more accurate

---

* GWP, or Global Warming Potential, was developed to allow comparisions of the global warming impacts of different gases. It is a measure of how much energy the emissions of 1 tonne of gas will absorb over a given period of time, relative to the emissions of 1 tonne of carbon dioxide (CO_2). The larger the GWP, the more a given gas warms the earth compared to CO_2 over that time period. The time period usually used for GWPs is 100 years. CO_2, by definition, has a GWP of 1 regardless of the time period used because it is the gas being used as the reference. (From 'Understanding Global Warming Potentials', EPA.)

indication of the impact of short-lived pollutants on global temperature.[86] (Note that the asterisk in GWP* is part of the denotation, not a link to a footnote.) This measure was featured in the IPCC special report on 'Global Warming of 1.5 Degrees'. The practical implications of this are best explained in terms of a single cow that belches out 100 kilos of methane every year.

> Under conventional GWP [GWP100] this methane would be equated with 2.8 tonnes of CO_2 per year, or a large SUV being driven 15,000km per year. But if that cow is part of a herd built up in the last century and now stable, its actual CO_2 warming-equivalent emissions calculated using GWP* are only 0.7 tonnes of CO_2 per year, equivalent to a plug-in hybrid.[87]

This means that the warming-equivalent emissions from cattle could be a quarter of the level that is implied by current carbon-equivalent metrics.[88] The LEAP scientists warn that a failure to adopt the more accurate GWP* metric 'could be putting at risk efforts to limit warming to a particular goal because it doesn't reliably account for the different impacts of long and short lived gases'. Any policy decisions which increase methane from agriculture or industry would be extremely detrimental to achieving the Paris Agreement temperature goal.[89]

The calculations underlying GWP* are very much dependent on a stable herd of cows, however. As long as herds are stable – that is, not increasing (as they are in the developed world) – methane from livestock contributes very little addition to global warming. If herds can be reduced by more than 10 per cent over thirty years, a cooling effect would be set in motion.

More advanced and efficient livestock management and

feeding systems have been proven to reduce methane per cow still further, thus inducing a cooling effect. Mitloehner reports that California's methane-reduction projects have already reduced GHGs per year by 2.2 million tons, which is approximately 25 per cent of California's inventory for dairy and livestock manure methane emissions, and equivalent to removing more than 460,000 cars from the road.[90] Experiments at Mitloehner's UC Davis have shown that feeding seaweed to cattle can reduce methane emission by 82 per cent.[91] In the UK, environment secretary George Eustace has expressed the view that developments like this could eliminate a significant proportion of methane emissions, and has asked scientists to evaluate competing technologies.[92]

The regenerative farming techniques discussed earlier represent an additional means of mitigating the climate impact of methane. They can help to restore the liquid carbon pathway that was in evidence when the world was full of wild ruminants, rebuilding soil that has been destroyed by industrial farming techniques.[93]

Thus far in this chapter we've seen how the emissions story has been distorted by misleading maths pertaining to both carbon and methane. Next, we need to understand how the story has been coloured by a reluctance to account for meat's true value as a nutrient in our diet.

What really matters – calories or nutrients?

You'll likely have heard the oft-repeated claim that red meat accounts for a huge amount of greenhouse gasses relative to the calories it provides. It's always about the calories, as if every calorie was the same and there was no such thing as nutritional value. For plant-based advocates on a mission, it's as though the concept of nutrition (including protein quality) doesn't even exist.

In his opinion piece titled 'The end of meat is here', Jonathan Safran Foer asked the question 'Don't we need animal protein?' He then quickly answered 'No', citing a single source, which turned out to be the film, *The Game Changers*.[94] (We'll take a closer look at the claims made in this film in Chapter 13.) *Guardian* environment editor, Damian Carrington, writing a piece titled 'Why you should go animal-free: 18 arguments for eating meat debunked',[95] also glossed over the protein question, saying, 'There is no lack of protein.' But he didn't provide a source for this claim or acknowledge the fact that plant proteins are incomplete and reduce the bioavailability of many vitamins and minerals. (See Chapter 2 for a refresher on this.) Carrington also dismissed concerns about vitamin B12. He did at least mention the word 'nutrition' while discussing the sodium (salt) in plant-based burgers but brushed any concerns aside, claiming that a plant-based burger 'is *most likely* to still be healthier than a meat burger when all nutritional factors are considered' (italics mine). He said nothing further about what these 'nutritional factors' might be.

In his televised attack on meat, *Apocalypse Cow*, George Monbiot's only reference to nutrition was a throwaway line about how we would all still need to eat some vegetables in a future dominated by lab-grown meat. He certainly didn't ask about amino acids, vitamins or bioavailability when marvelling about the slabs of fake flesh lying in the petri dishes.

Often, when health or nutrition is mentioned at all in the media, it's in the form of an assumptive close. This is an old sales trick whereby a salesperson forces a sale through by assuming that the buyer has already agreed to buy. Those selling the plant-based diet have perfected a clever two-handed version of this trick. When defending the health benefits of plant-based diets, they often assume that you've bought into the environmental benefits, wrapping up their argument with claims such as 'a plant-based alternative is *certain* to be less damaging to the environment'[96] (Carrington, italics mine). When proclaiming about the harm meat-eating does to the environment, they often assume that you've already bought into the health benefits of eliminating meat: 'We can live longer, healthier lives without it', wrote Safran Foer, as if this was a given. The idea of backing up environmental claims with apparently self-evident health claims, and vice versa, creates a neat, impenetrable package.

One would have expected better from Project Drawdown, with its comprehensive plan to reverse global warming based on the inputs of a coalition of researchers and scientists. (A generally superb piece of work that I applaud.) But even they seemed to take the healthfulness of a plant-based diet as a given. In a chapter titled 'The plant-rich diet', the authors claim that 'overconsumption of animal protein comes at a steep cost to human health', and that eating too much animal protein 'can lead to certain cancers, strokes, and heart disease', as well as 'increased morbidity'. This statement is not backed up by any source, likely because there isn't one, unless you count decades' worth of weak epidemiology (of the sort covered in Chapter 1) and dogma repeated ad nauseam. The Drawdown folks go on to say that 'a diet primarily of plants can easily meet the [protein] threshold', while failing to say anything about the lower quality of plant proteins or the fact that they inhibit the absorption of vitamins and minerals. They also say that 'the case for the plant-rich diet is robust' when we know (and as we saw in Chapter 2) that this is not the case. Like the salesperson deploying the assumptive close, the Drawdown authors seem to have concluded that we're already on board with their self-evident arguments about the relative health benefits of meat-inclusive versus plant-based diets. The point being overlooked is that some calories are cheaper, both economically and environmentally, but that doesn't make them good for us.

Because the greenhouse gas-to-calories ratio that is so often used to damn animal foods tells us nothing useful, some are pushing for a new way of thinking about the environmental impact of different foods. Alison Van Eenennaam, specialist in animal genomics and biotechnology at UC Davis, has urged us to stop viewing the consumption of animal products through the focused lens of the environmental crises of the urban Western world, a lens that obscures the ongoing problem of hunger and micronutrient deficiencies that still affect millions of poor people worldwide and fails to acknowledge the nutritional importance of high-quality animal protein in the diets of the rural poor, and the numerous non-nutritional benefits of livestock production in developing countries.[97]

Professor Leroy echoes Van Eenennaam's views, reminding us that the global challenge is to provide nutrient-dense foods – quality protein and foods with essential micronutrients – not just calories or carbohydrates. Leroy rightly says that an assessment of the environmental impact of plant proteins versus animal proteins would look entirely different if the metrics were based on DIAAS scores (the digestible indispensable amino acid score) for protein, as opposed to the crude measure of grams of protein.[98]

Professor Alice Stanton has also argued for a reassessment of the environmental impact of different foods based not on the emissions-to-calorie ratio but on the emissions-to-nutrients ratio.[99] At an address to the Oxford Farming Conference 2020, she highlighted a study by Drewnowski and colleagues in support of her case. The study analysed 661 foods in five major food groups (meat and meat products; milk and dairy products; frozen and processed fruit and vegetables; grains; and sweets) and demonstrated, firstly, that the GHG (greenhouse gas) cost of different foods varied dramatically depending on the choice of functional unit (kilograms or calories).[100] When foods were assessed based on GHGs per 100 grams, meat and dairy had a significantly higher GHG score than other foods. However, when foods were assessed using GHGs per calorie, processed fruits and vegetables came out worst, with higher GHG scores than both meat and dairy, and significantly higher scores than grains and sweets. Both of these analyses suggested 'that sweets, chocolate, sweet rolls, snacks and chips, and candy and cakes had the lowest carbon costs per calorie and per gram'. This is problematic, as the authors point out, because 'though sugar and sweets may have a low environmental impact, they cannot be viewed as the most sustainable foods because the FAO definition of sustainable diets makes a direct reference to population well-being and health'. The authors conclude that 'some trade-offs in balancing nutrition with the environmental impact and cost of diets may need to be made'.

Another analysis by the same authors demonstrated that when nutrient density was factored in, meat, dairy, eggs, cheese and fish delivered comparable nutrients for a given GHG cost to many commonly consumed foods. Processed vegetables, while high in nutrients, were off the scale in terms of GHGs per calorie, rendering their nutrients to GHG ratio similar to that of meat and eggs. It should be noted, also, that the GHG numbers used for meat and dairy products in this analysis will likely be overstated (because they do not use the GWP* metric or account for carbon sequestration by livestock), meaning that meat and dairy likely deliver more nutrients for a given carbon cost than many other foods.

A UK study assessing livestock production systems for the nutritional quality of their product, stressed that 'product quality' (that is, nutrient density) needs to be factored into discussions about the value of farming to society and the environmental consequences of different food systems. The researchers found that 'the relative emissions intensities associated with different [meat production] systems can be dramatically altered when the nutrient content of meat replaces the mass of meat as the functional unit'.[101] Reviewing the available research, van Vliet and colleagues concluded, similarly, that when environmental footprints are calculated to consider amino acid content and nutrient density 'the footprint of animal foods may be more similar to plant foods'.[102]

Simple substitutions of low GHG foods for high GHG foods may be counterproductive, not just in terms of nutritional impact but in terms of overall GHG reductions. A French study found that 'substituting fruit and vegetables for meat ... is not necessarily the best approach to decreasing diet-associated GHGE'. [103]

These sorts of analyses make one thing abundantly clear. Simplistic emissions-to-calories or emissions-per-kilo ratios should not be guiding decisions about which foods are best for human and planetary health. As Leroy and other researchers have asserted, 'dietary policies that aim at reducing GHG emissions but are nutritionally harmful or incomplete should be dismissed as unacceptable'.[104] We need more sophisticated metrics and more nuanced analyses. We're unlikely to get these things, however, if we continue to rely so heavily on the conclusions of a couple of much-quoted studies that are silent not just on matters of nutrition but many of the other issues discussed in this chapter. We'll take a look at these studies next.

How food systems studies make meat look bad

When *Guardian* environment editor Damian Carrington penned his lengthy article debunking all the arguments for eating meat, he opted to cite the work of six scientists. Two of these – Joseph Poore and Marco Springmann – were cited in almost every paragraph. Poore and Springmann are both from the University of Oxford, where they work alongside two of Carrington's other sources, Tara Garnett and Hannah Ritchie. Springmann and Garnett also worked together on the EAT-Lancet report. Ritchie's report for Our World in Data (OWiD) drew heavily on a study by Poore. Carrington's article thus drew on the work and views of a small group of researchers, at the centre of which sit Poore and Springmann.

Carrington isn't the only one to have relied heavily on the work of Poore and Springmann to score points against animal foods. Poore was featured in the 'Go Vegan for Lent' video produced by Million Dollar Vegan (discussed in Chapter 3). And his was the study ('Reducing foods' environmental impacts through producers and consumers') cited on the Jeremy Vine show, as we saw in the previous chapter. *The Economist* based its headline on Springmann's study, 'Multiple health and environmental impacts of foods'. Jonathan Safran Foer's claim (discussed in Chapter 6) that eating a plant-based diet is the most important contribution any individual can make to reverse global warming turned out to be based on the Poore study. George Monbiot then used Poore's work to support his claims in *Apocalypse Cow* and, as already mentioned, Hannah Ritchie and her team at OWiD used it to build a case for reducing meat consumption. Numerous scientists have cited Springmann's study as a starting point for their own work, one group asserting, for example, that 'the environmental costs of the current food system and the disproportionate contribution of animal-based food items to these costs are *by now firmly established*' (italics mine).[105] Recent reports by both the UK Health Alliance on Climate Change and the Global Panel on

Food Systems for Nutrition also relied heavily on the Poore and Springmann papers.[106]

The immortal words of Butch Cassidy and the Sundance Kid as they were being pursued by a group of unknown horsemen – 'who are those guys?' – come to mind. We must ask, who are *these* guys, and should we swallow their conclusions whole?

Joseph Poore, a researcher with the Department of Zoology in the School of Geography and the Environment, Queen's College, Oxford, was a student until 2016. Most of his citations have come since 2019, based on the aforementioned study, 'Reducing food's environmental impacts through producers and consumers', written with Thomas Nemecek.[107] This study assessed different foods according to five environmental impacts (GHG emissions, land use, soil acidification and eutrophication, and water use), consolidating data for over 38,000 farms and 1,600 types of processors, packaging types and retailers. The abstract highlighted the most striking finding, which was that 'the impacts of the lowest-impact animal products typically exceed those of vegetable substitutes, providing new evidence for the importance of dietary change'. The nature of that change (conversion to plant-based diets) is strongly implied (and stated overtly by Poore elsewhere), despite the authors' advocating an approach to change which allows producers some flexibility.

Marco Springmann, a senior researcher in population health at the Oxford Martin School, is one of the brains behind the EAT-Lancet Planetary Health Diet. His 2019 study, 'Multiple health and environmental impacts of foods', was co-authored with M. Clark, J. Hill and D. Tilman. The study, which we'll look at in more detail later, assessed fifteen foods in terms of their impact on health and the environment. The authors reported that 'of the foods associated with improved health (whole grain cereals, fruits, vegetables, legumes, nuts, olive oil and fish), all except fish have among the lowest environmental impacts', whereas 'foods associated with the largest negative environmental impacts – unprocessed and processed red meat – are consistently associated with the largest increases in disease risk'. The conclusion? 'Dietary transitions toward greater consumption of healthier foods [that is, plant foods] would generally improve environmental sustainability.'

In the space of just a couple of years, Poore and Springmann's studies have become the go-to resources for anyone who wants to argue for drastically reduced meat consumption.

Both studies have commonalities with what is an emerging multidisciplinary field known as 'food systems'. The limitations of the work in this field are summarised by Professor David Montgomery, professor of earth and space sciences and author of the book, *Dirt: The Erosion of Civilizations*: 'work in this field tends to focus on the environmental impacts of food production, with less attention to economic and social implications, or to links between farming practices, soil health and the nutritional quality of food. Many studies narrowly focus on greenhouse gas emissions from agriculture when addressing soils and sustainability, without including the many ecological benefits that healthy soils provide.'[108]

Professor Leroy offers a similar critique of many of the current wave of vegan-friendly studies that characterise the 'food systems' field, asserting that 'their manuscripts read more like roadmaps to a pre-set destination than as an impartial and critical analysis of the data' and that the metrics selected tend to tell the story they favour, while metrics that might tell a different story are omitted: 'So, they may talk about total land and water use, but not much about the *types* of land and water, and all the complexities involved. They prefer to focus on calories, not nutrients. And they rely on studies that make use of weak and confounded associations, but can never prove causation, to create these supposedly definitive models that spit out calculations as to the numbers of lives saved.'[109]

Poore and Springmann's research is prominent and, as we've seen, frequently referenced. It is also open to criticism on many of the grounds laid out by Montgomery and Leroy. Let's take a closer look.

'Reducing foods' environmental impacts through producers and consumers': a critique

Poore and Nemecek's paper, and the model on which it is based, is complex, as many papers relying on extensive modelling are. This may explain why journalists tend not to probe beneath the study's headline conclusions. But when a little probing is done, the study and the model are found to be far from perfect or conclusive.

As previously noted, Poore and Nemecek based their study on the assessment of 1,530 other studies against 11 criteria and covering 38,700 farms in 119 countries. But analytic scale may not have translated into accuracy. The study's headline conclusions stand in stark contrast with what we already know about what can be achieved by individual farms (White Oak Pastures being just one example) likely because, in aggregating such a vast array of different farm experiences and trying to make them fit into a neat model, all nuance and insight has been lost. Important details are also obscured: while the study covers five environmental impact indicators (land use, freshwater withdrawals, GHGs, soil acidification, and eutrophication), it does not consider the detrimental impact that monocropping has on soil health or fully account for the positive sequestration effect of livestock agriculture. And where is the differentiation between the use of green water (rainwater and other water contained in plants and soil) and blue water (lakes, rivers and groundwater)?

The paper also reiterates a familiar claim, which is that animal foods contribute about 57 per cent of 'different food emissions' while providing just 18 per cent of our calories. The nutrition word is stark in its absence, and there's not a whisper of a hint about the difference in quality between plant and animal proteins.

I wrote to Joseph Poore outlining my concerns and questions but received no reply. Reading other critiques of his study only served to deepen my concern about its limitations. Professor Frédéric Leroy labelled it 'reductionist'.[110] An agronomist and farmer, who goes by the name Bondevett, wrote a comprehensive online article detailing his concerns.[111] Bondevett analysed both the OWiD paper, 'Environmental impacts of food production',[112] and the Poore and Nemecek paper that the author of the OWiD paper had used as her primary source. His 28-page article is well worth a careful read, but the gist of his critique is this:

> The source paper [Poore and Nemecek's] seems to be based on a mix of actual data, assumptions and projections ... with data deficiencies and wide error margins, misinterpretations about land use, omittance of carbon sequestration and stock in grasslands, and calculations by an erroneous GHG metric (GWP100). Scaling the results up to a global level makes no sense ... since the results might already be basically skewed, scaling them up would easily increase errors and bias.[113]

Bondevett's concerns about the treatment of land and land use in the Poore model are best discussed in the next chapter. Suffice to say that he deemed the paper's conclusions as conflicting 'with both common agricultural practices and their related emissions and climate impact'.[114]

Bondevett was particularly critical of Poore and Nemecek's

use of the GWP100 metric for methane, which, he said, 'grossly overstates the warming impact of ruminants'. When methane is calculated using GWP* (as explained on page 245), the charts comparing GHGs from different foods look very different. Poore and Nemecek 'ignored all possibilities for accurate GHG accounting enabled by GWP*'.[115]

Frank Mitloehner echoes these concerns about the misuse of GWP metrics: 'Poore and Springmann have used CO2e for methane and by doing so you assume that methane behaves in the same way to CO2, but it doesn't. The other thing they do is use global numbers to depict the impact of meat and dairy, because these are much larger ... and they like to use the water footprint of beef but they are calculating rainwater as part of that footprint. That water goes into the grass, is eaten by the animals, and comes out as urine, [then goes] back into the grass. So they really distort the picture.'[116]

Richard Young of the Sustainable Food Trust has also criticised the Poore study's reductionist conclusions. He cites the observation that 'the highest impact 25 per cent of producers represent 65 per cent of the beef herds' GHG emissions'. A simplistic take on this observation would be to advocate the elimination of the '25 per cent of producers who are causing such a large part of the problem'. But this simplistic conclusion would be entirely wrong, says Young: 'This 25 per cent of producers mostly live in dryland regions, such as sub-Saharan Africa: areas which often have very poor soil and low rainfall. As such their animals grow very slowly, but it is claimed, still produce a lot of methane because they have to eat very poor quality herbage. No doubt, people living in the Global South could reduce their carbon footprint from food significantly if they gave up meat and dairy, but they would also very quickly starve.'[117] (They would starve because their land cannot be used to grow anything else. This challenge of using marginal land is something I'll discuss in detail in the next chapter.)

Young also notes that the Poore and Nemecek study underestimates the carbon-sequestering potential of grasslands. Although their model is based on grassland offsetting a maximum of 22 per cent of emissions, 'since they cite no specific UK data in their study it is not clear whether this has any relevance to the UK or whether it is simply a global average'. Young maintains that 'heavily stocked grasslands do have the potential to sequester more carbon if their management is improved, while all croplands could steadily regain carbon if they were converted to grass or to rotations including grass breaks. Since a third of soils globally are significantly degraded and another 20 per cent moderately degraded, the global potential for carbon sequestration is considerable.' There are many studies that support Young's assertion.[118]

'Multiple health and environmental impacts of foods': a case that's far from watertight

If we should be sceptical about the accuracy and universal applicability of Poore and Nemecek's model, we should also be wary of the uncritical acceptance of the conclusions of Marco Springmann's study, 'Multiple health and environmental impacts of foods'. In a press release for the study, Springmann said, 'imbalanced diets, such as diets low in fruits and vegetables, and high in red and processed meat, are responsible for the greatest health burden globally and ... for more than a quarter of greenhouse gas emissions'.[119] A chart in Springmann's paper would appear to support this statement. It compares different foods in terms of their impact on risk of death and their average environmental impact. Vegetables and nuts are in the left-hand corner of the chart (low risk of death and low impact on the environment), whereas meat sits on the right (high risk of death and high impact on the environment).

Eggs and dairy sit somewhere around the middle, worse than vegetables but not as bad as meat. But closer analysis reveals Springmann's claim about diets high in red and processed meat being 'responsible for the greatest health burden' to be far from watertight.

As in the case of Poore's work, if the assumptions underlying a model are incorrect or incomplete, the model and the conclusions drawn from it are likely to be incorrect too. And many of Springmann's assumptions are wide of the mark. For example, the study is based on an examination of linkages between and among five different diet-dependent health outcomes – type-2 diabetes, stroke, coronary heart disease, colorectal cancer and mortality – and five different environmental impacts of producing foods. But in most cases, the assumed linkages made between foods and health outcomes are crude or even incorrect, being based on epidemiological studies showing extremely small relative risks, the validity of which has been called into question: case in point, the study deems whole grains to be entirely good for health, and red meat to be entirely bad for health, despite the fact that recent meta-analyses have exonerated red meat and raised important questions about the healthfulness of grains. It also assumed vegetable oils to have 'health benefits similar to those of olive oil',[120] when much evidence (some of which we saw in Chapter 4) speaks to the inflammatory effects of omega-6-rich vegetable oils and possible associations with cancer. Moreover, the study did not assess the potential health implications of consuming more calories as a result of the substitution of a given food (say, meat) with another (say, rice), despite evidence that obesity and diabetes could be fuelled by just such a substitution.[121] And, like the Poore study, this one gave scant consideration to nutrition, and to the nutritional deficits and resultant diseases that would be caused by a wholesale swap from the authors' list of 'bad foods' to their list of 'good foods'.

The environmental outcomes considered were similarly skewed towards a favourable score for plant foods. The study included similar environmental outcomes to Poore's study. Conspicuously absent from this list is any proper consideration of soil depletion and degradation, one of the most pressing issues we face, and almost entirely caused by industrial mono-crop agriculture. Also absent is an adequate consideration of the carbon-sequestering, soil-improving characteristics of live-stock farming or an appreciation of the differences between biogenic methane and that from fossil fuels.

The nutrition question debated: Team Springmann versus their critics

After Robin White and Mary Beth Hall published their com-peting study demonstrating that a conversion to a vegan diet in the US would result in a tiny reduction in GHGs (2.6 per cent), and this achieved at the cost of significant nutritional deficien-cies, a war of words between these authors and the Springmann team ensued. Letters were exchanged about various aspects of the White–Hall study. White and Hall responded by demon-strating that even if they altered their assumptions to account for the criticisms, the reduction in GHGs was still small.

A telling comment was made by the Springmann team during these exchanges. It was said that 'nutritional ade-quacy is a poor marker for healthiness', a point to which White and Hall responded with profound disagreement.[122] If nutritional adequacy is a poor marker for healthiness, what is a better marker? Calories? Crude macronutrient content? Weak associations between food intake and disease seen in epidemiological studies? None of these markers can or should displace nutritional considerations.

Food systems models: the undisputed truth or just one point of view?

It's worth remembering that the models underlying the Poore and Springmann studies are just that – models. And, as Professor John Ioannidis has pointed out (about the limitations of scientific models in general): 'models are interesting and occasionally they are even useful, but they may also be totally wrong, especially for complex problems'.[123] Much that's useful has emerged from the Poore and Springmann models – the understanding that agricultural practices and their associated environmental impacts vary so widely around the world, and that there is much to be gained from encouraging best practices to be adopted. But, because they are imperfect and do not give adequate consideration to factors like soil health, carbon sequestration and human nutrition, we should not allow them to be positioned as providing a definitive road map to an ideal future food system. They represent just one perspective among many in the global debate about an extremely complex problem.

Livestock – not blameless, but unfairly charged

As we've seen, plant-based advocates have a host of weapons in their armoury: exaggerated GHG emissions numbers, failure to fully account for carbon sequestration, a methane metric that overestimates the methane from livestock, a downplaying of nutritional considerations, and an over-reliance on two highly reductionist studies, the influence of which is arguably disproportionate to the quality of the evidence they provide. It's no wonder that the world is hearing one message, and one message only: the only way to reverse climate change is to eliminate meat, dairy and other animal foods from our diets.

If we know that the data about livestock's imprint on the planet has been – to use Mitloehner's words – 'whipped until it confesses', that doesn't mean that livestock and livestock farming should be let off the hook entirely. There is enormous potential for methane mitigation through the widespread application of both feeding practices and regenerative farming approaches. The authors of Project Drawdown have identified CO_2 mitigation possibilities of up to 71 billion tonnes from the widespread implementation of extending managed grazing, silvopasture and other regenerative practices.[124] Researchers have documented the potential of other mitigation possibilities in addition. These include encouraging all producers to adopt the practices used by the 10 per cent most efficient, and focusing on feed strategies, veterinary care, smart use of manure and herd management.[125] Chapter 10 will focus on all that is already being done to capitalise on these mitigation possibilities.

If we must not let livestock off the hook, neither should we be making them a scapegoat. Doing so will get us nowhere in our fight against climate change. We risk sabotaging human health for the sake of negligible reductions in emissions. We also risk the destruction of our soils. The threat to soil is real, and a global vegan diet would exacerbate it. We'll dive into this in the next chapter, as we consider the accusations against livestock pertaining to land use.

8

Greedy, Thirsty Cows:
Answering the Charges About
Land and Water Use

This is how the land and water story usually goes: livestock occupy a lot of land while delivering a small number of calories, and it takes thousands of kilos of water to produce a single kilo of beef. Much land and water is also used to grow crops that are then fed to the animals. As a result of all these resources being devoured by livestock, biodiversity is being destroyed before our eyes. The answer? Get rid of the cows and feed the crops directly to people, then turn much of the free land over to forest, rewild the rest, and watch the wildflowers, bees, butterflies and insects come back.

If only it were that simple.

But of course, it isn't. Like the emissions story, the story of how livestock impacts land and water has been skewed in a way that makes livestock look bad and the plant-based diet look like the only solution to our environmental ills. The real story is complex and multi-layered, as all the best stories are. Once you've heard it, you may feel less inclined to heed the call to go plant based.

Assessing the lie of the land

About 77 per cent of all agricultural land is devoted to live-stock farming (including the land devoted to growing animal feed).[1] This high land-to-livestock ratio is said to mean that cows are much less efficient producers of calories and protein than plants.[2] An oft-cited statistic is that livestock take up almost 80 per cent of agricultural land while producing just 18 per cent of global calories.[3] George Monbiot has called the UK's farming practices the most wasteful in Europe, since 'vast tracts of land produce negligible amounts of food'.[4]

The land-to-calories ratio is as unhelpful as the emissions-to-calories ratio discussed in Chapter 7, since it says nothing about the relative delivery of *quality* protein and nutrients for any given unit of land. In fact, we get almost 32 per cent of our protein from grasslands in the UK.[5] The Food and Agriculture Organisation (FAO) estimates that livestock supply 37 per cent of the global protein supply.[6] If you account for the vastly superior quality of animal proteins, acknowledged by the FAO, the land-to-protein ratio suddenly looks quite different. Livestock might indeed take up 77 per cent of agricultural land, but if it provides almost 40 per cent of our protein, and if that protein is vastly more complete and bioavailable than the protein derived from plant sources, the land devoted to livestock begins to look like an investment, not a waste.

The authors of a 2020 report on regional land use efficiency, Ilkka Leinonen and colleagues, stress the importance of factoring the superior quality of animal proteins into the land-use equation. They warn that 'plant protein quality is distinctly different from that of animal protein', and that among the main global food crops, 'many cereal species have a relatively low concentration of the essential amino acid lysine, despite their relatively high protein content'.[7] High-protein legumes such as beans and peas are rich in lysine but contain low levels of the essential sulphur-containing amino acids (as we saw in Chapter 2). This, say the authors, 'poses a challenge when legume grains are considered as a direct replacement for animal protein'. Moreover, variable production environments around the world mean that there would be regions where plant-protein production would be restricted to low-quality or non-human-edible protein that could only be used as animal feed.[8]

While acknowledging that livestock products are a major contributor to land use, particularly in Europe and the US, an earlier report by Peters and colleagues also warns against simplistic thinking about dietary change.[9] Firstly, there's a 'wide range among individual livestock products and among different systems producing the same livestock'. As importantly, 'The quality of the land required differs as well. Modelling suggests that the largest fraction of land needs for ruminant animals are from foraging and grazing lands, which are often [on] non-arable land. Thus, reducing the most land-intensive products does not necessarily equate to freeing up land for cultivation.'[10] Because land used for livestock is very often unsuitable for growing crops, eliminating livestock would reduce the carrying capacity (the number of people who can be fed per unit of land). Modelling the impact of ten different diet scenarios, the authors found that 'the carrying capacity of the vegan diet was lower than two of the healthy omnivore diet scenarios'.

The Peters study highlights a fact rarely acknowledged by those who rail against the amount of land used by livestock: most agricultural land cannot be used for growing crops. Around two-thirds of the UK's 17.2 million hectares of agricultural land is pasture and rough grazing because it isn't capable of growing arable crops.[11] A similar percentage of the world's agricultural land cannot be used for growing crops due to unsuitable terrain, poor soil or lack of water.[12] An FAO report estimated that of the two billion hectares of grassland (as opposed to agricultural land) globally, 65 per cent cannot be converted to cropland.[13]

Understanding the UK's land

British farmer Joe Stanley paints a similar picture of much of the land in Britain, which can be farmed with no other crop but grass because the slopes are too steep, the soils too thin or the rocks too numerous:

> Broadly speaking, a line can be imagined which bisects the country from north-east to south-west: to the right of this line is the nation's breadbasket ... These are our prime arable and horticultural lands, level expanses with deep, rich soils and a pleasant, temperate climate suitable for growing crops. To the left of our imaginary line are the grasslands; rolling hills and valleys, the thinner soils of which are bountiful with lush, green grass, regularly watered by the ample rainfall blowing in from the Atlantic. It's these grasslands which are the basis of our sustainable livestock industry.[14]

It is in the grasslands of Devon that farmer Andrew Owens raises his cows, pigs, sheep and goats. Swapping his livestock for crops would be impossible because in Devon 'there is not a lot of arable land to speak of'. 'The hills are too steep for tractors, the wind is too strong, and there's too much rain. But it's an amazing place for grass. Humans can't eat that grass, but cows and sheep can. What the environmental movement is generally missing is that you do actually have to grow food, and you have to grow it in the right place. What grows in Devon is grass and cows and you can't have one without the other.'[15]

Despite these realities, land devoted to livestock is frequently deemed to be a waste of resources. This bias against land use by livestock extends to pastoral rangelands around the world. Rangelands are mostly arid or semi-arid lands, not suitable for any other use, including crop farming. Pastoralists move livestock across these lands, transforming vegetation into highly nutritious foodstuff such as meat and milk. Although these lands support the culture and livelihoods of some five-hundred million people, and account for up to 30 per cent of the world's terrestrial carbon storage, the idea that pastoralism is an inefficient form of land use, and that rangelands are wastelands, is still common among land-use planners and policy-makers.[16] And yet UNEP (the UN Environment Programme) has noted that 'pastoralism is increasingly recognised as one of the most sustainable production systems on the planet and plays a major role in safeguarding ecosystems and biodiversity in natural grasslands and rangelands'.[17]

Given that rangelands, grasslands and pasture mostly occupy land that is unsuitable for growing crops, and given that these lands play a valuable and proven role in carbon capture, it could be argued that the land-use accusations regularly lobbed at livestock are not just overblown but irrelevant. Can we say the same about the claims that meat production uses a disproportionate amount of water?

Water use: what's in a colour?

The charges against livestock pertaining to water use are many and various. According to the accusers, producing a kilo of beef takes anything from 2,500 to 110,000 kilos of water.[18]*

---

* I use both kilos and litres when referring to water use because some studies talk in terms of kilos whereas others talk in terms of litres. Conveniently, 1 kilo of water equals 1 litre of water.

Outliers aside, the most commonly cited number for the kilos of water required to provide a kilo of beef is that calculated by the Water Footprint Network (WFN): around 15,000.[19]

Even this number is a distortion of the picture (as is acknowledged by the WFN authors themselves) because it lumps all beef production around the world into one category and fails to take into account the differences between harmful and beneficial practices. One academic study found that beef requires 15,415 kilos of water, whereas another, looking at six different beef-production systems, found that it took just 221 kilos of water to produce a kilo of beef, which is comparable to the amount of water required for cereals.[20] Similar discrepancies were found for lamb (10,412 kilos versus 44 kilos). Other research has estimated water use to be around 500 kilos of water per kilo of beef if green water and feed sources are taken into account.[21]

Green and blue water

Accounting for the differences between green and blue water is critical. Green water is water from rainfall which is then stored in the soil and transpired (exhaled) by plants. The rain would fall on the land occupied by livestock (land that probably cannot be used for growing crops) regardless of whether the livestock were there or not. As such, green water is 'free' water. Blue water is sourced from surface or ground-water resources and incorporated into a product or used for irrigation. The Water Footprint Network has calculated that of the 15,000 litres of water required to produce a kilo of beef, 93 per cent is green (although there is 'huge variation around this global average').[22] In the UK, the NFU (National Farmers Union) has pointed out that of the 17,000 litres of water that are said to go into a kilo of British beef, just 0.4 per cent is blue water, whereas 84.4 per cent is green. (The rest is grey water, which is fresh water required to dilute pollution.[23]) For British lamb, more than 96 per cent of the water used is green.[24]

Analysis by Professor Frédéric Leroy shows that when water use is separated into blue and green water, beef is suddenly seen in a completely different light, requiring less blue water than nuts, and comparable amounts to fruits, vegetables and sugar.[25] Beef looks more efficient still when the amount of water used is expressed relative to protein rather than kilos. According to data provided by the NFU, beef requires 112 litres of water per gram of protein, compared to the 139 litres required to produce a gram of protein from nuts. And although beef uses six times more water than pulses per gram of protein, we know that beef protein is vastly superior in terms of amino acid content and digestibility.[26]

Of course, it's important to reduce water use, whatever the level, and farmers should be encouraged to put in place the water conservation practices that are used by the best. A study by C. Alan Rotz and colleagues notes that 'in areas where irrigation is required, efficient use of that water for crop or pasture production is critical for reducing blue water consumption'.[27] Incentivising and supporting more farms in the UK and around the world to transition to fully pasture-raised livestock systems would lead to more efficient water use by reducing the proportion of crops fed to animals. Critically, this would also halt the destruction of the rainforests to accommodate the demand for soya.

If reducing the volume of crops fed to animals is the goal, it's important to understand where we're starting from. As with claims made about land and water use, those made about the feed consumed by animals are often overblown. Some separation of fact from fiction is in order.

Grains of untruth in the grain story

Impossible Foods CEO Pat Brown has gone on record to say that 'a cow needs to eat about 30 pounds of corn and soya for every pound of beef they produce', giving meat a 30:1 feed-conversion ratio.[28] Other studies have estimated the grain required per kilo of beef at between 6 and 20 kilos.[29]

How accurately do these claims represent reality? Not very well. According to FAO estimates, livestock consume 6 billion tonnes of feed annually – including one-third of global cereal production – of which 86 per cent is made up of materials that are currently not eaten by humans.[30] Producing 1 kilo of boneless meat requires an average of 2.8 kilos of human edible feed in ruminant (cattle) systems and 3.2 kilos in monogastric systems (chickens and pigs).[31] These ratios – 2.8:1 and 3.2:1 – are a far cry from the 30:1 ratio suggested by Pat Brown.

Higher estimates, such as those put forward by Brown, may be based on feedlot beef production (though the numbers would have had to be ramped up further to reach his figures). But this method of production accounts for just 7–13 per cent of global beef output. The estimates do not apply to other forms of beef production, which produce between 87 and 93 per cent of beef.[32] Beef from non-feedlot systems is from cows that are pasture raised for at least two-thirds (and in the case of fully pasture-raised animals, 100 per cent) of their lives. While on pasture they eat grass, which, at the risk of stating the obvious, humans cannot digest.

The distinction between human edible and human inedible feed is an important one. Human-inedible materials include grass and leaves, fodder crops and crop residues such as the chaff, stems, cellulose and hulls that are left over once crops have been exploited for human consumption. As stated earlier, 86 per cent of what livestock consume globally consists of this food waste, with just over 13 per cent of livestock's total life-cycle feed being made up of grains.[33] For the average US steer, around 90 per cent of their feed over a lifetime is not human edible.[34] The NFU estimate that the average British cow's diet is 70 per cent grass, 23 per cent silage (grass cut in summer and stored) and by-products from crops, and just 5 per cent grains.[35]

FAO analysis shows that when edible protein (as opposed to edible feed) is set against the edible protein produced, the feed conversion ratios for ruminants look even better. In ruminant systems, 0.6 kilos of human-edible protein are required to produce 1 kilo of edible protein, whereas for monogastrics (pigs and chickens) the comparable number is 2 kilos. In other words, for monogastrics, protein inputs exceed protein outputs, whereas for ruminants the opposite is true. Analysis by the NFU in Britain also shows that ruminants produce more protein than they consume: for every kilo of human-edible plant protein consumed by dairy cows and beef cattle, 1.41 and 1.09 kilos of human-edible protein, respectively, is produced.[36]

Alison Van Eenennaam calls this ability of livestock to upcycle plants that are inedible for humans into high-quality protein its 'magic superpower'.[37] To take full advantage of this superpower, we need to raise more animals fully on pasture (that is, for the entirety of their lives) and reduce the percentage of cereals that are fed to livestock (currently around 30 per cent). According to Robert Barbour of the Sustainable Food Trust: 'dietary change will be an important factor in transitioning towards a more sustainable food system, and key to this will be dramatically reducing our consumption of grain-fed livestock products, with our meat and dairy thereafter coming principally from livestock fed on grass and other human-inedible feeds'.[38]

Getting more animals onto pasture – provided it's the right kind of pasture – could also influence the nutrients in meat.

A 2018 study in the UK showed that the omega-3 (EPA and DHA) content of meat from pasture systems was about nine times that of beef produced in concentrate systems.[39] And research by van Vliet, Provenza and Kronberg suggests that the nutritional benefits of grass-fed beef extend far beyond its potentially higher omega-3 content:

> Emerging data indicate that when livestock are eating a diverse array of plants on pasture, a wide variety of phytochemicals – terpenoids, phenols, carotenoids and anti-oxidants – with known anti-inflammatory, anti-carcinogenic, and cardioprotective effects are concentrated in their meat and milk. Some of these phytochemicals found in pasture-raised meat and milk are in quantities comparable to those found in plant foods.[40]

A wholesale swap from animal foods to plant foods would not likely reduce the amount of grains we grow or the amount of land devoted to growing grains. The aforementioned Leinonen study looked at land use in Scotland and found that the land requirement for pulses grown to produce a similar quality of protein to meat (with similar amino acids) 'would be similar to the land required for human-edible feeds needed in cattle production' and that 'reducing the current use of agricultural by-products in livestock feeding would considerably *increase* the land-use demand for other, potentially human edible crops'. The authors concluded that 'the potential changes in dietary protein source have, after all, rather limited effect on the overall requirement of land use for food production'.[41]

Neither will plant-based meat replacements reduce the demand for grains grown in mono crop systems. 'The problem with many plant-based burgers is that they still use conventionally produced ingredients that do nothing for improving soil health, water quality and farmer or worker livelihoods,' says Pete Huff. 'They're dressing up bad practices as a good alternative.'[42]

One way to reduce the volume of human-edible grains fed to animals would be to swap grain-fed chicken for grass-fed beef. This will be counter intuitive to most people, and in particular to those who have tried to have red meat banned from campus cafeterias but seem happy to see chicken served. We now eat five times as much chicken per person as we did in 1961, whereas consumption of beef has hardly changed.[43] Grains constitute more than 50 per cent of the diet of industrially produced chickens (and pigs) in developed countries,[44] and the biggest user of crop-based feed globally is the poultry industry.[45] (The production of cereals for monogastrics – including pigs and chickens – occupies 65 per cent of all land devoted to growing grains for livestock.[46]) As we saw earlier in this chapter, this has led to edible feed-to-meat conversion rates (and edible protein-to-protein conversion rates) that are inferior to those for beef. Grain-free chickens are hard to find whereas grass-fed and finished beef is more widely available. And if you do eat pasture-raised beef, you know that you are not contributing to the continued destruction of the rainforest for the purpose of growing soya. You can also rest assured that you are eating food from a system that enhances biodiversity.

Cows and biodiverse landscapes: an intimate relationship

There are two schools of thought about how best to protect biodiversity. Land 'sparers' insist that we need to spare land from agricultural use, and livestock production in particular, and convert it back to wild land and forest. Land sharers, on the other hand, believe that the best way to encourage biodiversity is to integrate livestock and crop farming into the land in a sensitive manner. The silvopasture techniques discussed in Chapter 7 are an example of a land-sharing strategy, as are well-managed grazing lands.

For farmer James Rebanks, the choice between 'wild' and 'farmed' is entirely false. Farmed land can be both. We can 'create something more biodiverse and healthy by thinking about how we've changed it and about how we can utilise our inevitable intrusions and power to shape it in ways that create these habitats for nature'.[47] Moreover, land sparing, or rewilding, could have unintended consequences. Rewilding comes with its own emissions, via the digestive processes of wildlife (which can be less efficient feed converters) and decomposition of plant matter.[48] And rewilding in the absence of the creation of complete ecosystems can be disastrous, says Dr Allen Williams.

> Regarding wild ruminants, we have seen disaster after disaster in many areas of North America where there are not complete ecosystems in play. Without predator pressure sufficient to keep the wild ruminants in check, they severely overgraze. In addition, with the towns, cities, roads, fences and other infrastructure in place, it makes normal migratory routes almost impossible. This means that in today's world, the wild ruminants must be managed just like livestock or they will do more damage to the environment than the livestock.[49]

Rewilding plans for Exmoor – which would see a reduction in the land available for grazing – have been criticised by farmer Joe Stanley on the grounds that they are part of a growing trend that could have the unintended consequence of leading to more beef imports from Brazil, where agriculture is fuelling deforestation.[50] In January 2022, others, including gardening expert Monty Don and Professor Chris Elliot, founder of the Institute for Food Security, issued warnings about the potential downsides of new plans to give millions to UK land-owners to plant trees and restore wetlands.[51] On a global level, there are fears that the commitment (by the attendees of the Convention on Biological Diversity) to turn 30 per cent of the earth into 'Protected Area' by 2030 will be 'the biggest land grab in human history and will reduce millions of people to landless poverty'.[52]

Research by scientists at the University of California, Berkeley, suggests that Rebanks and Stanley are right in deeming land sharing to be a more viable strategy. The research showed that 'rangelands provide an important "eco-system service" in farming by offering foraging and nesting habitat that supports populations of wild bees and other naturally occurring crop pollinators'. These habitats include 'undisturbed ground, cavities in the ground and trees, and hollow-stemmed grasses and reeds that are suitable for spe-cies of ground-nesting and stem-nesting bees respectively'. The report further notes that 'rangeland provide a diverse array of flowering forbs (herbaceous plants), shrubs, and trees that furnish successive blooms, supporting the needs of multiple bee species'.[53] Another study concluded that the cessation of grazing in historically grazed grasslands has far-ranging negative consequences for biodiversity and below-ground food webs which play a central role in ecosystem functioning.[54]

Cows on rangeland also produce dung, which plays an important role in supporting insect and bird life. A 2019 edi-torial for *British Birds* noted that 'one of the main ecological benefits derived from domestic livestock stems from their dung which, when deposited naturally on pasture, can support huge numbers of insects. These insects in turn may serve as food for birds.'[55] Each pat of cow dung can feed hundreds of insects and other organisms, and each cow leaves in its faeces enough food material in a year to support an insect population equal to a fifth of its own weight. Many bird species in Britain exploit these insects – species such as wagtails picking flies off the surface, others like jackdaws, starlings and lapwings digging into the dung pats and turning them over to expose the larvae and beetles within. But insect populations are currently at risk. A 2019 study found that over 40 per cent of insect species are threatened with extinction.[56]

If you want to better understand how cow dung and adaptive grazing work together to benefit both the land and the cows, it's worth spending an hour watching a series of short videos produced by the US-based Pasture Project, during which Dr Allen Williams explains that the ideal pasture is a diverse mix of different grasses, legumes (such as white clover and alfalfa) and forbs (plants such as horse nettle and lamb's quarters).[57] Seeing Williams walking through such waist-high forage, remarking on the sounds of abundant insect life and surrounded by contented cows, it's impossible to come to any other conclusion than that livestock on well-managed grassland is good for biodiversity. This is farming poetry.

More farming poetry can be found in the 2019 film *The Biggest Little Farm*, which tells the true story of how John and Molly Chester transformed a patch of Californian dirt into Apricot Lane Farms, a flourishing organic farm, through years of hard work and commitment to the principle of diversity – diversity of both crops and animal species. Apricot Lane Farms is proof positive of how diversity creates a thriving farm while contributing to the health of the land and wildlife on and around it.

If diverse farms such as Apricot Lane and adapted grazing

lands are good for biodiversity, there's something else that isn't: industrial monocrop farming. The post-war Green Revolution solved one problem (food supply) but created others, churning out enormous amounts of industrially farmed, calorie-dense foods such as refined wheat, sugar and vegetable fats, and leading to rising levels of consumption and obesity while doing untold damage to biodiversity. As wheat yields doubled between 1970 and today, the number of farmland birds decreased by 54 per cent.[58] The birds were just one of the species to go. According to Henry Dimbleby, architect of the new UK National Food Strategy: 'as we increased the amount of food we grew on our land, we drove out nature and increased our carbon emissions'.[59] Dimbleby would like to see a much more nuanced discussion about what food we produce and how we produce it, as well as an attempt to better 'understand the role that ruminants play in our diet, in improving soils, and in the broader farm ecosystem'.[60]

Like Dimbleby, researchers Fred Provenza, Cindi Anderson and Pablo Gregorini urge us to recognise the damage done by intensive agriculture:

> During the past century, agriculture declared fossil-fuel-based warfare on land mechanically (ploughing soil), chemically (herbicides and pesticides), and biologically (GMO technology). By separating rearing livestock from growing crops, we de-coupled bio-and geo-chemical cycling of carbon, water, nitrogen, phosphorus and sulfur, and increased emissions of methane and nitrous oxide, as well as eutrophication and contamination of water sources.[61]

Patrick Holden, founding director of the Sustainable Food Trust and a firm believer in the land-sharing approach to protecting the environment, takes the view that:

if we are to reverse the relentless decline of biodiversity and natural ecosystems ... we need to change the way we farm. We must move away from chemically-intensive and exploitative approaches and towards food production systems which quite literally work in harmony with nature, avoiding chemical inputs, producing less but higher quality food – and doing so in ways that do not compromise the capacity of nature to co-exist with food production.[62]

The authors of *Sacred Cow* have echoed Holden's view, pointing out that anything that shifts the food system further towards cereal monocrops and encourages the use of artificial inputs and soil tillage will have disastrous ramifications for plants, animals, insects, and the microbial populations in the soil.[63] This brings us to the all-important topic of soil, that extraordinary and life-giving natural resource where 95 per cent of life resides.[64]

Soil: crisis and opportunity

Soil is, says Dr Allen Williams, the foundation of everything. Healthy soil provides nutrient-dense food, sequesters carbon, protects biodiversity and soaks up heavy rain, preventing flooding while continuing to provide moisture for crops. It has also been said to be the foundation of lasting civilisation. In his book, *Dirt*, Professor David Montgomery writes that 'we can avoid the common fate of ancient societies as long as we do not repeat their grand folly of stripping off fertile topsoil at an unsustainable rate. Unfortunately, that is exactly what we are doing, only this time on a global scale.'[65]

The degradation of our soils is a genuine catastrophe in the making, and one that is largely being ignored amidst a popular discourse that is almost entirely focused on the emissions from livestock. It has been said that there are just sixty to one hundred harvests' worth of soil remaining.[66] Ethnobotanist James Wong has questioned the validity of the one hundred harvests claim, maintaining that the study on which it is based never actually used this number.[67] But regardless of the exact number of harvests that are left, experts are agreed that our soils are under threat. In 2015, the UN warned that soil was being eroded (washed or blown away) at a rate of some 24 billion tonnes every year, and degraded (losing its organic matter and structure) to such an extent that around 30 million acres of food-producing land was being turned into desert every year.[68] In the same year, the CCC (Committee on Climate Change) estimated that the UK has lost 84 per cent of its fertile topsoil since 1850, with the erosion continuing at a rate of 1–3cm a year.[69]

The destruction of the soil microbiome (the community of micro-organisms such as bacteria, fungi, archaea and protozoa that reside in the soil) has massive implications not just for biodiversity but also for water retention, flood and drought control, carbon sequestration rates and crop-nutrient density. Several studies reveal that the nutrient density of our fruit, vegetables and grains is in decline; one showing that the nutrients in forty-three fruits, vegetables and grains have fallen by between 5 and 40 per cent in the past forty years.[70] In his book, *Nourishment*, Fred Provenza explains the reasons for this decline in nutrient density. They include the widespread practice of picking produce while it's still green, but high up among them is the decline in soil health and phytochemical richness caused by the use of artificial sources of nitrogen, phosphorus and potassium.[71] Artificial nitrogen fertilisers damage not just soils but water too: when nitrogen-heavy topsoil runs out to sea via rivers it ends up in the ocean, creating dead zones such as that seen in the Gulf of Mexico.[72]

From chemicals to agro-ecology

Chemically intense industrial agriculture is bad for the soil, and, by extension, for biodiversity. Most concerning to those focusing on the decline of insect populations are the water-soluble pesticides known as neonicotinoids and fipronil, which currently account for around a third of the world insecticide market.[73] These pesticides are highly toxic to bees and other pollinators, and as little as one neonic-coated seed is enough to kill a songbird.[74] Like other pesticides, these ones poison the soil alongside the wildlife. But they don't just stay in the soil. Aided by rainwater, they flow into rivers and streams, and out to sea. The waters of North America, Japan and Canada are completely contaminated with neonicotinoids.[75]

The use of glyphosate (the health implications of which were discussed in Chapter 4) has also contributed to soil degradation and biodiversity loss. Glyphosate is the world's most used herbicide (the most well-known form of which is Roundup, produced by Monsanto, now Bayer) and is routinely sprayed on, and absorbed, by most cereal crops (including genetically modified crops) before harvest.[76] Some 18.9 billion kilos of this chemical have been sprayed across the world's fields since 1974, and use has increased fifteen-fold since genetically modified crops were introduced in 1996.[77]

Soil is also damaged by ploughing, or tilling, however, and glyphosate can help farmers to transition to no-till (no plough) systems. (Some believe tilling to be more destructive of soil health than any amount of artificial plant-protection products.) Going cold turkey on glyphosate use can therefore be challenging to farmers who want to use regenerative, no-till practices. Some are managing the transition to glyphosate-free farming by using less and less each season, and farmers can wean their farms off glyphosate successfully by first implementing a range of regenerative agricultural practices.

Freedom from glyphosate

British farmer George Young has written about both the necessity of moving towards glyphosate-free regenerative farming and the challenges involved:

> certain pesticides and artificial fertilisers are still necessary in this no-till method of farming ... As it stands, I still use glyphosate, pesticides and fertiliser on my farm. But my first field is going into organic conversion imminently, and the rest of my farm will follow suit as and when I can afford it. Farming should be as close as possible to a natural process.
>
> The excuse many farmers will make is that we need to feed the world. So I would pose the question: what does feeding the world really mean? Is it about producing nutritionally poor processed foods which are cheap, make consumers ill, prevent social mobility, increase mental health problems ... or should we be creating a diverse range of nutritional products in a way that does not cost the earth, either from a carbon or an ecological standpoint?[78]

When I visited George on his Essex farm, he took me to see his first organic field, and showed me how he was applying regenerative principles to build soil health and create an environment in which wild animals, birds and insects can flourish. George is thinking big. He talks not just about regenerative farming but also about the broader concept of agro-ecology, an approach that seeks to transform not just farming techniques but the wider food and agricultural system of which they are a part.

The FAO has specified ten elements of agro-ecology.[79] On his farm, George is taking action on every one of them, with projects that include creating a local food retail and education hub, assisting in the development of fully compostable food packaging, and helping to develop clothing materials based on natural plant fibres.

Like George, forward-thinking farmers around the world are thinking big and applying a wide range of regenerative principles to restore soil health. Within two years of applying these principles – which Dr Williams insists can work anywhere, 'no matter the climate, no matter the environment, no matter the scale' – water infiltration rates can go from 1cm per hour to 25cm or 50cm per hour. The implications for fire and flood management are enormous. Soil health also has implications for carbon sequestration rates,[80] and, as we saw earlier, the nutrient density of food. Preliminary results of studies being done by Understanding Ag, with Duke University, suggest that foods can have dramatically different nutritional profiles – sometimes as much as an 85 per cent difference – depending on the kind of soil in which they are grown.[81]

Reviving degraded soil

British farmer and author Isabella Tree is famed for having used regenerative principles to revive the soils at her family's 1,400-hectare farm in West Sussex. Prior to 2000 the land was biologically dead, 'severely degraded after decades of ploughing and chemical inputs'. Then she 'turned the farm over to extensive grazing with free-roaming herds of cows and pigs and saw the life return – fruiting fungi and orchids, subterranean networks of mycorrhizal fungi, 19 types of earthworm, 23 species of dung beetle, as well as birds and butterflies'.[82] The idea, she says, was to 'put nature in the driving seat' – to allow large herbivores rather than meddling humans to shape the landscape.[83]

US farmer Gabe Brown came to the knowledge that 'our

lives depend on soil' after many years of following soil-destroying practices on his farm. Now, driven by the goal of continuing to grow and protect soil, he follows five principles developed by nature over 'eons of time': limit soil disturbance; provide armour in the form of cover crops; strive for diversity of both plant and animal species; maintain a living root in the soil for as long as possible; and integrate livestock into your operation to drive nutrient cycling and provide a home and habitat for pollinators, predator insects, earthworms and all the microbiology that drives ecosystem function.[84] This way of farming has delivered both healthier soils and a profitable enterprise. On one of his plots, Brown has taken soil organic matter from 4 per cent to 10 per cent in just six years, an increase of 50 tonnes of carbon (stored in the soil) per acre.[85]

Brown's thinking has been influenced by others in the regenerative agriculture space. Canadian rancher Neil Dennis showed him how mob grazing – achieving high stock density on his land and moving the cattle around frequently – could improve the land as well as production and profitability. Brown also took inspiration from his study of the work of Australian soil ecologist Dr Christine Jones (whose work we discussed in Chapter 7) and that of another hero of the land-management world, Allan Savory.

Savory had studied the grazing behaviour of wild animals in his native Zimbabwe, observing that herds would be constantly moving, providing plenty of resting time to allow soils to recover. This observation was consistent with what was known about how North American soils had been formed with the help of large herds of roaming bison.[86] He developed 'an entirely new approach to livestock management using a planning process that improved the land for wildlife, livestock, and people'.[87] Much of the Savory Institute's work has taken place in the desertified environments of Africa, where lands have been transformed by properly managed livestock grazing. Conservation biologist and CEO of Conservation International, M. Sanjayan, PhD, said that Savory's method of Holistic Planned Grazing 'could be the best thing, the absolute best thing, conservation has ever discovered'.[88]

Listening to Savory's 2013 TED talk is the best 30 minutes you might spend if you want to understand why and how grazing animals need to be part of our future. Like *The Biggest Little Farm* and the Pasture Project short films, this is pure farming poetry. Like all good poetry, it inspires us to see the world differently.

See differently, ask different questions

'If you want to make small changes, change the way you do things. If you want to make major changes, change the way you see things.'[89] So said Canadian rancher Don Campbell at a holistic-management conference attended by Gabe Brown. Brown never forgot this valuable piece of advice.

Faced with today's environmental challenges, we do need to change the way we see things and the questions we are asking. We need to put an end to what Joe Stanley has called the 'facile misrepresentation of the evidence' that has led to a 'binary narrative that switching to a "plant-based diet" is necessary to avert climate change'.[90] Rather than raging about the amount of land taken up by livestock, we need to ask, how can livestock be best managed to maximise the health of this land and the ecosystem of which it is part? Rather than simply counting the litres of water used by the worst livestock systems, we should ask how we can best manage livestock so as to maximise green water use. Instead of using claims about the amount of feed required to raise livestock as an excuse to eliminate meat from the diet, we should be looking at ways to move more cows onto well-managed grazing land, and to find ways of raising more monogastric animals without grain inputs. And instead of pointing the finger at livestock for damaging biodiversity, we need to ask how we can better integrate livestock into all farming operations in a way that capitalises its symbiotic relationship with other forms of life.

In Chapter 10 we're going to meet people who have asked these questions and found the answers. But first, I want to take a brief detour to examine the claim that plant foods, by their very nature, are better for the environment than animal foods. Does eating a plants-only diet really make you green?

9

The Secret Life of Vegan Foods, and Why a Plants-only Diet Isn't Necessarily Green

'The single biggest thing you can do to reduce your carbon footprint is to eat a plant-based diet', said virtually every mainstream article on the subject of food and the environment published in recent years. The claim that a plant-based diet is intrinsically best for the environment has taken on the quality of an irrefutable fact. And when the emissions from different foods are compared, meat and dairy are invariably shown to be off the scale. Taking this information at face value, you might easily be persuaded to give up eating animal foods, or to feel extremely guilty about continuing to eat them.

Simplistic comparisons can produce nonsensical results, however, and those results threaten to lead us down a slippery slope towards some bad food choices. This was aptly demonstrated by Dr Zoë Harcombe in her analysis of a 2020 paper (published in the *BMJ*) that claimed that adherence to the Eatwell Guide could lower your environmental footprint.[1] If you were to take your cue from the paper, basing your diet on the least offending foods in terms of emissions and water use, you would end up on a diet of manufactured buns, cakes and pastries, chocolate, pasta, liqueurs, spirits and wine, bread, bananas, soya milk, salad, soft drinks, sugar and sweets.

Moreover, although the paper claimed that adherence to the Eatwell Guide would enable you to reduce your environmental footprint, it failed to consider other aspects of the environment. The growing of plants impacts not just emissions and water use, but also soil health, biodiversity and pollution levels, and many foods that we think of as being squeaky clean are the worst offenders, whereas grass-fed beef might be the greenest item in your shopping trolley.

Beef versus plant favourites: how they really stack up

If the aforementioned *BMJ* paper is to be believed, the worst thing we can do is eat beef and lamb. But when the nutritional profile of different foods is taken into account, the matter is much less clear. Let's compare beef and beans, for example, as Diana Rodgers and Robb Wolf did in their book, *Sacred Cow*. They showed that in order to obtain the same amount of complete protein (containing all essential amino acids) as in 112g of steak, you'd have to eat 336g of kidney beans and 130g (a cup) of rice.[2] The carbon cost of the serving of steak from the UK is around 3 kilos. (As we saw in Chapter 7, there are a wide variety of estimates, some lower and some higher. I've used the number for a UK steak listed in the latest edition of Mike Berners-Lee's *How Bad Are Bananas?: The Carbon Footprint of Everything.*) The beans–rice combination comes in at around 1 kilo. This makes the beans–rice combination look three times more carbon efficient than the steak.

Taking the White Oak Pastures estimate for grass-fed beef, however, the beans–rice combination looks less carbon efficient. Moreover, there are things to consider in addition to emissions. According to Rodgers and Wolf, the beans–rice combo comes in at 628 calories and 122g of carbs, whereas the beef comes in at just 181 calories and no carbs. And gram for gram, the beef delivers many more vitamins and minerals than the beans. The 112g serving of beef delivers four times the vitamin B3, three times the vitamin B6, one-and-a-half times the zinc and almost nine times the selenium as a 336g serving of beans. It also delivers vitamin B12, which beans do not contain at all. Taking a list of twenty-two important nutrients, beans deliver lower amounts than beef, on a gram per gram basis, of all but six.[3] Then you have to factor in the bioavailability issue with beans: the anti-nutrient content of beans means that many of the nutrients in both the beans and the foods eaten alongside them will not be fully absorbed.

Not only does the beans–rice combination deliver less nutritional value but its lower carbon cost must be set against a potentially higher cost in terms of soil health and biodiversity. When all these factors are taken into account, the plant-based combination looks less certain to be the winner in the competition for most environmentally friendly meal.

If beans and rice aren't all they're cracked up to be, nutritionally or environmentally, what about some other plant foods? Let's start with almonds, the most popular nut in the world, with over a million tonnes being produced every year. The average American eats almost 1 kilo of almonds annually, more than the residents of any other country.[4] Growing a single almond requires 5 litres of water,[5] so a handful (about twenty-five almonds) would require 125 litres. Compare this with the 25 litres required to produce a small serving of sustainably raised grass-fed beef (based on the estimates discussed in Chapter 8). As for almond milk, the average litre requires 158 litres of blue water, nearly twenty times as much as dairy milk.[6]

Then we need to consider how growing almonds impacts on biodiversity. In California, for example, bees are dying in record numbers due to habitat loss, exposure to pesticides and the reliance on industrial agricultural methods, and a large part of the blame is being attributed to the almond industry.

Almond growers deploy a monocrop-style of production, and almonds are doused with greater quantities of glyphosate – known to be lethal to bees – than other crops. According to the *Guardian*, 'More bees die every year in the US than all other fish and animals raised for slaughter combined.'[7]

Tree nuts in general require enormous amounts of water – Joseph Poore estimates that about 4,000 litres of water are used to produce one kilo of nuts. Avocados, too, are water guzzlers. It's estimated that growing a single avocado can take anything from 140–272 litres of water.[8] In water-stressed regions such as California, Chile, Mexico and Spain, avocado crops put enormous stress on the local environment. And avocados aren't the only thirsty fruit. Mangoes require 686 litres per kilo and plums require 305 litres. In the UK, we import 42 per cent of our vegetables and 89 per cent of our fruit, predominantly from water-stressed countries.[9]

Factory-farmed fruits and vegetables

Some of the fruits and vegetables that we import are grown in giant greenhouses jammed side by side, dominating the landscape. From the air, they resemble a tight arrangement of concrete slabs laid flat, scarcely a patch of soil or a blade of grass between them. It's a stark contrast to the image we might carry in our minds when we think of plant-based agriculture – fruits and vegetables growing in rich soil, open to the air and the sun and presided over by free-ranging birds and insects. A factory-farming operation that produces plant foods can be as much of an insult to the soil, and to the eye, as a factory-farming operation producing meat is an insult to the animals (of which more later in this chapter).

Soya

Now let's look at soya, a staple of the plant-based diet that the *Sacred Cow* authors have labelled 'a horror show to nature'.[10] Over 300 million tonnes of soya beans were grown in 2019, the vast majority of them in the US, Brazil and Argentina. Over 99 per cent of the soya grown in the US is non-organic.[11] In 2019 the New Food Economy (now called The Counter) noted that in Iowa, the second largest soya-producing state in the US, the expansion of farmland had driven a steep decline in native grasses, which in turn had depleted the quantity and variety of food sources for honey bees, causing bee colonies to decline much earlier than usual.[12] This is to say nothing about the detrimental effects of soya and other industrially produced monocrops on soil health or the greenhouse gas emissions produced by any crop grown with artificial fertilisers. (The production of synthetic fertiliser accounts for 3 per cent of all global greenhouse gas emissions.)[13]

An estimated 75 per cent of the soya grown goes into animal feed in the form of crushed bean cakes or whole beans.[14] Soya is consumed by humans in the form of foods such as tofu, edamame, soya milk, textured vegetable protein (TVP), soya lecithin (which is added to many processed foods as an emulsifier) and soybean oil. Soybean oil, which accounts for 25 per cent of global vegetable oil consumption, is a by-product of the crushing of the beans, with the crushed matter going into animal feed. This means that even though more soya (by weight) is consumed by animals than by humans, the amount that *is* consumed by humans has a direct impact on the amount of soya that must be grown. Increased consumption of soybean oil by humans – directly or via processed foods – is therefore a direct driver of deforestation and damage to soil via the use of industrial farming practices and chemical inputs. (It is very difficult to find organically grown soya.) If you choose to eat soya, in whatever form, you have to face the fact that you are contributing to environmental harm. It's also important to recognise that grass-fed animals consume very little soya, and that by far the largest proportion goes into pork and chicken feed, which makes the scapegoating of beef in this context senseless.

What about tofu, a commonly consumed soya product? A study by Dr Graham McAuliffe found that tofu could be more harmful to the planet than chicken, beef or pork. McAuliffe said 'if you look at tofu, which is processed so there is more energy going into its production, when you correct for the fact that the protein in it is not as digestible [bioavailable] compared to meat-based products, you can see that it could actually have a higher global warming potential than any of the monogastric animals'.[15] (Because the protein in tofu is limited and less digestible than that found in meat, you would have to eat far more tofu than meat to get your daily protein allowance.) In addition, much of the tofu consumed in the UK comes from Japan and the US, with the attendant transportation emissions. Ask yourself, could a plate of tofu flown in from Japan really be better for the environment than a small serving of grass-fed beef from a local farm?

Pollution is another concern. It turns out that some of the tofu made in Indonesia (in the area surrounding the village of Tropodo) involves burning a mix of paper and plastic waste, some of which is shipped from the United States. The smoke and ash produced has far-reaching and toxic consequences; for example, eggs laid by chickens living close to the tofu production sites studied were found to contain several hazardous chemicals, including dioxin, a pollutant known to cause cancer, birth defects and Parkinson's.[16] If the tofu you're eating is from Indonesia, it may not warrant being labelled a clean, green food.

Alternative meats

Great claims are made about these products; primary among them is that they have a much smaller environmental footprint than real beef. But do these claims stand up? In Chapter 7 we saw that well-raised beef has a lower carbon footprint than the Impossible Burger. And real beef, if grass fed, is also undoubtedly better for soil health. As one commentator points out:

> If we are to replace meat with plant-based alt-meat, we still need to grow those plants. Whether to make the sugar syrup used to grow mushrooms in vats or the soya and potato proteins that form the basis of the Impossible Burger ... [and] if we abolish livestock farming altogether and rewild the hillsides, we remove livestock from the farming equation. That means no manure for the fields. How are we to fertilise all the soya, pea, grain and potato crops that form the raw inputs for alt-meat? It's not at all clear that swapping industrial beef feedlots for nitrogen-fertilised plant monocultures will do much to ensure long-term soil and ocean health and biodiversity.[17]

Farmer Will Harris of White Oak Pastures has stressed the environmental harm caused in the production of one brand of alternative meat which relies on monocrop farming for its key ingredients:

> Industrial monocrop agriculture utilises tillage, and chemical fertilisers and pesticides which harm our environment in many ways: degrading the soil; killing off the life-giving

microbes; allowing top soil to erode; causing flooding; releasing greenhouse gases; leaching chemicals into our streams, rivers, and oceans; and I'm not even getting into carcinogenic impact and other unintended (and unnoticed) consequences of their use.[18]

Even Marco Springmann, the vegan environmental researcher who rarely declines an opportunity to promote the plant-based cause, has gone on record to say that the environmental claims being made by plant-based meat companies might not stand up to scrutiny. 'Beyond and Impossible need to better assess their carbon footprint,' he said. 'These companies make claims about sustainability that they do not sufficiently back up with data.'[19]

In 2021, the *New York Times* reported that serious questions about the environmental credentials of plant-based meat companies remained. 'One investor tracking firm gives Beyond Meat a zero when it comes to sustainability measures. Another rates it a "severe risk", the paper reported. The problem, say the critics interviewed, is that 'neither Beyond Meat nor Impossible Foods discloses the total amount of greenhouse gases emissions across all of its operations, supply chains or consumer waste'. (Beyond Meat said that it would release its greenhouse gas analysis in 2022; Pat Brown of Impossible Foods admitted that current accounting and reporting standards for emissions and other climate data 'doesn't reflect the total impact of a company like his'.)[20]

Plant milk

Like plant-based meat substitutes, plant-based milks are not the environmental heroes that their producers would like us to think they are. (And, as we saw in Part One, many doctors and nutritionists don't rate them as nutritional heroes either.)

Some advertisements for Oatly claimed that by drinking oat milk you could save 73 per cent in greenhouse gas emissions.[21] Seeing these advertisements – and without seeking out the more detailed explanation on the Oatly website – many people might think it possible to reduce their entire personal carbon footprint by 73 per cent just by drinking oat milk.[22] In fact, the claim seems to be based on Oatly's estimate that their milk generates 0.44 kilos of CO_2 per litre compared to 1.58 kilos for dairy milk. Therefore, yes, *if* their calculations are fully accurate (which, one could argue, they are not, since they do not account for carbon sequestration by livestock on pasture and are based on methane metrics that have been shown to be biased against animal foods – see Chapter 7), you might be able to reduce the emissions from the milk you drink by 73 per cent. Given that emissions from all the food you eat amount to 10–16 per cent of your footprint, and milk represents a fraction of that food footprint, it would be more accurate to say that drinking Oatly instead of milk could reduce your personal footprint by 1 per cent or less. But that wouldn't make for very persuasive advertising copy. As it stands, the copy is very persuasive indeed. As one group of brand commentators pointed out, Oatly have cleverly distilled their climate advantage into a nine-word claim – 'Swap to oat drink and save 73% in CO2e'. They ask us to imagine where Oatly would be right now without this simple claim.[23]

The GHGs/kilo metric used by Oatly oversimplifies what is a complex picture still further. The metric fails to account for the higher wastage level associated with the processing of plant proteins (that is, more raw material is needed to get the same amount of protein) or for the fact that plant milks are inferior in terms of protein quality (as represented by their DIAAS scores) and micronutrient content. When these factors are taken into account, dairy milk suddenly looks more sustainable than most plant milks. For example, when the carbon footprint is calculated in terms of kilo of CO2/kilo of available protein, dairy milk has a similar footprint to soya milk, a third of the footprint of almond milk and a quarter of the footprint of oat milk. When the metric used is CO2/micronutrient content, the footprint of dairy milk is similar to that of almond milk, half that of soya milk, and less than a third of that of oat milk.[24]

Another Oatly claim (made in a tweet accompanying an advertisement), that 'the dairy and meat industries emit more CO2e than all the world's cars, planes, trains, boats, go-carts, etc., combined',[25] is patently incorrect, as we know from the evidence presented in Chapter 7. *Farming UK News* reported that the Country Land and Business Association had joined 'a chorus of criticism, slamming the marketing campaign for "misusing statistics"'.[26] My guess is that few Oatly drinkers will have been aware of the criticism or been inclined to fact-check the company's claims. Oatly CEO Toni Peterson hasn't been deterred from reiterating the erroneous claim, telling *The Times Magazine*, in November 2021, that 'the impact of animal-based agriculture is higher than all transportation combined'.[27]

Palm oil

No discussion of the environmental impacts of different plant foods would be complete without the mention of palm oil. This oil, the popularity of which originally soared on the back of the campaign against saturated fats, has found its way into almost every processed or packaged food – plant-based or otherwise – on supermarket shelves. (It is estimated that palm oil is found in half of all packaged foods in the US.[28]) Just try to find a box of crackers or a packet of biscuits that doesn't list palm oil as an ingredient. It's a particularly important one for plant-based packaged foods because it's the only hard fat that's not animal based.

OWiD statistics put palm oil as the largest emitter of greenhouse gas emissions after red meats, chocolate, coffee and prawns.[29] Given that the OWiD number for beef is likely overstated (because it does not account for the effects of the biogenic methane cycle or the full effects of carbon sequestration), palm oil could be a bigger emissions offender. Then you need to factor in the nutrient density of products made with palm oil versus that of animal foods; the emissions-to-nutrients ratio of animal foods emerges as vastly superior to that of this ubiquitous oil.

Palm oil production also has devastating effects on land and biodiversity. The World Wide Fund for Nature (WWF) estimates that an area equivalent to three hundred football fields of rainforest is cleared each hour to create space for palm oil production, endangering habitat for orangutans and Sumatran tigers.[30]

There's a human impact, too. Children carry heavy loads of palm fruit, suffering injuries and heat exhaustion.[31] The problems associated with palm oil production are such that Unilever – which uses palm oil in many products such as Hellmann's mayonnaise and Ben & Jerry's ice cream – is now using a tracking system to detect mills that are sourcing from plantations on land illegally deforested or owned by companies linked to deforestation.[32]

Food waste

When thinking about how our diet impacts the environment, we must think about the food we waste as well as the food we eat. Previously, it has been estimated that we waste almost 40 per cent of the food produced, accounting for around 3.3 GT (gigatons) CO_2-eq[33] (6 per cent) of annual global emissions and 2 per cent of emissions in the US.[34] A recent report by the WWF and Tesco suggests that the problem of food waste could be even bigger than previously estimated, contributing 10 per cent of all greenhouse gases.[35] In the developing world, most wastage happens at the production stage, caused by problems such as drought and poor refrigeration technology, whereas in the developed world it occurs mainly at the consumption stage.[36] Cereals and vegetables contribute 34 per cent and 21 per cent of food waste emissions respectively, with meat contributing 21 per cent and other animal-sourced foods contributing 12 per cent.[37] Whether we eat all plants, mostly plants or an omnivore diet, we generate significant emissions via the food we waste, but the biggest source of waste is plant foods.

The how versus the cow

The fact is that *all* foods impact the environment in one way or another, and apportioning blame to individual foods on the basis of simplistic estimates as to the emissions generated or the land and water used isn't particularly helpful. If the how (the method of beef production) is more important than the cow (beef production, per se), the same principle should be applied to plant foods: the how and why of plant-food production is more important than a simplistic assessment of emissions or land and water use, or a crude 'plants are good, animal foods are bad' judgement. What impact does the food have on soil health and biodiversity? Is it grown in a sustainable way, without artificial fertilisers and pesticides that kill insects, poison and deplete the soil, and cause run-off into rivers and oceans? Does it cause pollution or harm to the workers involved in producing it? Is it transported over long distances? Does its importance to local economies or cultures justify its production and transport, or does environmental harm outweigh these considerations? Does its nutritional value justify all or any of the resources used to produce it?

For each food, the answer to these questions will be different. Scientists and policy makers aiming to guide consumers in the complex business of choosing what to eat do us a disservice if they fail to consider the full range of relevant factors that drive a given food's benefit-to-impact ratio.

Food labelling systems: can they capture this complexity?

A consumer wishing to understand the environmental impact of their food choices can call on resources like Sarah Bridle's book, *Food and Climate Change: Without the Hot Air*, and Mike Berners-Lee's aforementioned *How Bad Are Bananas?: The Carbon Footprint of Everything* to guide them. But these kinds of resources can only ever be a starting point. They tend to focus on carbon emissions at the expense of other considerations, such as a given food's contribution to soil health, carbon sequestration, biodiversity and human nutrition, all of which must be considered. Moreover, assessing a food's carbon footprint is, in the words of Dr Luca Panzone, a senior lecturer in consumer behaviour at Newcastle University's School of Natural and Environmental Sciences, 'extremely complicated'. Panzone observes that 'we aren't even close to standardisation'.[38] Berners-Lee warns that 'carbon foot-printing is a long way from being an exact process, whatever anyone ever tells you or whatever numbers you might see written on products', adding that all his numbers are 'best estimates and nothing more'.[39] (Recall Frank Mitloehner's comments about the difficulty estimating the carbon cost of beef, and how some estimates could be wrong by as much as twenty times.)

A new environmental labelling system being piloted by Foundation Earth, an independent not-for-profit organisation (and backed by some notable corporations, including

Sainsbury's, Co-Op Food, Nestlé, Greencore and Meatless Farm) will attempt to capture foods' environmental impact beyond carbon emissions. Products will be rated according to their farming, processing, packaging and transport footprints.[40] It's not clear, however, whether the carbon footprint will use GWP100 or GWP* for methane calculations, recognise the effects of the biogenic methane cycle or account for carbon sequestration. Neither is it clear whether water use calculations will account for the differences between blue and green water. And nutrition is not mentioned as a consideration. Unless a full and honest appraisal of a food's nutritional value (in terms of vitamin and mineral content as opposed to crude macronutrient content) sits alongside its environmental rating, consumers could be encouraged to make food choices that damage their health. A given bundle of plant foods may warrant an A* rating in environmental terms, while being nutritionally vacuous.

Changing the narrative

The average UK per person's food emissions are 6,027 grams CO2e per day, with the emissions generated by all the meat, fish, eggs and dairy consumed being only marginally more than those generated by the combination of sugar, sweets, chocolate, cakes, desserts, soft drinks, alcohol, rice, bread, pasta and cereal (all nutritionally vacuous foods) and food waste.[41] You have to ask, then, why the narrative has been so skewed towards an insistence that we reduce or eliminate consumption of meat and animal-sourced foods. An alternative narrative could easily have been, and could still be, 'cut down on sweets, empty carbs, junk food and food waste to save the planet'. (Some studies support this narrative absolutely, with one concluding that in some parts of the world the greatest reductions in per-capita carbon footprints would be achieved by reducing the consumption of sweets and ultra-processed foods alone,[42] and another, by an Anglo-Brazilian research team, finding that the eating of processed foods makes climate change worse[43].) Given that sweets, carbs and junk food are obesogenic and have little to no nutritional value (while animal-sourced foods in their real, whole form are nutrient rich), this would seem to make more sense. Such is the predominance of the plant-based message, however, that this alternative narrative is rarely proffered.

What about the animals?

You might now be thinking that there is surely one way in which a plant-based diet is undeniably superior to one that includes meat and other animal foods: it spares animals from suffering and death. But does it eliminate all suffering and death? In February 2020, Californian farmers John and Molly Chester (of *The Biggest Little Farm* fame) were interviewed about the philosophy and practicalities underlying the running of their farm. John said this about growing crops: 'For me to grow 214 acres' worth of stone fruit and avocados on this farm requires me to kill at least thirty-five to forty thousand gophers a year, thousands of ground squirrels, thousands of bees, thousands of butterflies, thousands of hummingbirds, those last three things completely by accident, the other two are predators or pests that I would kill intentionally.'[44]

Chester stressed that this kind of thing happens on all farms. Farming to produce plant foods involves death – a lot of it – and, as Chester says, 'if you're eating, you have blood on your hands'. In 2017, the US Department of Agriculture killed 1.3 million native animals to protect agriculture. Australian farmer Matthew Evans documents the animal deaths caused by plant-based agriculture in his 2019 book, *On Eating Meat: The Truth About its Production and the Ethics of Eating It*.[45] To grow 400 tonnes of peas on a single farm in Tasmania, for example, some 1,500 animals have to die each year: deer, possums, wallabies and ducks. Looking further afield, every year in Australia a billion mice are poisoned to protect wheat, around 40,000 ducks are killed to protect rice production, and every apple grower will kill around 120 possums to protect an orchard. Over a five-year period up to 2013, rice farmers in New South Wales killed nearly 200,000 native ducks to protect their rice crops. It has been estimated that producing wheat and other grains results in at least twenty-five times more sentient animals being killed per kilo of useable protein when compared to meat production. And it has been reported that 50 billion bees were wiped out in 2018–2019 alone, this high mortality rate attributed to pesticide exposure, disease from parasites, habitat loss and overuse of industrial farming methods.[46]

Death happens not just because farmers are forced to protect their crops, or because creatures get caught up in combine harvesters, but because we destroy habitats when we create spaces to grow food. Environmentalist and former vegan Lierre Keith reminds us that when we eat rice this is what we're eating:

> dead fish and dead birds from a dying river. It takes anywhere from 250–650 gallons of water to grow a pound of rice ... picture rice, tropically lush with green – and up to its neck in water. Where does that water come from? Now substitute 'home' for 'water'. Long-nose gar and roseate spoonbills, American alligators and piping plovers. There's death on your plate, and an entire ecosystem's worth, but it happened out past the asphalt, far, far, out, in a world we will never know.[47]

Around 80 billion land animals are slaughtered for food every year.[48] If you factor in all the small and large animals, insects and bees killed to protect crops, you very quickly arrive at comparable numbers for animal lives lost to the cultivation of plant foods. Then consider that each tablespoon of soil contains more than one million living organisms, and that a square metre of topsoil can contain a thousand different species of animals, including nematodes, springtails, enchytraeidiae (worms) and molluscs.[49] Clearly, tilling the soil to grow crops ratchets up the numbers of animal deaths from plant-based agriculture into the many trillions.

Plant-based advocates are apt to downplay the collateral damage from plant-food production. But they shouldn't. As Matthew Evans points out, 'what is it about the animals in our care that make them more important than every mouse, rat, locust or starling that will cop it if they stand in the way of vegetable production?'[50] Evans continues, 'I'm happy for all kinds of people to believe all kinds of things in life, although in my view, simple slogans such as "Meat is Murder", and viewing large, domesticated mammals as somehow intrinsically more "worthy" in the world ecosystem than insects, mice, snakes and birds, could be described as misguided, or even delusional.'[51]

Vinnie Tortorich has expressed a similar view about the vegan mindset with respect to animal death: 'Vegans look at a cow and say, "I can't eat that". So, you have to ask, but you're okay with the field mice and the rabbits and the deer dying? Because they are dying for your crops, and you don't even eat them. They don't count?'

Is the life of a cow worth more than the life of a mouse? Should we feel better about the death of a mouse than we do about the death of a cow, simply because the mouse is smaller, or because we don't witness the mouse being killed?

Or because we don't intend to kill it? In the context of the health of the broader ecosystem and a rational approach to ethics, you would have to say no to all these questions.

Diana Rodgers addresses the question of intent in her *Sacred Cow* blog: 'I have heard people say that as long as they didn't intend to kill the bunnies for their soya burger, then it's morally ok. The idea of intent is complex, but if you know that your actions will cause death as a side effect, and you do it, then you are still causing a death.'[52]

Rodgers goes on to assert that if you're looking to kill the least number of creatures, killing one cow on pasture causes less death than the number of animal lives lost by row-cropping techniques (where machinery harvests the crop), and that 'the principle of least harm may actually require the consumption of large herbivores'.

In a piece titled 'The least harm fallacy of veganism', another commentator questioned vegan claims that 'it's somehow okay that animals are maimed, injured and killed in cropland agriculture because none of those deaths were intentional': 'Let me argue this: There's nothing unintentional about a farmer going out to buy a jug of insecticide or a bunch of poison to kill a bunch of vermin animals going after his crops and his grain stores. A farmer doesn't accidentally shoot some squirrels who are finding their way into the grain bins, or pigeons who are shitting all over the place.'[53]

To eat is to cause animal death. Full stop. Simply to live is to cause animal death, as Matthew Evans explains:

Why do we suddenly think that putting up housing developments, growing copious amounts of cotton, digging up the ingredients for cement, or iron or bauxite – why do we think that having a human population that is growing exponentially and expects more leisure, greater comforts and a higher standard of living, is going to produce a world that is free from animal suffering, so long as we don't eat meat?[54]

The circle of life includes death

Few have written more eloquently about this difficult concept – that in order for humans to eat and live, animals must die – than Lierre Keith. Like most vegetarians and vegans, Keith hoped that her life would be possible without death. She writes that this 'prayer pulses in me like a heart', but that what now separates her from vegetarians and vegans isn't ethics or commitment, but information.[55] This information was gleaned, in part, from her experience of trying to grow her own food. She was determined to avoid tilling, bare soil and double digging (a process historically adopted for preparing beds for growing vegetables, which in more recent years has been found to disrupt the soil structure and the organisms and insects that live in the layers). But she was soon faced with knowledge that was difficult for her to accept: she wasn't the only one eating. The plants were hungry, too. 'Feed the soil,' the garden books urged. Was the soil actually eating? What was soil? Was it, too, alive?'[56] She would learn that the soil was indeed alive – with millions of living organisms, and that, yes, every one of them was eating. How far down did she need to dig to stop finding living creatures? Because if it was alive, she couldn't kill it. Here was the beginning of a realisation that her life might require death:

> I had bet my whole moral system – and built my whole identity – on the idea that my life did not require death. The more I learned, the more questions I had to ignore if I wanted to save this ethical directive that claimed to be about facing the truth. Did the lives of nematodes and fungi matter? Why not? Because they were too small for me to

see? Because they were on the other side of an intellectual Maginot line of us/them? But I was supposed to be one of the brave ones who refused to draw that line, who didn't put humans above animals in a hierarchy, who reverenced the natural world and all capital-H Her creatures.[57]

Keith describes how this new information flickered, signalling a dark forest that she refused to enter. She turned, instead, to information that had always comforted her as a vegan – information about the pounds of grain or the gallons of water consumed by cows, or the hungry bellies that would be fed if the world stopped eating meat. But she couldn't escape the fact that 'the soil wasn't a thing, it was a million things, and they were alive ... they broke down dead matter from plants, animals, fungi, bacteria and made the constituent elements available for more life'.[58]

The first commandment of organic farming was 'feed the soil, not the plant'. She had to feed the soil because it was alive. How was she to do this? She needed nitrogen, and no nitrogen-fixing plant could make up for all the nutrients she was taking out. She couldn't use synthetic fertiliser, created from fossil fuels, because it would eventually destroy the soil. She realised, reluctantly, that 'the soil wanted manure. Worse, it wanted the inconceivable: blood and bones ... My garden wanted to eat animals, even if I didn't.'[59]

Keith eventually found some solace in a book called *The Apple Grower* by Michael Phillips, which recounts the story of an apple tree near the graves of Roger Williams, the founder of Rhode Island, and his wife. The roots of the tree were found to have grown into the graves, and the graves were later found to have been emptied of every particle of human dust. The story eased Keith's mind because the tree ate the humans. Humans were therefore not sitting at the top of the hierarchy of creatures but were a part of the cycle of life and death:

We're not at the end because it's not a line. It's a circle, and if it ends anywhere it's with the degraders feeding the producers ... Our animal bones, our human blood: we belong here too, if we're willing to accept our place. We are eaten as well as eaters; raw material for an endless feast. That would have been the solace: a place at the table. We aren't above, just one among many beings embraced by carbon that one day will let go. I had to accept death before I could take my place.[60]

Acceptance of the fact that we, as humans, do not sit apart from nature but are part of it, eaten as well as eaters, dead as well as perpetrating death, is not readily or comfortably attained. It's easy to forget, as we fly around the world on jets, manage our lives with smart phones, and allow technology to seep into every last corner of our existence, that we are, at the heart of it, just animals. Animals with big brains and sophisticated rational and sensory capabilities, but animals nonetheless. As animals with a particular physiology, we – like Keith's garden – require certain nutrients to survive and thrive. Many of those come from other animals. Zoologist Colin Tudge expressed this idea beautifully in his 2004 book, *So Shall We Reap*:

we don't as a matter of habit think of ourselves in the raw biological form – as animals ... we like to think we are above mere flesh, and that with our rational minds and our technologies we can do whatever we want ... but whatever else we may be, whatever our aspirations and pretentions, in the end we are animals, and big and voracious animals at that; the greatest mistake humanity has made these past few thousand years is to forget this most elementary fact.[61]

For Tudge, when answering the great questions we face – and in particular the question of what we should eat and how it should be produced – we need to think biologically. 'Ignore the beating drum of biology and we and our fellow creatures haven't a prayer.'[62] Fred Provenza also reminds us that biology connects us with other living creatures and the plants and creatures that they in turn eat. He describes the universe as 'a restaurant that consumes itself', life feeding on life. The fact that we might be uncomfortable with this notion doesn't make it any less true.

Another inconvenient truth

Al Gore's 2013 film, *An Inconvenient Truth*, attempted to raise public awareness of the dangers of global warming. For those who are committed to eating a plants-only diet, the truth about our relationship with the animal world, and about how plants come to our table, may be even more inconvenient, and uncomfortable to confront, than the facts about global warming. A kind of cognitive dissonance can set in, as it did among vegans responding to the recent film, *Kiss the Ground*. The film makes the case for building soil health, and for the power of regenerative farming to restore degraded lands and facilitate carbon drawdown. It acknowledges the role of live-stock in this regenerative process, and it features interviews with prominent regenerative farmers such as Gabe Brown. Cows are definitely part of the picture. Yet a positive review of the film on a vegan website called totallyveganbuzz.com is followed by an invitation to watch Billie Eilish and Woody Harrelson talk about how 'everyone should go vegan to save the climate'.[63] Another website, plantbasednews.org, adver-tised the fact that vegan activist Harrelson had narrated the documentary and that it had featured a 'revolutionary group of activists, scientists, farmers and politicians', but neglected to mention that many of those farmers were cattle ranchers, and that cows are essential to the solution.[64]

Brian Sanders, host of the Peak Human health, fitness and nutrition podcast, and producer of the forthcoming film, *Food Lies*, commented on the cognitive dissonance that seemed to lie at the very heart of the film: 'They know soil health is important, but they can't let go of the idea that plant-based is best. So, they are trying to hold these two ideas in their heads at the same time – plants are best, and we shouldn't eat animals, but also, we need the animals to feed the soil to grow the plants.'[65]

The same kind of cognitive dissonance underlies a book by Christina Figueres, former UN executive secretary for climate change, and Tom Rivett-Carnac, *The Future We Choose*. Figueres has gone on record as saying that meat eaters should be treated like smokers, and her book paints a vision of the future in which animal protein and dairy products 'have practically disappeared from our diets'.[66] But she also talks about the need to revolutionise industrialised farming and transition to regenerative farming practices that include sustainable grazing.[67] Therefore, on the one hand she wants to get rid of livestock, but on the other she wants to use livestock to restore the soil and the landscape.

Plant-based advocates have a hard time accepting that animals, and animal death, are integral to the way we feed ourselves, whether we eat meat or plants or both, but we need to learn to accept our own and animals' place in the circle of life and death – or as Molly Chester puts it, 'learn to be more attached to grief'.[68] This acceptance does not absolve us of responsibility for the animals on which we depend or give us carte blanche to treat them any way that suits us. Instead, it demands that we put respect and compassion at the heart of food production. That we make sure the 'how' does justice, not just to the cows, but to all the animals that end up in our care and on our tables. As Tudge says, 'animal welfare matters, in short; and should be built into the grand strategy'.[69]

Factory farming: the worst-kept secret within our food system

We owe a debt to organisations such as Compassion in World Farming (CIWF), the Royal Society for the Prevention of Cruelty to Animals (RSPCA), and vegan activists who were motivated to give up animal foods because of concerns about animal welfare. Without their activism, we, as consumers, might never have learned about the cruelty inflicted on animals kept in intensive-farming environments, and we might not have known to demand organic eggs and chickens or pasture-raised beef. John Chester says that he'd be 'right there with any vegan marching against an industrial CAFO [Confined Animal Feeding Operation]'.[70]

Those involved in intensive farming operations are reluctant to let us see what goes on inside those overcrowded feedlots, pig pens or chicken sheds. Despite his many attempts to gain access to these sorts of farms in Australia, Matthew Evans – the farmer we met earlier in this chapter – saw very few. He describes what he did manage to see with unflinching honesty. If you want to educate yourself as to what intensive farming looks, sounds and smells like, what it really takes to get that cheap meat to your plate, his book, *On Eating Meat*, is essential reading. For now, I'll give you his first impressions of an intensive-farming operation. Evans doesn't specify whether he's talking about a cattle feedlot, a pig farm or one of the chicken factories he describes later, where thousands of birds are kept in cramped quarters, snatched in the night and stuffed into crates that are loaded onto conveyor belts to pass through gas chambers before being clipped to a conveyor belt swinging past rotating knives. For him, all intensive operations are the same – they simply stink:

> I smell ammonia. Something that hits you high and hard in the nostrils and causes an almost involuntary gag ... It's the smell of intensive animal confinement, one that can lead to ammonia levels in pig sheds to be over four times the recommended 25 parts per million set by Safe Work Australia ... The saying, 'Smells like Money', is the difference between the owners of these farms and me. I smell toxins. They smell profit.[71]

The stench of intensive animal farms signifies everything that's wrong with them – the way the animals are managed, the substances that they are fed, the hormones and other drugs used to stimulate growth, the polluting practices, wasted resources, long-distance transport of live animals and slaughter practices.[72] Most importantly, these farms are places where animals cannot display their natural instincts to root, graze, move or play. They lead terrible lives. By raising animals in this way we are in breach of what food writer Michael Pollan has called the unspoken 'bargain' between domesticated animals and humanity: humans 'agreed' to provide essentials to animals – food, shelter and protection from predators – in exchange for the animals providing human foods in the form of eggs, milk and meat. As Nicolette Hahn Niman points out, torture was never supposed to be part of the deal, and 'by raising animals in factory farms, humans are violating their age-old contract with domesticated animals'.[73]

Our 'contract' with pigs and chickens has been breached more than any other. 'Pigs have the worst life of all; most live a life of total horror,' says farmer Andrew Owens, 'whereas most sheep, and most cows in this country, have a content existence.' Many chickens, too, live a life of horror. The rising demand for cheap chicken has driven the rise in intensive chicken farming, and an estimated 70 per cent of chickens raised for meat globally are now raised in intensive-farming systems.[74] Chickens raised in these conditions are arguably worse off than any cow raised either in a CAFO or on pasture.

Renowned animal behaviour and welfare expert Temple Grandin has found some of the worst examples of animal cruelty at poultry farms. Grandin, professor of animal science at Colorado State University and a consultant on animal welfare to farmers and corporations within the beef and fast-food industries, credits her autism for her ability to see, hear, feel and think like the animals she helps. She has spent most of her life trying to improve the welfare of domesticated farm animals, one of her claims to fame being a squeeze chute (a narrow corridor with sides that restrain the animal, enclosing them for treatments or procedures) that enables cows to feel calm when being vaccinated. Today, half the cattle in the United States and Canada are handled in systems that she has designed for meat packing plants, systems that ensure the animals are treated calmly and with respect. She has witnessed how well-managed farming operations benefit the animals: 'The animals were happy and healthy. They can live better lives on the ranch than most animals live in the wild. And I'd rather die in a good slaughterhouse than be eaten alive by a coyote or a lion.'[75]

Nicolette Hahn Niman and her husband, Bill Niman, have strived to implement Grandin's principles on their ranch, and Hahn Niman has laid out her own prescriptions for a more humane animal farming system. She advocates eight specific improvements, including better grazing management, an end to feeding cattle drugs, hormones and other junk, an end to young calves being placed in feedlots and slaughtered, an end to long-distance transport, and improved slaughter practices.[76]

End-of-life care

Slaughter isn't something that most of us like to think about. But slaughter practices are key to the welfare of both the animals and the humans who do the work of killing on our behalf. Smaller and more local is better. The difference between the welfare at an organic operation such as Daylesford's in Gloucestershire, which has a maximum capacity of 10,000 chickens per week, compared to a huge processor that kills up to 10,000 chickens an hour, is hugely significant.[77] Slaughter is less concentrated in the UK than it is in the US, and less reliant on large operators, but small, local slaughterhouses are fast disappearing.[78] The Sustainable Food Trust reports that in England, for example, small, local abattoirs are 'at a critical point and in danger of collapse', with their number having fallen from 1,700 in the 1970s to just 63 in 2018. The Trust have campaigned, with some success, for improved support for small abattoirs. But policy makers must ensure that greater and continued support is forthcoming. We, as consumers, can help too, by buying our meat from suppliers such as Daylesford and others who uphold high standards of animal welfare.

Better abattoirs and other practices like those laid out by Hahn Niman would undoubtedly improve animal welfare, enabling us to fulfil our unspoken contract with farm animals. But there would be a price to pay, and meat-eating consumers would have to pay it. Evans calculates that the cost of pork from pigs raised the way he raises them is twice or three times as expensive as pork from intensive farms. Grass-fed and finished beef is more expensive than standard feedlot beef. The same is true of chicken. Here in the UK, top-quality organic, free-range chickens can be four times the price of intensively reared ones.[79] But, says Evans, 'You do, really, get what you pay for – but what's also worth remembering is that the chicken gets what you pay for too.'[80] Richard Smith, farm manager for Daylesford Farm, agrees. 'Yes, there's a price difference, but everybody wins – the animal, the farmer, the customer and the environment.'[81]

If we manage to make a wholesale shift from intensive farming to regenerative, pasture-based operations, the cost of our meat will likely increase, and some kinds of meat will be in shorter supply.[82] For most of us in the big meat-consuming nations that will likely mean that we eat less meat. Meatless Mondays, or smaller portions of meat at each meal, will be driven, not by the notion that meat is intrinsically bad for health and bad for the environment, but by our commitment to eating food that has been produced in a humane and sustainable way.

As we make that commitment, we shift the debate. Instead of being centred on the question of which foods cause the least harm according to a narrow set of criteria, it becomes a debate about which foods do the most good according to a broad set of criteria. Those criteria include the minimisation of emissions, yes, but also the practical and efficient use of land and water, soil health, biodiversity enhancement, animal welfare, local availability, cultural and gastronomic traditions, and human nutrition. This is a good deal more complicated than deeming all plant foods to be superior to animal foods on the basis of a few statistics about emissions.

10

The Future of Food: Lab Coats and Factories or Regenerative Agriculture?

The food future depicted in *Apocalypse Cow* (George Monbiot's film for Channel 4) looks like this: animal agriculture will have been eliminated and most grazing land will have been rewilded or converted to forest; both our flour and protein will be manufactured in labs using hydrogen pathway technology; these factories will be located in a few selected hot, dry areas where they can be powered by solar panels, and their products will be shipped around the world; as for fruits and vegetables, these will be grown on organic farms that somehow manage to thrive without the application of either manure (since there won't be any) or chemical fertilisers.[1]

If you like the sound of this future you can join those who are pushing for the kinds of policies that will hasten our journey towards it – policies that encourage the uptake of plant-based diets in schools and other institutions, impose taxes on meat consumption, lend support to start-ups involved in the race to develop affordable lab-grown meat, and bring to life the UN's New Deal for Nature. You might find that you'll be promoting a future that's more about technology and industry than nature, however.

Or maybe you prefer the vision of the future provided by John and Molly Chester, the founders of Apricot Lane Farm and the creators of *The Biggest Little Farm*[2] referenced previously. In 2011, the Chesters took a large patch of dry, useless soil in California and turned it into an organic, regenerative farm that produces more than 100 different crops and animal foods. Like other farms of its type, Apricot Lane is a carbon sink (explained on pages 233–4). Diversity is the key to its success. The more varieties of plants and animal foods you produce in one place, the more you are able to replicate a naturally self-contained and self-perpetuating ecosystem. The natural cycle of life and death generates efficiencies that outstrip any large-scale industrial type of operation: the ducks eat the snails that plague the plum trees; the coyotes ravage the gophers that attack the avocado trees. Yes, the coyotes kill some chickens, too, but then the farm dogs do a pretty good job of protecting the chickens most of the time.

This kind of farming is hard work. (It took the Chesters eight years to turn that patch of dry soil into the thing of beauty it is today.) But there are many who think that this represents the best way of farming in the future – one that combines respect and reverence for animals with a system that acts to restore soil health and draw carbon down from the atmosphere.

In this chapter I'll examine these two competing visions of food production in some detail, starting with the vision presented in *Apocalypse Cow*, not because it's more credible but because, I confess, I don't want to end with it. I'd rather end this section of the book on a high, talking about a system that works in harmony with nature rather than about one that actively repudiates it.

Apocalypse Cow: a dystopian vision of our food future

Apocalypse Cow was roundly criticised. I was among the critics, writing an article for the Real Food Campaign in which I detailed the many errors of fact and distortions of logic underlying the programme. These included an exaggeration of the carbon cost of meat, a failure to consider the carbon sequestration potential of livestock agriculture, a distortion of the facts pertaining to land use relative to protein delivery, a failure to consider the nutritional implications of the proposals being made, and a whitewashing of the challenges we would face in trying to produce organic fruit and vegetables without the organic matter from livestock.[3]

Independent journalist Cory Morningstar (who, like George Monbiot, eats no meat, fish or dairy) scripted an extensive rebuttal to Monbiot's claims via a series of tweets. Morningstar criticised Monbiot's obsession with efficiency, an obsession that led him to favour industrial farms over farms where livestock range free and live quality lives, simply because they take up less land. He also warned that lab-produced flour (produced using hydrogen-pathway technology) is a 'dangerous concept'. Valuing the science of hydrogen over nature's process of photosynthesis only serves to feed what is already a broken relationship with nature. Furthermore, 'this path would deepen our dependence on the global industrial capitalist system that is killing our natural world'.[4]

Monbiot is not the first or the only person to hail the advent of artificial and lab-produced food. Colin Tudge reminds us that scientists were talking about the need for 'textured vegetable proteins', and meat spun from bacteria raised on oil, back in the 1970s.[5] And today, the organisation RethinkX is campaigning for an even more radical and dystopian food future than that presented in *Apocalypse Cow*. The organisation predicts that by 2030 demand for cow products will have fallen by 70 per cent, the US cattle industry will be effectively bankrupt, and the 'current industrialised, animal-agriculture system will be replaced with a food-as-software model, where foods are engineered by scientists at a molecular level and uploaded to databases that can be accessed by food designers anywhere in the world'.[6]

Wow! All this is the space of ten years. This scenario seems to me to be as unlikely as it is repugnant. Even more unlikely is the utopia that RethinkX believes would ensue: a distributed system based on abundant resources as opposed to a centralised system dependent on scarce resources. I'm not convinced that concentrating power and resources in the hands of a few large companies using patented technologies to design and produce our food will result in the right amount of food being made available to the right people at the right price at all times. Or that it will, in the process, free up billions of hectares of land for rewilding – as opposed to, say, massive land grabs by property developers and industrialists.

The new meat technologies

Others might not share RethinkX's certainty that the current food system will be completely overturned by 2030, but they are betting on a different food future and on new meat technologies. Richard Branson and Bill Gates are two of the high-profile names who have invested in cell-cultured meat companies, alongside dozens of venture capital firms. Gates' motive seems to be one of providing global food security; he doesn't believe that it will be possible to provide enough real meat to feed the world.[7] Disappointingly, for a man famed for reading extensively on the issues that interest him, his public pronouncements, highlighting the land and water needed to raise meat, reflect none of the nuances and mitigating factors covered in earlier chapters.[8]

The cell-cultured meat industry now comprises some thirty start-ups, including JUST and Memphis Meats in the US and Aleph Farms in Israel. Since 2015, venture capitalists and existing food giants have invested more than 100 million dollars in these start-ups.[9] The costs of producing the product, while still well beyond that of real meat, have fallen dramatically. In 2013, cell-cultured meat was going for 1.2 million dollars per pound, but by 2019 JUST's cell-cultured chicken nuggets were down to 50 dollars per nugget, and Israel-based Future Meat Technologies said it was on track to have cell-cultured meat on the market in 2022 for about 10 dollars per pound.[10]

The fascinating story of how this happened is told by Chase Purdy in his book, *Billion Dollar Burger*.[11] Purdy does an excellent job of documenting the trials, tribulations and dramas that have engulfed the main players in the cell-cultured meat market. To a certain extent, he also manages to remove the 'yuck factor' from the topic. After reading his book, I definitely viewed cell-cultured meat as less creepy than I did initially. There's a great scene in which Purdy takes his mother – a trained nutritionist and a big believer in locally grown, organic food – to a taste test at JUST's laboratories. She finds the various meats completely delicious and ends up trying to reassure JUST's people that consumers will eventually come around to the idea of eating their products, in just the same way that they warmed to the idea of plant-based meats substitutes such as the Impossible Burger.

Purdy's mother's enthusiasm aside, the cell-cultured meat industry faces some big challenges, the navigation of the regulatory process being primary among them. Important questions about the product also remain outstanding. We know, for example, that a living animal moves around as it grazes, and that this affects the quality of the protein.

We don't know whether cell-cultured meat can replicate the effects of that movement.[12] And, says Purdy, 'while cell-cultured meat manufacturers market their product as "cleaner" and as having an identical nutritional profile to the meat it mimics, for all of 2018 and 2019 it was impossible for the beef industry or consumers to know if this was true. We take the cell-cultured meat start-ups at their word.'[13]

Will faux meat be our future?

Might cell-cultured meat be the new margarine, a product once marketed as better for health than butter, and later found to be detrimental to health? We don't yet know. Neither do we know whether cell-cultured meat actually consumes dramatically fewer resources than real meat, says Purdy, highlighting the work of researcher Hannah Tuomisto. The lead author of a much-cited 2011 Oxford University study on cultured meat sustainability, she later found that total energy consumption by cell-culturing meat would be about four times higher than previously shown in the 2011 study.[14] As for land use, this would undoubtedly be lower for cell-cultured meat than it is for real meat. But given what we know about the land used for livestock (most of which is unsuitable for growing crops), would freeing up that land really create the benefits that cell-cultured meat firms claim? Can we be assured that any land freed up would be rewilded, or might it fall into the hands of industrialists who would put it to uses far more detrimental to the environment than the raising of livestock? And what about the foetal bovine serum (blood drawn from the foetus of a cow), which has been used to feed the stem cells? This is expensive and implicates the cultured meat manufacturers in the kind of exploitation of animals that they profess to deplore. Companies such as JUST have searched for an alternative to material from actual cows, but these plant-based mediums aren't yet perfect, and might not prove viable.[15]

A more fundamental concern was expressed by Alice Waters, head chef at the Chez Panisse restaurant in California and a leader of the slow food movement: 'It just frightens me that scientists believe they know more about it than Mother Nature does,' she said to Purdy. 'I really think of my food as deeply connected to nature. It has to do with seasonality, it has to do with a complexity of the soil that grows the vegetables that the animals eat. I think that's what nourishes us.'[16]

Pete Huff, project director at The Pasture Project, expressed a similar concern to me: 'A lot of it comes down to the human struggle with humility – appreciating just how limited is our knowledge around soil and ecosystems and the profound relationships that bring nutrients from soil and give them to us in a form that we can digest and be healthy.[17]

Huff is also concerned about the prospect of a small number of companies controlling the intellectual property behind lab-based foods, whether they be made from cultured meats or plant-based meat substitutes, particularly in a world in which communities have already lost so much control over their food. The cultured meat solution is also an inadequate response to climate change, as farmer George Young pointed out. 'Technology from Silicon Valley isn't a fix for climate change. There are natural systems that we've broken and we need to repair.'[18] That Silicon Valley cannot provide the answer to our environmental problems is abundantly clear to researchers Provenza, Anderson and Gregorini, who despair of those who are 'in the midst of convincing themselves that plant-based faux meat is better than the real thing and that nature is a feeble-minded nitwit compared to the "time-tested wisdom" of Silicon Valley technologies'.[19]

Purdy concludes that cell-cultured meat is definitely coming, whether we like it or not. But will cell-cultured meat end up replacing real meat, bringing RethinkX's vision to fruition? That is less certain. Meat is not purely a commodity, as Purdy points out. It has a value that it 'possesses by virtue of its history and place in human culture'.[20] Moreover, there are people with a competing vision of how we might feed the world and save the planet. These are the proponents of regenerative agriculture.

Regenerative farmers: saving the planet one cow at a time

We glimpsed the power of regenerative agriculture in earlier chapters, but what does it mean at a practical level? Understanding Ag, the agricultural consultancy organisation founded by Gabe Brown, Allen Williams, Ray Archuleta and Shane New, deals with the practicalities on a daily basis as it seeks to improve human, animal and soil health simultaneously, starting with the soil. The group uses a model based on six principles of soil health and three rules of adaptive stewardship to explain the practicalities to the farmers with whom it partners. The six principles are: knowing your context; not disturbing the soil; building surface armour with cover crops; mixing it up; keeping living roots in the soil; and growing healthy animals and soil together. (You'll recognise these principles from an earlier chapter, as the methods Gabe Brown learned to apply on his own farm.) The three mutually reinforcing rules of adaptive stewardship are: recognising that everything on the farm produces compounding and cascading effects; striving for diversity at all levels, from the plants to the soil to the animals; and introducing periodic planned disruption to keep things moving forward.[21]

Frank Mitloehner uses a different but complementary approach that he calls 'good farm stewardship', and the

Savory model is called 'holistic farm management'.[22] Whatever the model, well-managed livestock is an essential element. Research by the Rodale Institute has shown that farmers and ranchers who have the highest soil carbon levels are, without exception, applying some form of managed grazing – whether they call it multi-paddock, AMP, mob grazing, high-intensity rotational grazing, holistic grazing or regenerative grazing – as part of a holistic approach.[23] Having examined the peer-reviewed evidence, the authors of a recent white paper by the Rodale Institute declared, with confidence, that 'the global adoption of regenerative practices across both grasslands and arable acreage could sequester more than 100% of current anthropogenic emissions of CO_2'.[24]

US farmers Will Harris, Gabe Brown and Joel Salatin have proved that regenerative techniques work. Research done at Will Harris's White Oak Pastures (home of the zero-carbon burger discussed in Chapter 7), has demonstrated that White Oak's soils are ten times as rich in organic matter as the soil of surrounding farms. The results of Gabe Brown's efforts to improve the environmental impact of his farm were documented by an exercise that compared his farm to three others that relied on different levels of tillage and synthetic fertiliser application, none of which had integrated livestock into their operation. Brown's farm – which uses no tillage or synthetic fertilisers and does incorporate livestock – had dramatically higher levels of soil nutrients, organic matter and carbon content as well as a higher water infiltration rate.[25]

Joel Salatin, farmer, lecturer and author, raises livestock on Polyface Farm in Virginia. Where the farm was once in poor shape, full of rocks, gullies and bare soil, Salatin and his family transformed it by applying regenerative principles, critical among them the stacking of diverse enterprises and the closing of the carbon cycle loop (that is, ensuring that animals are raised in such a way that they sequester as much CO2e as they emit).[26] The soils are now so healthy that if you walk out on the land at the right time of the morning, 'you can catch the sound of the earthworms moving across the fields'.[27]

Harris, Brown and Salatin have inspired, educated and mentored farmers all over the world. Although they represent the high-profile face of regenerative agriculture, the UK is not short of its own advocates. The regenerative approach is well established at Isabella Tree's Knepp Estate, while George Young, who we met in Chapter 8, is in the early stages of implementing plans to regenerate his farm. There are farmers all over the UK at different stages of their journey towards regenerative agriculture. That journey can be filled with trepidation, says Joe Stanley, partly because of the 'unfamiliar buzzwords that are increasingly bandied about to describe the change we are seeing. "Regenerative", "agroecological", "silvopasture", "mob grazing", "min-till", "net zero", "rewilding"'. While not every farm will become a 'regenerative, net-zero, agroecological exemplar', says Stanley, 'there are things we can all do – from precision application of inputs and metering of grass growth to the planting of field margins and digging of sedimentation ponds – that are good for the environment and, ultimately, our bottom lines'.[28]

Holkham Estate

Jake Fiennes, conservation manager for the Holkham Estate in Norfolk, home to Thomas Coke, the eighth Earl of Leicester, was interviewed about his work in *The Times Magazine* in March 2020. Fiennes has been charged with promoting biodiversity, carbon sequestration, general all-round sustainability and the phasing out of pesticides.[29] Fiennes and Coke are moving away from the traditional intensive agribusiness model of the past century on their home farm and encouraging tenant farmers to do the same. They are most definitely in the business of farming (food production) as opposed to wholesale rewilding, but there are wild areas – a nature reserve, wetlands and woods – on the estate.

Fiennes describes what they are doing at Holkham as multifunctional farming, in the best Gabe Brown tradition. (Fiennes presented Coke with a copy of Brown's book when he first arrived on the estate.) He extols the virtues of hedges, floristic margins and cover crops that attract wildlife and pollinators and capture carbon. He insists that this biodiversity also increases yields, and that mixing arable land with livestock (as was common in the past) is preferable to monoculture farming.

Smiling Tree Farm

Smiling Tree Farm is a seventy-acre, pastoral, regenerative farm occupying steep land that's unsuitable for growing arable crops. The traditional Hereford beef cattle and Jersey dairy cows that farmer Christine Page raises on this land feed on diverse pastures and browse among trees. The way Page raises her cows is vital to the health of the soil and the health of the cows' microbiome and it provides a habitat for invertebrates and small animals. It's also good for the food they give us. Page cites studies showing that organic milk and meat contain 50 per cent more beneficial omega-3 fatty acids than conventionally produced products. She believes that all flavour starts in the soil, too, and that flavour and nutrition are inextricably linked.

The specific techniques that Page uses at Smiling Tree are laid out in her presentation, 'Smiling Tree Farm: Why what we feed animals matters'.[30] They include: over-sowing herbs into pasture, which keeps cattle healthy without the need for wormers and vaccinations; choosing diverse species of grasses and forbs for their root depth; providing shelter, shade and browsing spaces using diverse hedgerows; using trees as part of the pasture (the silvopasture technique referred to in Chapter 7) to provide wildlife habitat and help the cows to self-medicate; and using the kind of mob-grazing systems that Gabe Brown learned about from his Canadian farmer friend, Neil Dennis.

Page also talks elegantly about utilising the cow 'poop loop' to maximise photosynthesis and root exudates (see page 233) and provide plants with micronutrients. Citing grazing expert Dr Christine Jones, she also explains that the right sort of grazing is necessary for carbon sequestration, soil health and water retention. 'Right' means 'put them in when the grass is up to their knees and take them out before you see their feet'.

Cholderton Estate

Award-winning farmer Henry Edmunds farms a thousand hectares at Cholderton Estate, where the soil is classified as grade 4, meaning that it has severe limitations which restrict the range of crops that can be grown there and is mainly suited to grass with occasional arable crops. Edmunds uses a mixed farming system with beef and dairy cattle plus sheep, all of which graze on rich leys of mixed grasses and legumes. Most grassland in the UK is planted with simple combinations of Italian and perennial ryegrass: shallow-rooted grasses that demand high levels of nitrogen fertiliser and are vulnerable to drought. The more sophisticated mix of grasses and legumes at Cholderton, however, produces higher yields without the need for artificial fertiliser. Above ground, these plants provide nectar opportunities for invertebrates, which have led to fields full of bees and the return of a formerly rare species of butterfly and other wildlife. Below ground, the deep-rooted plants draw carbon from the atmosphere and fix it within a soil matrix that's rich with nitrogen-fixing nodules. The result: good yields, enriched soils, moisture retention, crop resilience and an avoidance of the environmental damage done by nitrogen fertiliser, of which 25 per cent is routinely lost to groundwater and another 25 per cent leaked into the atmosphere, where it is four hundred times more powerful than CO_2 as a warming agent.[31]

Devenish Lands

At Devenish Lands at Dowth, Ireland, part of the global network of Lighthouse farms, John Gilliland and his team are working towards delivering carbon-neutral beef and lamb by 2025. They have active projects to improve soil fertility and optimise biodiversity and are measuring carbon sequestration both above and below ground. They use a 'whole farm, annual carbon balance sheet' to visualise their journey. Peer-reviewed studies have shown that Dowth currently sequesters 665 tonnes of CO_2e per year.[32]

Devenish Lands are working closely with the Global Innovation Centre of the agri-tech company Devenish Nutrition, applying science and technology to increase knowledge about how to optimise farming methods. One project involves looking at how different types of swards (grasses), establishment methods and fertiliser (organic/inorganic) affect factors such as yield, carbon sequestration and soil-nutrient cycling. Results thus far have demonstrated that using multiple sward species leads to significantly lower levels of nitrogen inputs, improved soil structure, more insect and wildlife, and more efficient sheep and cattle production systems.

Fowlescombe Farm

When Andrew Owens bought Fowlescombe Farm in 2018, he was determined to farm in the best way possible – producing the best meat from the most beautiful animals in the most sustainable way. Owens and his farm manager, Rosie Ball, have created an enterprise that makes use of every inch of their land, using grassland for cows, sheep and goats, and woodland for pigs. 'You won't find better, happier animals or a more sustainable system,' says Owens. And each animal group is doing its bit for the land. The pigs have revitalised the forest, while the cows, goats and sheep have improved the quality of the grass and soils. 'You need the animals to poop and dig that into the ground,' Owens says. 'Without animals the grass decays and you need mechanical intervention and fertilisers.'

Owens' farm is organic, but he warns against making judgements based on the organic/non-organic divide. Organic isn't always better and doesn't necessarily mean regenerative. 'Some organic farmers are doing shocking things to the soil with tillage, and failing to do what's necessary to enhance biodiversity,' Owens said. Neither should a farmer be judged for raising cattle inside for part of the time. An inside barn does not mean 'industrial feedlot'. In the worst of the winter weather, some breeds of cattle need to be brought inside for their own comfort, welfare and health. This was something Trent Loos and Andrew Henderson were keen to stress during our tearoom meeting in London. Loos maintains that animals will sometimes choose to be inside rather than ranging free because that's where they're more comfortable. UK dairy farmer Neil Dyson has observed that cows kept indoors are happy and has begun an experiment that could prove it. Working with FAI Farms (a research consultancy) he has fitted each of his cows with a pedometer and an electronic collar. These will help him to work out how much time is spent eating and lying down, both indicators of well-being. The study is due to be completed by summer 2022.[33]

Andrew Henderson was also at pains to point out that not

all antibiotic use is bad: 'If an animal has an infection in the hoof, do you want to let the animal suffer, or chop its leg off, or give it the antibiotics it needs?' Henderson asked. 'Good farmers,' said Loos, 'can be trusted to make the right decisions about where to put their animals and how to maintain their health.'

James Rebanks' *English Pastoral: An Inheritance*

James Rebanks' journey to the more regenerative form of agriculture that has restored biodiverse life to his farm is recounted in his book, *English Pastoral: An Inheritance*. The word 'inheritance' is key. Rebanks not only inherited his farm, but also the destructive post-war model of industrial farming. He writes, 'the last forty years on the land were revolutionary and disrupted all that had gone before for thousands of years – a radical and ill thought-through experiment that was conducted in our fields. I lived through those years. I was witness.'[34] Rebanks has also been witness to the gradual restoration of his land through the application of regenerative, mixed-farming principles and the effort to bridge what he calls the 'historic animosity between farmers and ecologists'.[35]

Weston Park Farms

John Cherry and his brother inherited the same post-war model of farming which de-prioritises soil health. He says, 'we felt we ought to look after the soil, but we didn't really look after it. We did what everyone else did, which was cultivating and using fertiliser and thinking that was the right thing to do.'[36] John started seeing other farmers who were doing things in a better way and persuaded his brother that they should start using regenerative techniques on their mixed Hertfordshire farm, Weston Park Farms, in 2010. Not only have they seen massive improvements in the health of their soils and increased insect and bird life, but their workload has fallen dramatically. 'On the arable side it's much less work since we gave up tilling ten years ago. On the cattle side, they are all together in a couple of mobs and we move them every day. That's so much easier than having them spread out all over the place. It would take all morning to find them all! They do so much better with mob grazing.'[37]

A guiding hand for farmers

Cherry's plunge into regenerative farming was assisted by training he received from 3LM, the UK hub of the Savory network. 3LM, founded and run by Christopher and Sheila Cooke, has helped over three hundred farms to implement holistic, regenerative farm-management practices. In addition to running training courses and providing personal mentoring, they conduct farm Ecological Outcome Verifications (EOVs) to establish how well farms are doing in terms of improving such things as water cycles and energy flows on the farm and relationships with surrounding communities.

Farms such as John Cherry's now make up the membership of a UK-based organisation called the Pasture-Fed Livestock Association (PFLA). The association promotes 'the unique quality of produce raised exclusively on pasture, and the wider environmental and animal welfare benefits that pastured livestock systems represent'.[38] It provides the leading, and only, certification mark for 100 per cent grass-fed, grain-free ruminant meat and dairy in the UK, and a link to farms and retailers who sell meat from exclusively grass-fed animals.

One of those retailers is The Ethical Butcher, founded by Glen Burrows, a former vegetarian and photographer, and Farshad Kazemian, a meat trader with fifteen years' experience selling meat to the restaurant trade. Glen and Farshad's mission is to reconnect people with nature, and to change an industry that has gone badly wrong. To that end they source exclusively high-quality meat from farmers who are fully committed to farming in a way that is better for the animals, better for human health and better for the planet, and count both Andrew Owens and John Cherry as two of their twenty suppliers.

One of the achievements of which Glen is proudest is supporting farmer Mark Chapple at Redwoods Farms in working out how to raise 100 per cent soya-free chickens. Glen had searched the country for a soya-free chicken but had been told there was no such thing, and what's more, that raising chickens without soya couldn't be done. He was approached by Mark, who wanted to try Joel Salatin's technique of using mobile chicken tractors to transport chickens to land just vacated by cattle, where they could feast on the grass and the insects in the fresh dung. The experiment was a remarkable success, and Mark's chickens now get up to 40 per cent of their diet from the land, with the rest made up of scattered soya-free, organic feed. I can personally vouch for the fact that they are meatier and more delicious than any chickens I've ever tasted. I've tried meat from several Ethical Butcher farms, and it is invariably off the scale in terms of quality. Consumers will appreciate the fact that each piece of meat is stamped by a bar code that enables them to click through to a video about the source farm. Imagine the revolution in farming standards if all meat was required to come with such a link, and we were able to see what those organic and free-range labels really meant?

Making regenerative farming pay

Can farmers make money farming to Ethical Butcher-type standards? Both John Cherry and Andrew Owens say yes.

There are huge savings on the costs of inputs (artificial fertilisers, insecticides and pesticides) and higher revenues from the sale of premium-quality produce. Diversity also generates profits, as Gabe Brown has pointed out. Whereas Brown used to manage for yield, he now manages for profit per acre, and the key to generating profit is stacking enterprises, or diversity rather than specialisation.[39] Brown makes a healthy profit by taking the waste stream from one enterprise to fuel profit from another, for example: 'We feed the screenings from our grain, which we would be docked for if we sold our grains at the elevator, to our laying hens, broilers and hogs. Thus we convert waste into cash by running it through livestock.'[40]

Similarly, the livestock graze on the perennial forages from fruit and nut crops, the cover crops feed livestock and bees, and 'even the livestock guard dogs that protect the sheep and poultry make us a profit because we raise and sell puppies'. For Brown, as for John and Molly Chester at Apricot Lane Farm, diversity is king. It creates practical and financial resilience while serving one overarching goal: drawing carbon down from the atmosphere to create carbon-rich soil.

Gabe Brown and Allen Williams's work with farms across the US confirms that Brown's experience is not unique. Farmers who apply regenerative principles are seeing their soils improve, along with farm profitability. 'Regenerative farmers are clearing thousands per acre in profit margin' and experiencing freedom from subsidies and debt, says Allen, and once they start, 'very few go back'.[41]

A challenging journey

This is not to underestimate the many barriers to change. A myriad of factors stand in the way of more farmers being able to transition to regenerative agriculture. One of those factors is fear. Williams says that farmers can be fearful of both failure, and the scepticism and condemnation of doubting family and neighbours. Suppliers can stoke this fear, talking up the downside of moving away from their seeds, fertilisers and pesticides.

The economic risks are also real. Transitioning to regenerative agriculture requires upfront investment in new, more nimble equipment such as the seed drills that enable no-till approaches. In the US, for example, a simple thing such as the cost of perimeter fencing, essential for effective mob grazing by cattle, can serve as a barrier to change because it isn't currently covered by US government support programmes.[42] Farm subsidies, in general, tend to reward the status quo, including growing commodity crops on a large scale. Brown describes the US subsidy programme as something that was intended to minimise risk but has become 'a monster that now dictates most of the cropping decisions made in the United States'.[43]

In the UK, says Robert Barbour of the Sustainable Food Trust, many farmers 'are stuck in a system that they recognise as unsustainable from an environmental, financial or personal point of view but the economics make it difficult to break out from that. One of the key reasons for this is that the damage inflicted on the environment and public health by unsustainable farming practices is generally not included in the price that consumers pay at the till, meaning that food which should be the most expensive is, instead, the cheapest.'[44] Brexit and the new Agricultural Bill represent additional challenges for farmers, says Barbour. Farmers face the withdrawal of CAP (Common Agricultural Policy) subsidies, which make up as much as 61 per cent of average farm incomes, with little assurance of what funds will replace them. According to Barbour, 'it's hard to overstate just how difficult Brexit will be for agriculture'.

Joe Stanley echoes Barbour's views, believing that farmers

are trapped in an 'obscene cul-de-sac' born of Brexit, our collective obsession with cheap food, and policy makers' refusal to acknowledge what is required to improve farming and food systems: 'The subsidies were barely enough to prop up the cheap food system. More cash would be required to create the system we want. But existing levels of cash are about to be withdrawn. At the same time, farmers are expected to increase standards while facing more competition from abroad. These things don't add up. We have to do better than this. The government could replace the three billion pounds [that's needed] quite easily. It's within their power to do so.'

At the time of writing, a new agricultural bill had been passed into law in the UK, but its provisions did not look sufficient to help farmers escape the 'obscene cul-de-sac'. 'So much hinges on how much funding will be put in place to support all the things they [the government] say they want to support,' said Barbour, warning that the specifics of the Environmental Land Management Scheme (ELMS), which could be used to support farmers transitioning to more environmentally friendly forms of farming, will not be known for years.

Stanley worries that the mechanics of the ELMS might encourage large estates to force tenant farmers off the land so as to benefit from funds for 'landscape transformation' schemes. 'Small tenants will be worst affected; they will be unable to access the higher tiers of the ELM,' he said. 'And small tenants are most reliant on current subsidy payments and extensively [regeneratively] grazed livestock – the very farming we want to see – even more so.' In short, and on current projections, said Stanley, 'government policy will lead to huge dislocation and tragedy in our countryside with a greatly reduced proportion of our food being produced domestically'.[45]

Farmer John Cherry raised similar concerns. Writing in the *Financial Times*, he admitted that subsidies had been 'embarrassing to receive' but that many farmers relied upon them because they were 'trapped in a high-input/high-output/low-return system'. They would need more help in transitioning to a more sustainable farming system than the government seemed willing to give. 'The [government] document says it wants to transform the way it supports British farmers by helping them "produce healthy food profitably without subsidy", while also "taking steps to improve the environment, improve animal health and welfare and reduce carbon emissions". Will it? The tone is right but some of the specifics are hazy. The devil is in the detail.'[46]

If the tone is right, the detail is perhaps insufficient to shift what Cherry says is a fundamental misunderstanding in the UK 'about how important the soil under our feet is'. Although the new government report 'has encouraging elements', it needs to go much further. 'Why not pay farmers for the carbon they sequester in their soil?' Cherry asks. He also notes that the Swiss government is providing a more extensive, five-year support package for farmers transitioning to regenerative practices.

Corporations accepting the challenge

If governments cannot always be counted upon to provide sufficient support for farming's shift towards regenerative practices, might corporations play a role? In North America, there are signs that a more positive kind of corporate influence is beginning to exert itself, one that promises to serve as an antidote to what has largely been the negative influence of large manufacturers and retailers. (If you are in any doubt about the way UK supermarkets have reshaped our food chain, I urge you to read Joanna Blythman's *Shopped: The Shocking Power of Britain's Supermarkets*, in which she exposes how large supermarkets' sourcing, buying and pricing practices have rewarded and encouraged intensive farming and militated against smaller, more quality-conscious producers.[47]) A number of corporations are championing the regenerative agriculture movement by providing support to farmers to help them weather the time it takes to transition their operations to practices that promote healthier soil.[48] General Mills has committed to advancing regenerative practices on at least a million acres of land by 2030. The company began with a pilot programme with forty-five oat farmers in North Dakota and the Canadian provinces of Manitoba and Saskatchewan, later adding a project involving twenty-four wheat farmers in Kansas. General Mills provides funding for one-on-one coaching for farmers, in addition to paying for ecological services to monitor carbon sequestration rates, soil structures and biodiversity gains.

The one-on-one coaching is provided by Gabe Brown and his partners at Understanding Ag. Brown says that he was first approached by General Mills in 2015, when its sustainability director, Jerry Lynch, brought a team from the company out to his ranch. Brown told Lynch that his company had to find a way to put more nutrients back into the foods they produced, and that the only way to do that was through healthy soil. Lynch absorbed the message and became an immediate advocate of regenerative farming as a means of improving both soil health and the nutrient density of food. Brown has been impressed by the company's continuing commitment to the cause. 'They are really bending over backwards to make this work, and Mary Jane Melendez [who replaced Lynch on his retirement] is 100 per cent on board.'

Danone, in the US, has also shown itself to be a champion of regenerative agriculture. Its pledge to invest six million dollars in soil health research was the catalyst for a biodiversity consortium announced in 2019, and the company has since stepped up its support for regenerative agriculture with two new sources of funding. The company makes funding available through long-term procurement contracts with farmers. Soil research is already being carried out with twenty-three dairies across ten states, and two new programmes announced in January 2020 will help farmers to invest in the new equipment and seeds required to switch to regenerative practices.[49]

The Pasture Project team engages with corporations and other private companies to explore how they can shift their meat and dairy supply chains towards regenerative practices. The Pasture Project takes an agro-ecology approach, looking for a wide range of positive outcomes besides soil health. 'The economics are important,' says Pete Huff. 'We don't want to lead farmers towards a cliff that they fall off because they can't sell their product. So, we look at how to maintain fair prices for farmers, as well as social values like good conditions for workers, racial and gender equity, benefits to local communities, and food sovereignty.'[50]

3LM's Sheila Cooke believes that much of the impetus for change could come from the clothing industry. The Savory network is supporting clothing brands such as Patagonia and Eileen Fisher, who seek to buy their raw materials from sustainable-farming operations. And a shift away from fast fashion, promoted by groups such as Sustainable Edge, has the potential to give a boost to natural products sourced from regenerative farming enterprises. But this potential will only be captured if natural fibres win out over vegan synthetics:

The problem with fashion is that their direction has thus far been towards vegan products – vegan leather, and fabrics made from apple skins, that sort of thing. That's okay as long as the properties of those fabrics are replacing plastic-based products. But if they replace real leather and natural fibres, that impacts negatively on the environment. The process of making artificial fabrics uses a lot of energy and chemicals that producing leather does not. And while we need livestock on the land, we also need to use the whole animal or that's disrespectful and a waste in its own right.[51]

Impetus for change could also come from the hospitality industry. A restaurant-led effort in the US called Zero Foodprint provides a model that others could follow.[52] The fifty plus restaurants and other food businesses who've signed up agree to add a few cents to the cost of a meal in order to provide funds to help farmers implement carbon-reducing farming projects. One farmer who benefited from funding planned to use it to create more silvopasture, which he said would provide a windbreak for the grass that would help keep moisture in the ground during a drought.[53] Imagine what could be achieved if those restaurants who've declared meat to be off the menu opted, instead, to join this kind of initiative and encouraged others to do the same.

You can't keep a good revolution down

Corporate support like that provided by General Mills will play an important role in establishing regenerative agriculture as mainstream practice. Currently, it's estimated that fewer than 5 per cent of farms in the US are truly regenerative, and the percentage is likely to be lower in the UK, according to Cooke. But interest is snowballing according to the folks at Understanding Ag. Williams says that ten years ago he and his team might deliver four workshops a year, each one attended by fifty to a hundred people. In 2019, he and his partners spoke at over four hundred workshops and to a total of around 93,000 people, not including the millions they reached online.[54]

Brown says that he spent 280 days on the road in 2019, supporting farmers involved in the corporate projects such as that funded by General Mills and delivering general education on regenerative principles. 'My partners and I feel like we're strapped to a rocket ship,' he says. 'We've no idea where it's going because we literally can't keep up. But we've all realised that we were called to do this.'[55]

Hard data and farmers' stories are winning people over to the regenerative cause, says Pete Huff at the Pasture Project:

> We have increasing data sets that show the benefits of regenerative practices and these help to generate funding and resources to support farmers to adopt these practices. The data matter. You can say to an agency like the USDA's NRCS [National Resources Conservation Service], look, these methods have a soil-health benefit and they serve your conservation goals, they should be prioritised. And then we have the stories of the individual farmers who have seen the benefits on their farms – these accounts are just as important as the data. These are the people who we need as active and vocal advocates for grazing cover crops and other regenerative practices.[56]

All indications are that interest in regenerative agriculture is snowballing in the UK, too. Inspired by his experience attending a No Till on The Plains event in Kansas, John Cherry founded Groundswell, a regenerative agriculture festival, in 2015. Reaction to the first festival was 'embarrassingly effusive' and attendance has been growing year on year. Delegates come from all over the UK and the world to listen to regenerative experts, meet the suppliers of no-till equipment, and swap stories about their own regenerative experiments. Cherry says that there are 'green shoots happening all over the place', and that 'we'll suddenly get to the point in the farming world where this will be the norm'.[57] But he would like to see the government do more to make this happen. 'Some farmers find it hard to change because they can't afford to sell their ploughs and buy new drills, for example. The government could help people with the transition. The pay-offs would be enormous because no-till and mob grazing has the potential to dramatically improve soil health and take carbon out of the atmosphere. It's crucial for fighting climate change – it's the only way we'll sort it out.'[58]

What Cherry calls 'green shoots' are growing up all around the world. Diana Rodgers showcases some of them in her wonderful film, *Sacred Cow*. Other examples can be found in the science library of the Savory Institute (https://www.savory.global/science-library). Evidence of the positive effects of regenerative and holistic approaches is documented on farms in a number of countries, including Argentina, Australia, Kenya and Mexico.[59] Those who watched *Rick Stein's Cornwall* series will have learned about many Cornish farmers who are deploying regenerative practices. Even Extinction Rebellion appears to have become open to the regenerative agriculture message. A blog featured on its website in March 2021 described regenerative agriculture as something that both heals ecosystems and strengthens food security.[60]

The consumer also has a role to play in propelling the regenerative movement forward. 'Consumers will lead the grassroots movement by being more vociferous about what they want to eat,' says Cherry. Christine Page is encouraged by the fact that 'more and more enlightened consumers are looking for high quality, ethically produced food, [and] they appreciate its value and wish to support small-scale, local producers'.[61] Every time a consumer makes a choice in favour of foods produced by sustainable, regenerative farming systems they send a signal to retailers, encouraging them to provide more.

But can we feed the world this way?

Ah yes, regenerative agriculture is all well and good, but we can't feed the world that way. This retort has become commonplace, uttered by everyone from Bill Gates to the *Guardian*'s environment editor. We need to challenge it. As Lierre Keith points out, those closest to the ground say differently.

> The activist-farmers have a very different plan from the polemical-writers to carry us from destruction to sustainability. The farmers are starting with completely different information. I've heard vegetarian activists' claims that an acre of land can only support two chickens. Joel Salatin, one of the high priests of sustainable farming and someone who actually raises chickens, puts that figure at 250 an acre. Who do you believe? Frances Moore Lappé says it takes 5.4–7.25kg (12–16lb) of grain to make 450g (1lb) of beef. Meanwhile, Salatin raises cattle with no grain at all.[62]

Gabe Brown insists that farmers do not need to chase ever-increasing yields, delivered to the world at commodity prices, in order to feed the world.

> We need to wake up and realise that there is no shortage of food in the world. There are political and social factors that prevent foods from reaching the hands of people who need it. And there are increasing problems with the nutrient density in the foods produced. But there is no shortage of food. Several recently released reports showed that worldwide food production in 2016 was enough to feed ten billion people.[63]

The authors of the aforementioned white paper for the Rodale Institute concur, calling the notion of food shortage a myth and the 'continued use of the trope that we "will soon need to feed nine billion people" as justification for seeking ever greater yields' duplicitous. 'Hunger and food access are not yield issues,' they say. 'They are economic and social issues.'

Back in 2004, Colin Tudge came to the same conclusion: there is no shortage of food in the world. His analysis suggested that the global population would reach its peak (around ten billion) by 2050 but would then stop increasing, and that there was little reason to fear that we would not be able to feed those ten billion people.[64] 'The broadest statistics suggest that there is still scope for us to do very well indeed. But there is no case for euphoria, or excessive bullishness, or risk, or putting faith in any one particular technology – whether civil engineering or biotech – no matter how commercially attractive it might seem in the short term. Traditional farmers the world over know this. They've known it for centuries. They are worth listening to.'[65]

Farmers like Brown know that not only is an absolute shortage of food not the issue but regenerative agriculture does not, in any case, have to lead to a fall in output: 'This ranch used to run 65 calves and 20 yearlings along with some monoculture wheat and barley. Today we run 12 times as many cattle on the same land, plus sheep and hogs and 1,400 laying hens and broilers, plus barley, oats and wheat and a myriad of other products. I'm producing 15–20 times as much human edible product as my father-in-law did before me.'[66]

Joel Salatin says that he now 'makes as much off one acre as we used to make off 12'. To the naysayers who insist that regenerative farming can't feed the world, he says 'don't talk to me about that. I've seen it work.'[67]

Allen Williams has done the maths and shown that grass-fed systems can be scaled up to produce more food. In the US, there are 29 million grain-fed cattle finished in feedlots every year. By using idle grasslands, including existing USDA

Conservation Reserve Program land unsuitable for farming but good for grazing, and converting corn and soya mono-crops used for fattening cows, over 50 million grass-fed head of cattle could be produced a year, which is almost double what is produced in feedlots today.[68] The widespread application of regenerative principles could then increase the carrying capacity (sometimes called the stocking rate) of any grassland by as much as 50 to 70 per cent, according to several studies.[69] And there is evidence of 'increased carrying capacity from multi-species grazing . . . for instance mixing cattle with sheep or goats, which improves productivity of both animals and vegetation when compared to grazing either animal alone'.[70]

Farmer Henry Edmunds believes that a return to regenerative, mixed farming will help to rectify harmful imbalances within the food and farming system:

> The UK is currently growing an excess area of cereals. The surplus grain is being exported; frequently even dumped on the world market where prices for third-world farmers are then depressed. Yet, we import 60,000 tonnes of beef, this often a product of despoiled rainforest. Restoring pastures to our arable farms should result in self-sufficiency in dairy, beef and lamb products but in a sustainable way that will protect our ability to crop the land into the future.[71]

Robert Barbour of the Sustainable Food Trust is also cautiously positive about the potential for regenerative mixed farming systems to produce enough food: 'If we return to a mixed farming system [involving a wider variety of livestock and crops within the same farm] with animals raised primarily on pasture, there will be a decline in some crops and some types of meat. But we need to counteract this by changing our diets, and by reducing the amount of grains fed to animals. This will likely lead to some reduction in meat consumption, and in particular the consumption of chicken and pork ... the key is to look at the systems of production and only eat the amount of meat that can be supplied by the most sustainable systems.'[72]

Barbour also insists that a reduction in food waste is critical. As we saw in Chapter 9, we produce enough food, but we waste almost 40 per cent of it. Eliminating food waste must become a priority for policy makers, manufacturers, retailers and consumers alike.

Listen to the farmers

The latest IPCC report (2019) maintains that mixed farming systems, including properly managed livestock, can heal damage done by years of continuous arable cropping reliant on mechanical and chemical inputs. But the naysayers insist that converting our industrial model of agriculture to a regenerative one would take too long and is too big a task. Yes, it's a daunting undertaking. But is it more challenging than the proposed alternative, which is eliminating all animal agriculture from the face of the earth and replacing it with cell-cultured meat designed to mimic the exact taste, texture and nutritional content of meat, grown in a few large labs and shipped to every corner of the world? A wholesale shift from animal agriculture to lab-based food would be neither straightforward nor without enormous risks, the greatest of which would be to separate food production from the ecosystem of which it is part, bringing about disastrous unintended consequences that could be difficult, if not impossible, to reverse.

Listening to and supporting the farmers – many of whom are already successfully doing what needs to be done – seems an infinitely better idea.

Part Three

Who is Advocating for the Plant-based Diet, and Why?

'In researching this subject, you come to realise that it takes on a multitude of vested interests. Not just vegans and vegetarians who are passionate about their choices but also well-funded animal rights activists, Big Pharma, Big Food and Big Ag, plus environmental groups and many of the wealthiest foundations, as well as multinational global leaders, including the United Nations and the World Health Organization. You're also unlikely to find a sympathetic media, because many top journalists lean vegetarian, so they're no longer doing what they would normally do, which is to dig around, follow the money, and find the truth.'

NINA TEICHOLZ, best-selling author and science journalist

'Rather than ending up as a wholesome approach, it [veganism] risks being hijacked by vested interests and totalitarian schemes. It would be particularly difficult to reverse such a situation, once established.'

FRÉDÉRIC LEROY, ADELE HITE and PABLO GREGORINI,
'Livestock in Evolving Foodscapes and Thoughtscapes',
Frontiers in Sustainable Food Systems

'Why is this lying bastard lying to me?'
20th-century journalist, LOUIS PHILIP HEREN
and, latterly, JEREMY PAXMAN

11

How a Serving of Religion
Ended Up on Your Plate

Often we need to make connections between seemingly unrelated events, people or organisations in order to appreciate the full extent to which the debate about food, health and the environment is being distorted. The connection I want to make here is between a recent study by Marco Springmann and fellow authors Clark, Hill and Tilman ('Multiple health and environmental impacts of foods', discussed in Chapter 7) and a twelve-year-old American boy who, in 1864, was given the task of typesetting a manuscript titled *An Appeal to Mothers*. The manuscript spoke of the responsibility of mothers to deter their children from masturbating and made it clear that 'children who practice self-indulgence to puberty, or during the period of merging into manhood and womanhood, must pay the penalty of nature's violated laws'.[1] The penalty would come in the form of diseases such as headaches, loss of memory and sight, weakness in the back and loins, spinal illnesses, the decaying of the head and the ruination of the mind.

What does a 2019 study have to do with the twelve-year-old

boy who later devoted his life to preventing intemperance and masturbation? They are connected by the teachings of a woman named Ellen White, and the church she formed in 1863, and by an antipathy towards meat and a fondness for cereals that is being played out in today's diet wars.

To fully understand the connection, and why it matters, we need to go back to when Ellen White founded the Seventh-day Adventist Church and follow the church's evolution through the next 160 years, tracing its involvement in the development of dietary guidelines, its commercial power and its alliances with corporate giants, until, finally, we arrive back at the 2019 study, co-authored by a long-standing advocate for plant-based diets and peer-reviewed by an academic at a Seventh-day Adventist university that champions plant-based diets for religious reasons.

Follow me back to the early nineteenth century and we'll see how it all started. The credit for piecing this tale together belongs entirely to Belinda Fettke, who has written brilliantly and extensively on the topic, and whose work can be found at www.isupportgary.com and on YouTube.

Ellen G. White and the temperance reformers

The Temperance Reform Movement became a national movement in the United States during the 1820s, and the 1830s saw tremendous growth in temperance groups in the US, the UK and British colonies.[2] Temperance Reformers believed that citizens were plagued by disease because of immoral behaviour and over-stimulation, and they set out to curb this stimulation via abstinence from alcohol, a 'vegetarian diet, sexual restraint, and a balance between rest, exercise and cleanliness'.[3]

Ellen G. White was born in 1827, just as the Temperance

Reformers' ideas were becoming popularised. Growing up, it's likely that she would have been influenced by their teachings. At age seventeen, she claimed to experience visions and dreams from God.[4] The particular vision, allegedly given to her in 1863, led her to pronounce that the Garden of Eden diet of fruits, nuts, vegetables and seeds constituted the 'diet chosen for us by our creator'. White brought this vision into the Seventh-day Adventist Church, which she co-founded in May 1863 in Battle Creek, Michigan.

The Garden of Eden diet helped to create an identity for Seventh-day Adventists, giving them something tangible around which they could rally, an easy route to purification, and a way of demonstrating their faith in God. It was a way of taking the Gospel to the people, and a way for people to demonstrate their love of the Gospel.[5]

This is where our twelve-year-old boy comes into the picture. He was John Harvey Kellogg, the son of John Preston Kellogg, the man who helped White to establish her church in Battle Creek. John Harvey was given the task of typesetting White's book about the dangers of masturbation, and continued to typeset, edit, print and publish monthly journals for the church until he was sixteen. Thus, for four years, during which he was at his most impressionable, he was immersed in Adventist health reform. Temperance reform became his life's purpose, a purpose that led him to invent bland-tasting cereals and prescribe vegetarian diets.

Kellogg went on to establish the cereal company of the same name and became one of the most influential promoters of the Western diet. By 1882, he had perfected gluten foods, flaked wheat and corn. He went on to patent thirty different soya- and vegetable-based products, and to invent nut-meat analogues for the patients at his Battle Creek sanatorium. In 1896, Nuttose became the first commercial meat alternative in the Western world. We can safely say that Kellogg originated the plant-based burger, long before Linda McCartney or the Impossible and Beyond Burgers came on to the scene. I wonder if the modern-day newcomers realise that the origins of their offerings lie in a movement to prevent the sin of masturbation?

No meat = high carbs

The corollary of Kellogg's advocation of the removal of meat and other animal foods from the diet was an endorsement of a carbohydrate-rich diet. If people weren't going to eat meat and animal fats, they would have to fill up on something, and that something was carbohydrates. (I touched on this trade-off in Part One and will cover it further in Chapter 12.) Both Kellogg's religious beliefs and the profits from his health-foods company based at the Battle Creek Sanitarium depended on this trade-off being made. In this way plant-based diets and carbohydrates became intertwined, and anti-meat advocacy became synonymous with condemnation of LCHF and keto-genic diets. The anti-meat, pro-carb link is evident in articles such as this one, penned for *Spectrum* magazine in 2018: 'How to defend Adventist dietary principles in light of new diet trends'.[6] In it, the author condemns LCHF and keto diets that, he says, 'stand in direct contradiction to the Adventist dietary recommendations'. It's clear, he writes, that 'the diet given to Adventists is one that should abound in foods that are high in carbohydrates, high in dietary fibre and low in fat'.

When belief shapes science

You'll note that the title of this article is 'How to *defend* Adventist dietary principles' (italics mine). This retrospective 'defence' of religious beliefs about diet, a kind of shoehorning of scientific evidence into Adventist-shaped shoes, is charac-teristic of the effort to convert us all to their Garden of Eden diet. The history and results of this effort at persuasion are recounted in an official Seventh-day Adventist paper entitled, 'The global influence of the Seventh-day Adventist Church on diet'.[7] Adventists have secured appointments within dietary organisations and influenced the guidelines they produce, funded research designed to confirm the superiority of their diet, deployed their vast wealth to push the plant-based message via schools and hospitals, and formed relationships with large corporations that have a vested interest in promoting carbohydrate-rich, plant-based diets. Latterly, they've done this under the jaunty and inoffensive banner of Lifestyle Medicine, a brand that few would find reason to challenge. It's as ingenious as it is alarming.

How Adventists gained sway over the dietitians who advise us about what to eat

Adventist influence over dietary-advice organisations and dietary guidelines began with three women – Ella Eaton Kellogg, Dr Kate Lindsay and Lenna Cooper – who were early proponents of the Adventist health reform message. Ella Eaton Kellogg, John Harvey Kellogg's wife, supervised and taught at a school of cookery for homemakers, nursing students and the home-economics students who were forerunners of the dietetics organisations. Dr Kate Lindsay worked at the Battle Creek Sanitarium at the same time as John Harvey Kellogg. She went on to develop the first Adventist school of nursing and grew it into a nationally accredited course.[8]

The last member of this influential triumvirate, Lenna Cooper, was a dietitian of such influence that the Academy of Nutrition and Dietetics honour her memory with the Lenna Frances Cooper Memorial Lecture Award. After graduating from Kate Lindsay's nursing programme, Lenna became a protégé of John Harvey Kellogg and his wife and dean of the school of home economics at the Battle Creek Sanitarium, where she trained more than 500 dietitians. She went on to establish the American Dietetic Association in 1917, to serve on the staff of the US Surgeon General, and to create the department of dietetics at the National Institute of Health (NIH). She cemented her position as a leader in worldwide dietetics through her role as senior author of *Nutrition in Health and Disease*, a textbook that was used for the next thirty years in dietetic and nursing programmes around the world. In this manner, Adventist dietary principles, supposedly communicated to Ellen G. White via a vision from God, became firmly established as mainstream dietary advice.

Other Adventist influencers included Dr Harry Miller, a missionary who spent seventy years in China, founded the modern soya renaissance there, and brought infant soya milk formula back to the US. He established nineteen sanitariums, mostly in Asia, where he provided training for nurses doing outreach work, and founded the New Nutrition Research Laboratory in 1953, where he set about demonstrating that science could prove what had been ordained by divine inspiration. (In other words, science would somehow be shoehorned into those Adventist shoes.)

Then there was Dr Mervyn Hardinge, a strict Adventist and a technical expert in Dr Miller's research laboratory. Like Miller, he wanted to post-rationalise the diet that had been ordained by God, and so he set about investigating the health status of Adventist vegetarians. At first, administrators at Loma Linda University discouraged his work because they were afraid that if vegetarian diets were found to be deficient, it would embarrass them.[9] In the 1950s his doctoral dissertation at the Harvard School of Public Health was supervised by Dr Frederick Stare, who was later found to have strong ties to the sugar industry and had worked to downplay the harm done by sugar and blame saturated fat for heart disease. Hardinge went on to establish the School of Public Health at Loma Linda University in 1967, where he created the first official course of study on medical ministry and evangelism.

(A brief aside here to remind ourselves of that connection noted at the beginning of this chapter: a study by Marco Springmann and colleagues, hailed by many as groundbreaking evidence that there should be a global shift towards eating a plant-based diet, was peer reviewed by Joan Sabaté (of whom we'll hear more later), an academic at Loma Linda University,[10] an Adventist institution originally named the College of Medical Evangelism that offered the first course of study on medical ministry and evangelism and whose modern-day stated mission is to continue the teaching and healing ministry of Jesus Christ. Given the importance of the plant-based Garden of Eden diet within that ministry, it would be fair to ask those involved in the peer-review process how confident they are that unconscious biases did not creep into their work. Setting aside a whole belief system to concentrate on objective science is a tall order, but one that must surely be the target if we, the public, are to have confidence in the conclusions reached.)

Other Adventist influencers include U.D. Register, a food chemist for Madison Foods, an Adventist company founded by Ellen G. White herself. Register spoke at the White House in 1969 and at a 1972 meeting of the American Dietetics Association. Later, at the request of the ADA he co-authored a manual on vegetarian diets for dietitians. Like Miller, Register was determined to post-rationalise Adventist health-reform principles. Speaking to students at the College of Medical Evangelism he said that 'evidence will be presented here to show how science verified statements made over fifty years ago through the spirit of prophesy'.

Another Adventist influencer, Kathleen Zolber, went from her role as chair of the Department of Dietetics at Loma Linda to being president of the American Dietetics Association (ADA) in 1981, giving her influence over some 42,000 professional dietitians and nutritionists. Within a year, the first vegetarian position paper was written. Seven years later, in 1988, the ADA issued a formal acceptance of vegetarianism. Of the nine reviewers who issued the acceptance, five were vegetarians and Adventists, and three were vegetarian or vegan for ethical, health or environmental reasons.[11] The only non-vegetarian was a public trustee of the International Life Sciences Institute (ILSI), a Coca-Cola-funded organisation with membership made up of companies from the processed food industry (of which more later).[12] The reviewers were undoubtedly convinced by the science behind vegetarianism. But it's surely reasonable to ask whether their unconscious biases might have influenced the review process, allowing them to draw firm conclusions from science that is often weak, far from conclusive or even contradictory. We might also ask whether the position paper might have been different had the committee been made up of an equal number of vegetarians and omnivores.

Belinda Fettke asks about the dietitians who are members of the Australian equivalent of the ADA, the DAA (Dietitians Association of Australia): 'are they aware that their parent body puts a stamp of approval on vegetarianism and veganism which has been shaped by religious ideology and their own corporate partnerships with the cereal industry?' She points to the DAA's vegetarian position statements, which are supported by just four references, all of them papers written by Seventh-day Adventists and/or employees of two cereal companies, Sanitarium and Kellogg's. She also points out that all the research papers cited in an article in the *Medical Journal of Australia*'s supplement, 'Is a vegetarian diet adequate?', were sponsored by the Sanitarium Health and Wellbeing Company, wholly owned by the Seventh-day Adventist Church and the Adventist Ministries in the US.

In the US, Adventists were busy helping to shape the 2020 Dietary Guidelines for Americans. The chair of the guidelines committee was the aforementioned Joan Sabaté, former chair of the nutrition department at Loma Linda, co-author of the Adventist paper, 'The global influence of the Seventh-day Adventist Church on diet' (referenced earlier), and peer reviewer of the Springmann study.

In a piece written for the Nutrition Coalition, a charitable organisation founded by Nina Teicholz to ensure that the guidelines process is based on rigorous science, Teicholz revealed not only that the main guidelines were being steered by a known Adventist (Sabaté) but that the Subcommittee on Dietary Fat appeared to have been assembled to maximise partiality towards plant-based diets and against saturated fats. This committee included Sabaté and four other individuals with long-standing leanings towards plant-based diets as well as ties to the food and pharmaceutical industries. (I'll talk about the role of food and pharmaceutical companies in propping up the plant-based message in Chapter 12.)

Given the committee's membership, it's perhaps not surprising that it discussed reducing the caps on saturated fats to less than 7 per cent of calories. (In the end, they simply reaffirmed the existing 10 per cent cap, however.) This despite a wealth of recent evidence featured in peer-reviewed journals, and formally submitted to the USDA, supporting the conclusion that the caps on saturated fats are not warranted or evidence based.[13]

The 2020 US guidelines process represents just the latest example of many decades' worth of Adventist influence over the dietitians and nutritionists who formulate dietary advice. But the Adventist church doesn't rely on this single mode of influence; it also has a commercial empire of its own, and significant relationships with other commercial enterprises.

The Seventh-day Adventist Church: educator, healthcare provider, commercial operator

Today, the Seventh-day Adventist Church (SDA) boasts over 20 million members worldwide.[14] It is the biggest educator in the world after the Catholic Church, with 8,515 educational institutions under its management in 2016, and evangelist activities in countries throughout Africa, Asia and South America. The Adventist healthcare system is one of the largest non-profit healthcare delivery systems in the world, and includes more than 200 hospitals, 329 clinics, 133 nursing homes and 21 orphanages, providing some 17 million outpatient visits.

The SDA church is also a commercial animal, its empire including more than twenty companies that are wholly SDA owned. Prominent among them is Sanitarium, the largest cereal manufacturer in Australia (described by the Australian Charities Not-for-Profit Commission as a company 'established by the Church to promote and produce plant-based health foods in line with its beliefs that plant-based diets are designated by God).[15] Other companies are owned by practising Seventh-day Adventists, such as US companies Worthington Foods and Cedar Lake.[16] These companies produce breakfast cereals, meat analogues, soya foods, wheat gluten, peanut butter and a range of specialist vegetarian foods. Estimated sales of these companies is over 650 million dollars.

The SDA's Complete Health Improvement Programme (CHIP) offers vegan cooking lessons and promotes a wholefood, vegetarian/vegan eating pattern with daily physical activity. CHIP is now owned by the Sanitarium Health and Wellbeing Company, a subdivision of Sanitarium. And Sanitarium's links with the church give it tax-free status: all profits go back to the church.

All this information is on record, and a source of some pride to Adventists. They have described Adventist-owned companies as providing 'good opportunities for outreach'.[17] Outreach to millennials is going gangbusters. Sanitarium's Life Health Foods brand, Australia's largest alternative meat producer, anticipates 25 per cent annual growth, driven purely by a rise in vegetarianism among millennials, who are not only buying the church's plant-based products but also, it seems, buying into the research carried out by church-affiliated scientists and institutions.

Loma Linda University is perhaps the most well-known of these institutions. An early connection between Loma Linda and Harvard University was established in the 1950s in the form of a collaboration between two individuals: Adventist researcher Mervyn Hardinge (mentioned earlier in this chapter) and Dr Frederick Stare, chairman of the newly formed nutrition department at Harvard, who served as Hardinge's dissertation supervisor.[18] The full array of Dr Stare's interests is dizzying. Stare was a director and shareholder of the Continental Canning Company; he used a grant from General Foods to expand Harvard's nutrition research activities, and secured further grants from the Sugar Association, and commercial entities including Procter & Gamble, Kellogg's and Nabisco. Using all these funds, he produced research that was disseminated via *Nutrition Reviews* and the Nutrition Foundation. Serving as an advisor to the US government, Stare rejected the idea that the American diet (packed full of foods from the sugary processed food industry) was harmful, 'stating, for example – that Coca-Cola was "a healthy between meals snack" and that eating even greater amounts of sugar would not cause health problems'.[19]

In 2016, Dr Cristin Kearns and fellow researchers Laura Schmidt and Stanton Glantz revealed that Stare and a Harvard colleague, Mark Hegsted, had conducted sugar-industry funded research that downplayed the role of sugar in heart disease.[20] Hegsted also played a key role in the drafting of the first dietary goals for the United States, commonly known as the McGovern Report, which set the US and much of the rest of the world on a path towards eating low-fat, high-carb diets.[21] In other words, Stare's and Hegsted's (and therefore Harvard's) work served to advance the Adventist agenda by encouraging the widespread uptake of what was essentially a Garden of Eden diet.

That same diet has been promoted by scientists at another well-known institution, the Mayo Clinic. In 2019, a review conducted by the Mayo oncology and haematology fellow Dr John Shin and four Mayo Clinic Scottsdale colleagues rendered a timely, vegan-friendly conclusion that diets high in plant foods 'may be associated' with decreased prostate cancer risk. It turned out that Dr Shin is a Seventh-day Adventist who has served as a speaker in the Adventist Medical Evangelical Network (AMEN). In response to a journalist's question asking if Adventism seeks to move the public towards a plant-based diet in keeping with religious beliefs about the foods that promote health, Shin responded in the affirmative:[22] 'Yes ... because the original diet given to man in the garden of Eden as described in the Bible was a plant-based diet, [and] Seventh-day Adventists believe that this is the ideal diet for maintaining and restoring health.'[23]

Paul Scott, the journalist reporting on the Shin paper, pointed out that it was based on methodologically weak epidemiology that cannot prove cause and effect, and that most of the studies that Shin reviewed showed no effect for any foods in relation to prostate cancer. No matter. Dr Shin, by his own admission, already believed that the Garden of Eden diet was the 'ideal diet'. Scott asked, 'shouldn't being an Adventist while studying nutrition require a disclaimer?'[24]

Many would say yes. Commenting on this issue, Dr David

Klurfeld (the scientist who served on the WHO's working group on meat and cancer, whom we met in Chapter 1) said that intellectual biases can be stronger than financial biases but are usually undeclared: 'If you're a good Seventh-day Adventist you're a vegetarian. So, you have not only the scientific vegetarian approach but you have a religious reason to be a vegetarian ... do you need to declare that? I don't see any declarations like that in science.'[25]

As consumers of research, we have the right to know when what's being sold as scientific fact might actually consist of findings that have been viewed through the lens of a religious agenda. We also have the right to know when non-profit organisations seemingly dedicated to the advancement of health have other agendas – religious or commercial – besides.

Enter Coca-Cola and 'lifestyle medicine'

Coca-Cola's alignment with the ideas and objectives of the Adventists and the Temperance Health Reform Movement dates back to the 1800s, when the company marketed its product as the 'Great Temperance Drink'.[26] The alignment was given a more solid form over one hundred years later, in the early noughties, via Coca-Cola's active involvement with various Adventist health organisations.

The first of these Adventist organisations was CALM (the Christian Association of Lifestyle Medicine), founded by Adventist John Kelly Jr, MD, at Loma Linda University in 2003. This became ACLM (the American College of Lifestyle Medicine) in 2004,[27] an organisation that extended its reach via offshoots in Europe, Australia and the rest of the world. (Some affiliates, like the British BSLM, may be only loosely connected. While described by an ACLM representative as 'a sister organisation in our global network',[28] the BSLM states that it does not have any religious or political affiliations.)[29] Coca-Cola is an acknowledged financial sponsor of the ACLM and its network. Coca-Cola also partners with the ACLM in the LMEd (Lifestyle Medicine Education) Collaborative, and several executives involved with the ACLM are linked to a Coca-Cola-backed and funded initiative called Exercise is Medicine (more on this in a moment).[30] The LMEd receives funding from both Coca-Cola and the Adventist Church.

Both the ACLM's and Coca-Cola's influence has been amplified via an organisation described as having been 'birthed from under the ACLM's wing in 2015'.[31] This is the THI (True Health Initiative), founded by David Katz while he was president of the ACLM in 2014. Like the ACLM, the THI advocates for a diet comprised of 'generally plant-predominant foods', and in this sense its dietary views are well aligned with those of the Adventist Church.[32] If you've watched films like *The Game Changers* and *What the Health*, you may recognise Katz as one of the experts who regularly speaks out against meat consumption and in favour of plant-based diets.

Coca-Cola's efforts to promote its brand are additional to its own alignment with organisations such as the ACLM, the LMEd and the THI. The company has consistently tried to position itself as a health advocate. This effort began with the foundation of the International Life Sciences Institute (ILSI) in 1982, an organisation that took over the publication of *Nutrition Reviews* (a top nutrition journal), and later founded the ILSI Nutrition Foundation. Via ILSI and these other initiatives, Coca-Cola became associated with good nutrition. ILSI claims to be a non-profit science organisation, but others see it as a lobby group for an industry that wields great influence on global food and health policy. Given that its membership includes more than four hundred of the world's leading manufacturers of food and food ingredients, chemicals, pharmaceuticals and other consumer products, it certainly looks like a lobbying group. In an exposé written in 2019, The *New York Times* labelled ILSI a 'shadowy industry group' that 'shapes food policy around the world' and 'the most powerful food industry group you've never heard of'.[33] In emails exchanged between two former senior Coca-Cola employees who had been prominent within ILSI (analysed by Gary Sacks and colleagues in *Critical Public Health*), ILSI was repeatedly mentioned as providing a model for how the food industry can work to influence scientific, medical and consumer opinion in the industry's favour.[34]

In 2020, a campaigning group called Corporate Accountability, the advisors for which include investigative journalist and author Naomi Klein, produced a report titled 'Partnership for an unhealthy planet: How big business interferes with global health policy and science', in which it exposes the manner in which ILSI 'has insinuated itself into the health sciences and policymaking at every level of government'.[35] The report details how ILSI operatives have influenced the Dietary Guidelines for Americans by dominating the guidelines committee, and by using its nutrition publication, *Nutrition Reviews*, to circulate research that favours industry products, including research disparaging global recommendations to reduce sugar intake. The report also details how ILSI has influenced policy in ways that favour industry members in Mexico, Taiwan, Argentina and India.[36]

Another report documented how ILSI had been instrumental in Coca-Cola's efforts to sway obesity policy globally, with particular success in redirecting China's obesity science and policy to emphasise physical activity.[37] 'Beneath ILSI's public narrative of unbiased science and no policy advocacy,' wrote the author, 'lay a maze of hidden channels [that] companies used to advance their interests.'

ILSI has consistently rejected allegations that it works to

advance the interests of its corporate members. But others have begged to differ. Mars, for example, withdrew from ILSI in 2018, 'saying that it could no longer support an organisation that funds what a Mars executive described as "advocacy-led studies"'.[38] And, in 2015, the WHO withdrew ILSI's special access to its governing bodies because of concerns about its industry ties.[39]

Like ILSI, Exercise is Medicine (EIM) was a Coca-Cola initiative, founded with the American College of Sports Medicine (ACSM) in 2007. This was a global partnership dedicated to prescribing exercise as a medical treatment. Here was more marketing genius at work. Via EIM, Coca-Cola and other corporations involved with the organisation became associated with the idea of exercise. It is difficult to argue with the proposition that exercise is good for us. But what exactly are the motives of companies that stand to make a lot of money from consumers who are persuaded that any detrimental impact on their health caused by the consumption of highly processed, sugar-heavy products can be exercised away? Can we – should we – take their recommendations at face value?

Whether we're talking about ILSI, EIM, the ACLM, or one of its offshoots or strategic partners (Katz's THI), the messaging is similar: exercise, water, sunshine, temperance and nutrition (with an emphasis on plant-based diets). And the individual corporate members of ILSI and EIM have used similar messages: Coca-Cola talk of an 'active balanced lifestyle'; for Mars it's a 'well-balanced lifestyle'; and for Kellogg's, it's a 'balanced diet and active lifestyle'. Lifestyle, lifestyle, lifestyle. Don't worry too much about what you eat (and whether you consume sugary foods in particular) because what really matters is your lifestyle, that is, how much you move.[40]

This is clever marketing. But it is also misleading. As we saw in Chapter 1, a calorie is not just a calorie and the type of calories you eat matters. It is also increasingly accepted that you can't out-run a bad diet. (Unless you are spending many hours a day exercising, the calories you burn through exercise cannot do much to balance out calorie intake, particularly when some of those calories impact the body's hormonal system more than others.) But the messages emanating from these companies and the non-profit organisations of which they are members imply that we can consume lots of processed junk and take comfort from the misapprehension that we won't suffer any ill effects as long as we run, bike or gym it off later.

Coming to a screen near you

These lifestyle-enhancing organisations are funded and run by a group of interconnected individuals and organisations which, while proclaiming their interest in improving your health, have other objectives besides. And at the heart of it all is the Seventh-day Adventist Church. That religious organisation just strolled straight into your sitting room, or wherever it is that you stream content. In 2020, the Adventist ACLM endorsed the pro plant-based film, *The Game Changers*.[41] It also teamed up with George Washington University to offer course credits or course hour equivalents to medical students, nursing students, pharmacists and registered dietitians simply for watching it. The idea that a film so short on reliable scientific evidence will form the basis of educational material for health professionals is worrying, to say the least. (I'll discuss the film and the shortage of evidence for its assertions in Chapter 13.)

As worrying are the ACLM's recent endorsement of the call for a second White House Conference on Food, Nutrition and Health, and its position statement on the connection between diet and both human and planetary health. The position statement advocates a 'plant-predominant lifestyle' to protect human health, fight disease, 'rein in greenhouse gas emissions, and feed what will soon be over nine billion people on the face of the earth.'[42] (There's that 'feed the nine billion' trope critiqued by the Rodale Institute in Chapter 10.) The ACLM is entitled to advocate for whatever diet it wants, of course. But to do so without clearly and publicly acknowledging that the origins of its stance on diet are rooted in a religious ideology, and while piggybacking on current heightened concerns about the environment, is disingenuous.

When religious and commercial interests coincide, the result can be not just disingenuousness but something far worse, as Dr Gary Fettke, an orthopaedic surgeon practising in Tasmania (whom we met in Chapter 5), knows from first-hand experience.

Prophets and profits versus the doctor

To appreciate Dr Fettke's experience, we need to know a little about his backstory. At thirty-eight he was diagnosed with an aggressive pituitary tumour and endured several years of radio- and chemotherapy. In 2004, he required further surgery and ended up on a cocktail of medications. By 2009 he had gained a lot of weight, was pre-diabetic and had high blood pressure and cardiac arrhythmias. A friend suggested that he consider talking metformin, a diabetes drug that works by reducing blood sugars, as part of his cancer treatment. Gary thought, *Why take another drug to reduce blood sugars when I can just stop eating sugar?* He was working towards the concept that sugar played a harmful role in the proliferation of cancer cells. Thus began Gary's journey, exploring and researching the benefits of removing sugar from the diet with a low-carbohydrate approach. Over the next couple of years 'the jigsaw came together', as he realised that inflammation was driven not just by sugar but also by polyunsaturated oils.

When Gary gave up carbohydrates, not only did his blood sugars improve but his cancer stopped in its tracks. After eating a low-carb diet for a year, he came off chemotherapy under supervision. He has now been off chemotherapy for seven years, and his cancer is in remission. He does not believe that he could have achieved this if he had continued to eat a low-fat, high-carb diet.

This experience led to Gary's interest in nutrition, and the idea of food as medicine. He began to think about how he might help his patients, many of whom were coming to him with complications from diabetes. He had seen that living long term on a blood sugar rollercoaster came with real risks: diabetic neuropathy, kidney and liver disease, ulcers and, ultimately, amputation. And he was seeing diabetes affecting more and more young people. But in Tasmanian hospitals, the very places where patients were supposed to heal, they were being fed unlimited sugar and processed foods.

Inspired, he collaborated with a dietitian to create a starter sheet with simple low-carb swaps, a 'what to expect when you go low carb' printed resource, and 'teaspoons of sugar' charts. In 2013 he called for the removal of junk food from hospital vending machines. He tried to speak to the hospital's dietetic department about his ideas but found them distinctly unreceptive. They didn't seem to want to know that achieving healthy levels of blood glucose was possible with a low-carb diet.

Resistance wasn't all that Gary encountered, however. In 2014, three anonymous complaints from dietitians were brought against him, claiming that his advice was 'inappropriate and not evidence based'. On the back of these complaints, AHPRA (Australian Health Practitioner Regulation Agency) launched an investigation that lasted over four years, subjecting him to enormous personal strain and threatening to undermine his reputation and derail his career. At one point

The Medical Board of Tasmania, under the umbrella of AHPRA, issued a life-long, non-appealable ruling that Gary could not 'provide specific advice or recommendations on the subject of nutrition'. The actions taken against Gary, which he labelled 'bullying, mobbing and victimisation', eventually led to his resigning from the Tasmanian Health Service in 2018.[43]

The intricate web of competing interests

Belinda Fettke was anxious to defend her husband, a man she describes as a doctor who 'goes to work every day with the perspective of a patient, the spirit of an activist, and the heart of a healer'. Prompted by curiosity as to why AHPRA had called Mark Wahlqvist (an esteemed professor, former head of the International Union of Nutrition Science, and one of the most high-profile nutritionists in the South East Asia Pacific region) as witness, she embarked on two years of research into the links between Wahlqvist, Australia's leading cereal companies, the DAA, Coca-Cola and Sanitarium Health and Wellbeing Company, the commercial arm of the Seventh-day Adventist Church. She discovered that Wahlqvist had a long-standing association with Sanitarium. He had been chair of Sanitarium's ANAC (Australasian Nutrition Advisory Council) from 2000 to 2010 and was expert advisor to Santuary Sanitarium – described as a Centre of Influence based on the teachings of the Seventh-day Adventist Church – from 2010 to 2016.[44] He had publicly expressed the view that the best way to avoid cancer was to avoid meat and his textbook is used by nutrition students at the University of Tasmania and by the Seventh-day Adventist Church for their Health Ministry Training Course. These affiliations, and the impact that they might have had on the witness' testimony, were not openly acknowledged.

This fact formed the tip of the iceberg into which Gary had

crashed. Beneath the surface was a web of affiliations such as Belinda could never have expected to find. The DAA had been receiving annual funding from the Australian Breakfast Cereal Manufacturers Forum (ABCMF); the organisation also used their influence to protect and promote messaging in support of cereals, grains and sugar. Four major companies form the core of the ABCMF: Sanitarium, Kellogg's, Freedom and Nestlé. These corporations have an obvious interest in people sticking with cereals and grains for breakfast, and much to lose if the idea of low-carb eating takes off.

Belinda concluded that Gary's advice to patients to avoid carbohydrate-rich foods represented a genuine obstruction to Sanitarium's continued ability to manage its messaging to the DAA, and the DAA's messaging to patients. Her investigations showed that, previously, the messaging had been managed via people, research papers and funding. Sanitarium had become the go-to resource for diabetes information used by doctors, with branded pamphlets available at the press of a button. And, as previously discussed, Belinda had found that research conducted by representatives of the Seventh-day Adventist Church, its affiliated institutions and the cereal industry formed the basis of the DAA's position paper on vegetarianism.[45]

How is it that doctors and the DAA could get away with providing dietary advice based on research by Adventists and cereal companies with such a clear religious and commercial interest in promoting high-carb diets and foods? The reason is that, unlike the boards of professions such as psychiatry and osteopathy, which are officially overseen by AHPRA, the DAA appears to have been left to self-regulate. Herein lies a great irony of the case, that Gary Fettke was on trial with AHPRA for giving dietary advice, despite the fact that the dietary advice industry (in the form of the DAA) was, itself, completely unregulated.

Belinda pieced this messy, unedifying jigsaw together prior to 2017, and her suspicions were confirmed that year when she and Gary were given sight of an 845-page document submitted to AHPRA. In that document were two letters (from the then CEO of the DAA) asking that Gary be silenced.[46]

Thanks to Belinda's research and determination, Gary was finally exonerated in September 2018, after a four-and-a-half-year fight against organisations driven by what he calls 'prophets and profits'. He received an unprecedented written apology from AHPRA and was free to talk about the health benefits of low-carb diets. His exoneration also implies that other health professionals can do the same.

The less positive news is that the SDA, the DAA and those in the cereal and processed-food industries continue to endorse the high-carbohydrate, plant-based message – all wrapped up in a 'lifestyle medicine' cloak embellished with save-the-planet embroidery. You're free to buy that message if you want to, but you should do so in the full knowledge that both the message and the dietary advice that flows from it would likely look very different had it not been for the influence of the Seventh-day Adventist Church over the last century.

12

Follow the Money: Why Big Business Loves the Idea of a Plant-based Future

Most individuals who become vegetarians or vegans are in it for the animals, the environment, their health, or all three. But their message, and the apparent strength of the movement, has been amplified by the fact that corporations have entered the conversation in a big way, welcoming the plant-based future with open arms. Why have corporations become involved? For the most part – and allowing for some exceptions, because there are always exceptions – it's because the plant-based movement represents a profit-making opportunity. And for businesses operating within a global capitalist economy, seizing profit-making opportunities is what they must do.

For the food industry, the surge of interest in the plant-based diet represents an opportunity to make money by fulfilling demand for plant-based food products, and still more money by promoting the growth of that demand. For the pharmaceutical industry, the opportunity arises from the continued scaremongering around LDL cholesterol (an integral tenet of plant-based advocacy), and the consequent acceptance of the idea that LDL must be lowered via pharmacological solutions.

If you like, you could probably stop reading right here and move on to the next chapter, because that's the crux of why Big Business loves the plant-based diet.

Alternatively, you can indulge my more extensive exploration of how all this works. If you're still reading, let's start with the food industry.

Why much of the food industry backs the plant-based diet

Let's start with the obvious. Without doubt, the newly ubiquitous plant-based food companies that are pushing both their products and the plant-based message have at least one eye on the prize (assuming that the other eye is on making a difference). And the prize is big indeed. The rapidly growing plant-based 'meat' market alone is expected to be worth more than 30 billion dollars by 2026.[1] (In the event of the complete demise of animal agriculture, eagerly anticipated by some, that number would be significantly larger.) The leaders of these organisations might tell a convincing story about improving our health and saving the planet, and most probably believe that story, but you only have to look at the myriad of patent applications associated with the Impossible Burger, for example, to realise that profit through technology is also a key end goal for many companies. Impossible Burger, for example, has made over one hundred patent applications, including one to protect the 'expression constructs and methods of genetically engineering methylotrophic yeast'.[2] Nice.

It isn't just the Pat Browns (Impossible Foods) and Ethan Browns (Beyond Meat) who stand to make millions from the campaign to persuade us to exchange real meat for the fake kind. The financiers behind these companies and other meat-alternative start-ups are also set to get their share of the millions sitting in the pot at the end of the rainbow. Chris Kerr, founder of New Crop Capital, summed it up nicely when he said that the 'vegan revolution was upon us "and there are fortunes to be made"'.[3]

Some individual investors will benefit from the vegan revolution in ways that are not immediately obvious. James Cameron, the director behind the pro plant-based movie *The Game Changers*, is also CEO of Verdient Foods, an organic pea-protein company that aims to be the largest pea-protein producer in North America, in which he invested 140 million dollars.[4] It's been reported, also, that former US Vice President Al Gore – whose 2006 documentary *An Inconvenient Truth* alerted us to the extent of the climate disaster – is a partner in and advisor to Kleiner Perkins, Beyond Meat's big investor. Kleiner Perkins is, in turn, connected to Generation Investment Management, founded by Al Gore and David Blood. And David Blood is the co-chair of the World Resources Institute (WRI), the very same organisation that produced a report recommending eating less meat to save the planet.[5] Via his influence in the WRI, Gore is thus in a position to promote global policies that discourage meat consumption while potentially increasing the value of his own investment in Beyond Meat.

Of course, investments such as those made by Cameron and Gore could simply be examples of people putting their money where their mouths are. The trouble is that once the money has been put, the position taken by the mouths becomes harder to reverse. There must be a danger that intellectual positions become more firmly fixed, irreversible and impervious to new evidence. Persuading someone with a large financial stake in fake meats that regeneratively raised meat might be better for both the planet and their own health – and better still, persuading them to talk publicly about this – becomes difficult to say the least.

Large, established corporations also stand to gain from the vegan revolution. Consider the examples of DuPont, which has capabilities in making plant proteins and the texturants that impart a beef-like feel to them, and IFF (International Flavours and Fragrances), which offers features such as grill marks and antioxidants. IFF's purchase of DuPont's nutrition and biosciences business for 26 billion dollars resulted in an entity with enhanced know-how to serve the fast-growing meatless-meat market.[6]

What about the rest of the food industry? The Coca-Colas and the PepsiCos, the Unilevers and the Nestlés, the Tescos and the Greggs? These household names in the food industry look set to capture a slice of the profits from the vegan revolution: Unilever has a European vegan product range that is over seven-hundred strong, and purchased The Vegetarian Butcher (which, incidentally, piggybacked on Cop26 discussions to promote the idea of reduced meat consumption);[7] Tesco recently announced a new plant-based range to great fanfare; and Greggs boasted record 2019 profits on the back of its vegan sausage roll. For corporations such as these, the money will be easy because, at its core, the plant-based revolution is essentially about adding value to cheap raw materials through ultra-processing and charging premium prices for the end product.[8] Unlike real foods, such as meat and eggs, these ultra-processed foods are easily transportable and have long shelf lives. Profits are virtually guaranteed, even if the health-giving properties of the products are not.

Retailers are well aware of the profit advantage represented by processed foods, and plant-based processed foods within that category, as compared to meat, fish and poultry. A former retail manager confirmed that meat, fish and poultry would once have been one of the main profit areas, but it's 'very different these days'. Another retail manager, in charge of the meat category for a major supermarket, confessed to having a limited ability to promote the benefits – for both human and planetary health – of meat. Meat is a 'loss leader', he said, 'not where the profit margins are', and the marketing department would never allow him to promote meat at the expense of more profitable categories. Moreover, promoting the health benefits of eating meat just 'goes against the vibe'. Here we have the zeitgeist and the profit motive working in tandem to squash positive messaging about the very real health properties of well-raised meat. And the ordinary consumer is likely unaware that they are being encouraged to walk away from the meat aisle and towards those aisles stacked with more profitable, processed categories.

If retailers are conscious of the profitability of ultra-processed foods, so are manufacturers. The authors of the UK's National Food Strategy note that companies 'invest more money into researching, developing and marketing unhealthy foods' for 'sound commercial reasons'. Their investments are 'intended not just to help capture a bigger slice of the market, but to grow the market itself'.[9] Such is the underlying logic of commercial organisations in a capitalist economy.

The reason this commercial logic prevails, allowing processed food manufacturers 'to make their nutritionally poor yet highly palatable junk food and drink available to anyone, anywhere, anytime,'[10] says Dr Aseem Malhotra, is partly down to the failure of our policies to curb 'their excesses and manipulations'.[11] In fact, some company bosses have said that they would welcome legislation designed to improve the food they sell – 'they want to do the right thing, but they need a level playing field'.[12]

Why is this relevant to the discussion about the ascendant power of the plant-based movement? Because the movement has gifted to processed-food manufacturers a reason to produce more hyper-palatable, high-carb processed foods. What's more, they'll be able to stick 'heart healthy' and 'green' labels on the packaging to make consumers feel good about buying them.

How corporations shape the environment in which they operate

If food companies have been able to get away with producing hyper-palatable, nutritionally suboptimal, carbohydrate-dense processed food because we let them, we must also appreciate that some have actively deployed strategies to protect the environment in which they operate, and their freedom within it. Such activity – designed to shape government policy in ways favourable to the firm – has been labelled corporate political activity (CPA). The former Director General of the WHO, Margaret Chan, identified the CPA of the food industry as representing 'a substantial challenge to NCD (non-communicable disease) prevention efforts'.[13]

Researchers Mialon, Swinburn and Sacks describe six long-term CPA strategies that food companies can and do deploy to shape the world to their advantage: information strategy (disseminating information that is beneficial to their activities to influence health policies and outcomes); financial strategy (providing funds, gifts and other incentives to politicians and other decision makers); constituency building (gaining the favour of public opinion and other stakeholders such as the media and public health community); policy substitution strategy (proposing policy alternatives when threatened with regulation); legal strategy (suing opponents and challengers); and, finally, constituency fragmentation and destabilisation (preventing and counteracting criticism of their products or practices).[14]

Industry groups and initiatives are one powerful vehicle

for the deployment of these strategies. ILSI, the activities of which were discussed in Chapter 11, is a prime example. The organisation has actively worked to shape health and nutrition policy across the globe via a range of channels, including positioning themselves within government and nutrition bodies, cultivating allies within academia and government through sponsored conferences and recruitment to committees working on food issues, and publishing the academic journal, *Nutrition Reviews*.[15] There is also evidence that other organisations such as the International Food Information Council (IFIC), a trade group funded by large food and agrichemical companies, and Foodminds, a food and nutrition communications and consulting company, have taken action to promote industry interests and influence policy.[16]

The story of another Coca-Cola-funded initiative, the Global Energy Balance Network (GEBN), launched in 2014, is illustrative of how far corporations sometimes go to try to influence the environment in which they operate. The GEBN was pitched as an 'honest broker' in the debate about obesity and a 'premier world-wide organisation led by scientists working on the development and application of an evidence-based approach to ending obesity'.[17] Emails soon revealed that the motives behind the GEBN were considerably less upstanding.[18] One particular email from a senior Coca-Cola executive outlining a proposal for the GEBN positioned the proposal as a much-needed response to the failure of existing strategies to address the obesity crisis. But the email also revealed the importance of other, more self-serving motives. 'There is a growing war between the public health community and private industry over how to reduce obesity' the email began, going on to say that 'extreme public health experts' had focused on 'government regulation to limit, tax or ban foods they consider to be unhealthy' and that there was a need for a strategy that would 'aim to counter the unreasonable views' and 'change the conversation'. The GEBN would be the vehicle for that strategy, and would 'counteract their shrill rhetoric indirectly, but forcibly with reasonable voices and with science-based strategies'. The science on which those strategies would be based was of one particular type, however, focusing entirely on the energy balance theory of obesity (which, as we saw in Part 1, may be the type favoured by industry but is hotly contested). The proposed activities in which the GEBN would engage included advancing energy balance as the appropriate framework for addressing obesity via a 'multi-year advocacy "campaign"', and the deepening of 'ties to industry, government, and community organisations to connect and promote best practices that are effective in terms of *both policy and profit*'[19] (italics mine).

Subsequent emails were equally concerning, and evidenced that Coca-Cola was intimately involved in defining the scope and specifics of GEBN activities, and that research on energy balance would be 'very specific to coke [sic] interests'.[20] One email written by James Hill, the GEBN president, to a Coke executive about a research proposal stated that the research 'could provide a strong rationale for why a company selling sugar water SHOULD focus on promoting physical activity' and 'could be a game changer'.[21]

The GEBN folded abruptly in November 2015 not long after being exposed in the press as being a front for Coca-Cola's efforts to 'control the conversation over public policy and consumer choices pertaining to obesity'.[22] The story of its formation and demise should serve to remind us of the strategies that can be and sometimes are deployed by major players within the global food industry. It should alert us to the fact that whenever the food industry participates in the conversation about food and health, that participation almost invariably helps to shape the outcome in favour of their own financial interests. More often than not, the outcome will also favour carbohydrate-rich plant foods and play into the hands of plant-based advocacy. Let's take a look at this in the context of dietary guidelines.

The unavoidable anti-meat message embedded in the food guidelines

In Chapter 11, I raised questions about the extent to which the 2020 US guidelines process was subjected to religious influence in the form of Seventh-day Adventist representation on the committee, and industry influence in the form of committee members' affiliations with various corporations. This is a longstanding concern – questions were also raised about the 2015 guidelines. Some 29,000 public comments were submitted, compared with only 2,000 in 2010.[23] Writing in the *BMJ*, Nina Teicholz argued that the expert report underpinning the guidelines had failed to reflect the findings of some important studies, one of the consequences of which has been a reinforcement of the idea that plant-based diets are best for health.[24]

Dr Georgia Ede pronounced her own verdict on the guidelines process in her presentation titled, 'Brainwashed: The mainstreaming of nutritional mythology' (available on YouTube).[25] She calls the USDA guidelines (1977–2015) one-third of a 'Holy Trinity' of reports that are 'responsible for implanting anti-meat messages in our minds', the other two being the 2015 WHO report on cancer and the 2019 EAT-Lancet report (discussed in earlier chapters). These reports have many characteristics in common, says Dr Ede, including the fact that they are 'lengthy, impenetrable, and unwelcoming ... omit/misrepresent studies that challenge their recommendations, [and their] arguments are irrational, incomplete [and] internally inconsistent'.[26] 'These documents are biased against animal foods in general and red meat in particular', with 'the most extreme position being the EAT-Lancet report'.

The 2015 USDA guidelines encourage the consumption of several servings of *refined* grains (italics mine) per day on the basis of the fact that they are fortified with iron and B vitamins, while discouraging the consumption of those whole (animal) foods that are naturally rich sources of iron and B vitamins.[27] Referring to a table of iron-rich foods included in the report, Dr Ede says 'of all the iron-rich foods on this table to choose from, they chose fortified cereals as their choice, which makes you wonder what forces influence the recommendations process'.[28]

One might reasonably ask whether those influential forces include corporations who produce fortified cereals. We might also ask whether the unconscious biases of the committee's membership might have played a role in shaping its recommendations. (Nine of the fourteen members of the guidelines committee had previously 'conducted research or written books in support of plant-based diets', says Dr Ede.)

The fight for evidence-based eating guidelines
Via her role as head of the Nutrition Coalition, Nina Teicholz has spent several years campaigning for the US guidelines to be more evidence based and less subject to industry influence but has found those involved in the process to be largely resistant to change.[29] We cannot discount the possibility that industry influence has also overshadowed the evidence in the UK. The 2016 Eatwell Guide was formulated by a group, appointed by Public Health England, that included a large contingent from industry: four out of eleven of the authors were representatives of industry groups (the Institute of Grocery Distribution, the British Retail Consortium, the Food and Drink Federation, and the Association of Convenience Stores); another three were representatives of nutrition or dietetic organisations with members in the food industry.[30] The new Eatwell Guide

increased the segments of the plate allocated to starchy foods and fruits and vegetables and decreased the segment allocated to dairy; non-dairy protein stayed the same but was renamed, becoming beans, pulses, fish, eggs and other proteins, effectively giving plant proteins parity with animal food proteins[31] and giving the impression that animal-sourced proteins were now completely optional.

Unilever marked this outcome by placing adverts in national newspapers to celebrate the fact that unsaturated fats, including their own margarine brand, Flora, had been given their own 'dedicated section'.[32] If Unilever thought the plate a triumph, Dr Harcombe labelled it the Eat Badly Plate, as we have already seen,[33] a guide for wealth, not health, that was not in the least evidence based. Dr Kendrick asserted that the anti-fat guidelines on which the plate is based are 'complete nonsense' and 'based on absolutely no research at all'.[34]

Even if the industry representatives involved in the guide's creation did not actively seek to influence the plate in their own favour (and I have no evidence that they did), it remains a real possibility that their unconscious biases (underpinned by a natural inclination to view their industry's products in a positive light and an appreciation of the drivers of business profitability) steered them away from embracing a low carbohydrate, real food, omnivorous diet. Whatever the biases in operation, it remains a fact that the outcome suits those involved down to the ground, since the corporations they represent produce none of the animal-sourced foods and all of the carbohydrate-based, processed foods in other sections of the plate.

The longstanding bias against animal-sourced foods

It's important to remember that, quite apart from any possible corporate influence over guidelines such as the Eatwell Guide and the Dietary Guidelines for Americans, the bias against animal-sourced foods within those guidelines has deep historical roots.

As we saw in Chapter 11, that bias originated in Adventist principles and influence, and has been solidified by the relationships between health-advice organisations and the food industry. Registered dietitian, farmer and author Diana Rodgers notes that 'in America, there are still SDA [Seventh-day Adventist Church] influences behind our meat-phobic guidelines' and that these influences worked their way into the official position paper in vegetarian diets issued by the Association of Nutrition and Dietetics (AND). When Diana was a dietetics student she was 'repeatedly told that eating a Paleo-type diet was unhealthy because it "cut out food groups," yet being a vegetarian or vegan was perfectly acceptable'.[35]

Like Diana Rodgers, Dr Caryn Zinn has testified as to the bias against meat and animal foods within dietetics organisations. Zinn now uses LCHF in her practice for both adults and children and is an advocate for real food, but she says that she is embarrassed by the fact that, in her university days, she never questioned her university lecturers' biased teaching about diet and nutrition, and the fact that she took these early biases into her own teaching and practice. Her 'Damascene moment' came in 2011 when a colleague asked her to provide evidence that proved that LCHF was a dangerous diet, and she realised that there wasn't any. She was 'flabbergasted' to discover that most of what she had learned and thought about diet and nutrition was wrong and that 'the evidence that led to mainstream dietary guidelines was largely observational, correlation-based research'.[36]

The anti-meat bias that colours so much of the advice promulgated by mainstream dietetics organisations is echoed in the pronouncements of other influential health-advice organisations such as the Physicians' Committee for Responsible Medicine (PCRM). No surprise, perhaps, given that the committee is led by vegan activist Dr Neil Barnard and that its largest donor is People for the Ethical Treatment of Animals (PETA). The PCRM's anti-meat stance masquerades as objective, evidence-based advice in its magazine, its continuing education courses for nurses and doctors, and materials that these nurses and doctors can hand to patients. The PCRM's *Nutrition Guide for Clinicians* – a book that blames meat for virtually every disease known to man – is given to new medical students, many of whom likely take it to be undisputed scientific fact. This despite the fact that the American Medical Association (AMA) has described the PCRM as 'neither physicians nor responsible'.[37] In fact, fewer than 10 per cent of the PCRM's 175,000 members are physicians.[38]

Many dietitians still operate within the same tram lines as the PCRM – discouraging the intake of saturated fat and animal-sourced foods, encouraging carbohydrate consumption amidst a diet that prioritises fruits and vegetables, whole grains, nuts and seeds. For some, this will be because their views are entirely consistent with that line, and they believe that the evidence supports it (which, as I argue in Part One, it does not). But to what extent are others swayed by the food industry via its deployment of what Mialon, Swinburn and Sacks identified as a 'financial incentive strategy'? I'm not talking about political lobbying here (although that is a factor, with the food industry paying millions to lobbyists in the US, for example).[39] I'm talking about funding directed towards dietary influencers – dietitians and dietary experts, health-advice organisations and academics.

How funding shapes the conversation about food and health in favour of plant-based diets

Mialon and colleagues describe corporate financial strategy as being the provision of 'funds, gifts, and other incentives to politicians, political parties and other decision makers'. One form that these financial incentives take is funding for initiatives that appear to be neutral and exploratory in nature but actually turn out to be geared towards promoting industry products and/or points of view.

Many of the activities backed by ILSI, the IFIC and the GEBN appear to match this description. Consider, also, the specific case of a 'Breakfast Council', set up by cereal giant Kellogg's. It was billed as being made up of independent experts who were to guide Kellogg's nutritional efforts. But it actually consisted of individuals who were paid 13,000 dollars a year, were prohibited from offering media services for products that were competitive or negative to cereal, and were required to engage in 'nutrition influencer outreach' on social media or with colleagues. The council managed to publish an academic paper defining a quality breakfast, but a Kellogg's employee oversaw the editing and asked for the removal of a line deemed unfavourable to Kellogg's products.[40]

Financial incentives also come in the form of sponsorship of and representation at dietetic conferences. For example, the list of sponsors of the Academy of Nutrition and Dietetics' 2019 Food and Nutrition Conference and Expo exhibition – the world's largest annual meeting of food and nutrition professionals – consisted exclusively of corporations from the pharmaceutical and processed food and drinks industries, including Big G Cereal, Danone, GSK Healthcare, Premier Protein, Splenda sweeteners and PepsiCo.[41] PepsiCo sponsoring a nutrition conference? It's no wonder that conference attendees advise the consumption of a 'balanced diet' that includes processed and sugary foods at the expense of real foods, and the *American Diabetes Association Magazine* can be found promoting peanut butter and Graham Cracker sandwiches stuffed with sweets and chocolate chips as a snack.

The food industry also 'targets key thought leaders and nutrition experts, offering freebies and stipends', and employs dietitians as part of their marketing teams.[42] Dietitians have been paid by both Coca-Cola and PepsiCo, for example, to endorse their products as being healthy snacks. Even when disclosures are made, they are usually in the fine print that goes unnoticed by consumers.[43] In 2015, the Associated Press reported that fitness and health experts had been paid to write posts during American Heart Month, each one featuring a mini can of Coke as a healthy snack idea. The publication asserted that the posted pieces (on nutrition blogs and other sites, including those of major newspapers) offered 'a window into the many ways food companies work behind the scenes to cast their products in a positive light, often with the help of third parties who are seen as trusted authorities'.[44]

The problem of industry influence over dietitians is so widespread that American dietitians opposed to taking industry money were prompted to found Dietitians for Professional Integrity (DFPI) to counter corporate influence.[45] DFPI considers its main purpose to be raising awareness, since many members of the Academy of Nutrition and Dietetics (formerly the American Dietetic Association) may be 'unfamiliar with the various repercussions and consequences of corporate sponsorship'.[46] Marion Nestle, professor emerita of nutrition, food studies and public health at New York University, writes that 'DFPI has forced the Academy to at least go through the motions of dealing with the effects of its sponsorship history and the current problems caused by its food industry ties',[47] and that while the Academy 'may still be stumbling in these dealings', it 'has come a long way'.

The complicated business of sponsorship
Corporate financial strategy also includes the provision of sponsorship monies (or funds in kind) to health advice

organisations. Sponsorship is a double-edged sword, providing much-needed funds that enable these organisations to do important, impactful work, but exposing them to potential corporate influence that could limit their independence. The American Heart Association's first significant sponsorship arrangement came in 1948, in the form of a 1.7-million-dollar (17 million dollars in today's money) donation from Procter & Gamble. This massive donation transformed the AHA from small fry to a big player, enabling it to invest in research and to establish regional chapters. But it also created a potential difficulty: it would have been difficult for the AHA to take a stand in favour of saturated fats and against polyunsaturated oils, such as those made by P&G and used as ingredients in most processed food. (In 1961, the AHA formally came out against saturated fat and in favour of polyunsaturated oils, and its position remains the same.)[48]

We cannot discount the possibility that the official advice given by the UK's specialist health organisations are similarly impacted by sponsorship arrangements. The sponsors of Diabetes UK, for example (www.diabetes.org.uk, not to be confused with www.diabetes.co.uk), include BHR Pharmaceuticals, Boots, Britvic, Bunzl, Florette, Janssen, Merck, Novo Nordisk, Roche, Saladmaster, Sanofi and Tesco.[49] Here, in one place, you have insulin makers, sugary drinks manufacturers, food retailers and an international distribution company that can ferry their products around. This is not to say that these sponsors exert direct pressure on Diabetes UK to promote their own products as part of a diabetes management strategy, but we can't discount the possibility that the very fact of the financial connection makes it awkward for Diabetes UK to pursue any strategy that might bring their sponsors' products into disrepute or damage their businesses.

Let's unpick why this might be. Corporations provide

sponsorship for a variety of reasons. Among them may be the desire to do good, and the motivating effect that sponsorship has on the employees of those corporations. However, one of the reasons that corporations give money to charities, foundations and patient advocacy groups is to 'advance brand objectives', as is explained by the following quote from *Pharmaceutical Executive* Magazine. 'Product managers see advocacy groups as allies to help advance brand objectives, like increasing disease awareness, building demand for new treatments and helping to facilitate FDA clearance of their drug.'[50] Sponsorship contracts in other sectors have been known to require the sponsored organisation to avoid engaging in activity or making statements that might discredit or damage the reputation of the sponsoring company.[51] It is probably naive to think that the food sector is immune to any such pressures.

Corporate funding of nutrition research and the scientists who conduct it: to what extent is it 'capture'?

Like sponsorship arrangements, the funding of nutrition research by corporations is a double-edged sword. And corporate funding is extensive. According to UK scientist and author Tim Spector, 'in the US, the food industry provides 70 per cent of the funding for food research, and the picture is similar in other countries'.[52] Company-funded research is directed towards areas that suit the industry while distracting the field 'from addressing the real problem of additive-rich, ultra-processed food,'[53] says Spector.

Professor Noakes attests to the potentially negative influence of industry funding: 'Our research was once funded by the carbohydrate industry, and that is capture. You can't be objective. What you're looking for is continued funding for more research, so you write things up in a way that will serve that end. It's not that you cheat, but you might not conduct experiments that could disprove your hypothesis. It's so easy just to accumulate evidence that supports you.[54]

It was disclosed that even federally funded health researchers in the US have *at least* 188 million dollars in potential conflicts of interest (dating from 2012). These interests range from stock holdings in companies that might benefit from the outcome of the research to payments for royalties, consulting work and speaking engagements. Harvard University Professor David Sinclair, named one of the most influential people in healthcare by *Time* magazine, reported equity stakes of more than 600,000 dollars in two separate companies that would appear to benefit from research findings resulting from his studies. Yale, via its connection with David Katz, has been paid 15 million dollars for pro-nut studies, and Katz himself has been paid millions to defend and promote sugar, nuts and other plant-based foods.[55]

These examples are just two of many. One journalist, reporting on the surfeit of competing interests in the industry, asked 'can you trust their findings?'[56] Certainly, one can reasonably ask whether the research that results from such industry funding can ever be truly independent or taken completely at face value. Marion Nestle concluded that 'funding effects appear in nutrition research as well as drug research'.[57] In 2015, she collected and published food industry-sponsored studies on her blog, Food Politics, finding that seventy-five of the studies were favourable to the sponsors while just six were not.[58]

A small victory for transparency and independence in nutrition science came in late 2020, when the campaigning efforts of the Corporate Responsibility group resulted in Coca-Cola announcing that it would officially terminate its ILSI membership effective January 2021. This followed previous decisions by Mars, Inc. (noted earlier) and Nestlé to discontinue their memberships. ILSI, it seemed, had become a 'reputational liability' for these companies.[59]

ILSI has been rebranded AFSI (Agriculture and Food Systems Institute). Corporate Responsibility notes that it has the same team, trustees and corporate ties as ILSI, and 'is still backed by the private sector and supports research on topics such as nutrition and food'. It remains to be seen whether the AFSI carves a new path and behaves less like ILSI, which, you'll recall, the *New York Times* called a 'shadowy industry group'.[60]

Welcome to the Wild West of nutrition science

The financial links between corporations and researchers, and the potential conflicts that result, are just two characteristics of a field that Nina Teicholz has called the Wild West of nutrition science, 'a place where bullying is rife and epidemiological research amplifying weak associations by using relative risk in place of absolute risk is used to frighten the public unjustifiably'.[61] When the *Annals of Internal Medicine* published its papers (discussed in Chapter 1) showing that the evidence linking red meat consumption to heart disease and cancer is too weak to recommend that adults eat less of it (which Teicholz described as being like 'a bombshell' in the world of nutrition science), there was more than a whiff of the Wild West in the ensuing furore.[62]

That reaction consisted of some 2,000 emails flooding into the inbox of *Annals* editor-in-chief Christine Laine, most bearing the same 'caustic' message and apparently generated by a bot linked to the True Health Initiative (referred to on page 360). 'We've published a lot on firearm injury prevention,' Laine said. 'The response from the NRA [National Rifle Association] was less vitriolic than the response from the True Health Initiative.'[63]

You might recall that the THI is the non-profit organisation birthed from the Adventist-linked ACLM and founded and headed by well-known plant-based advocate David Katz MD. Walter Willett and Frank Hu from Harvard University serve on the THI council of directors. Katz, Willett and Hu 'took the rare step of contacting Laine about retracting the studies prior to publication', the timing of these demands suggesting that the journal's embargo policy had been violated. They subsequently accused the *Annals* researchers of having used inappropriate methodology (the rigorous GRADE method, which they deemed unsuitable for nutrition research) and of having conflicts of interest (of which more in a moment). Neil Barnard, head of the PCRM (the plant-based advocacy organisation mentioned earlier) launched a campaign to expose those conflicts.

The reaction to the papers by certain parties was undoubtedly driven by genuine differences of opinion about meat and health, and about what constitutes solid evidence. In addition, professional reputations were at stake: 'Some of the researchers have built their careers on nutrition epidemiology,' Laine said. 'I can understand it's upsetting when the limitations of your work are uncovered and discussed in the open.'[64] Dr Michael Eades put it more bluntly in a tweet, commenting that 'their lives' work goes up in smoke if it turns out meat isn't a killer'.[65] Revealing exactly how much was at stake, Katz himself likened the articles to '"information terrorism" that can blow to smithereens ... the life's work of innumerable careful scientists'.[66]

But we must ask whether something other than intellectual differences might also have been at play here. It happens that many of the individuals who objected so vehemently had a record of accepting funds (for research) from corporations in the sugar, nut and processed plant-based food industries; businesses that thrive on the promotion of plant-based diets and the corresponding notion that meat is bad for us. You don't have to draw a crude, direct line of influence to hypothesise that those corporate ties might have coloured the perspectives of the objectors. Could unconscious bias, formed over years of promoting, for example, carbohydrate-based packaged foods,[67] along with an acute awareness of the need to protect the hand that feeds, reasonably be suspected to have intensified what were longstanding intellectual positions?

In fact, unconscious biases based on industry connections may have affected both sides of the debate. It emerged that the chief author of the *Annals* papers had previously accepted funds from AgriLife Research (an arm of Texas A&M University that is partly funded by the beef industry) for a meta-analysis on saturated fat and authored a study on sugar funded by ILSI.[68] These competing interests were later acknowledged in a correction. As for the competing interests evident in the anti-*Annals* camp, these were dismissed by the parties involved. Katz played down his own and THI's conflicts of interest and, later, said 'we're not anti-meat ... we're just pro-science'.[69] His critics begged to disagree. McMaster University professor, and a leader in the development of evidence-based medicine, Gordon Guyatt called the Katz camp's response 'completely predictable' and 'hysterical'. Tufts University professor Sheldon Krimsky called it a 'political campaign' akin to those he had seen waged by Monsanto. Steven Novella, MD, a Yale neurologist, branded team Katz's response 'a total hit job' to dismiss scientific findings they don't like.[70]

At the heart of this case is an important fact of which we, as observers and laypeople, need to be aware. Nutrition research is an imperfect science, epidemiological research the most imperfect of all. As we saw in Chapter 1, Professor John Ioannidis of Stanford University has gone on record as saying that the field of epidemiological research is so flawed that it requires a complete reboot.[71] (Note that when epidemiological outcomes are tested in clinical trials, they are proven wrong over 80 per cent of the time.[72]) The necessary reboot may be on its way. 'People are realising that epidemiological studies that attribute something to one food are spurious,' says Stephan van Vliet. 'The critics are getting louder.'[73]

In light of the acknowledged imperfections in the field of epidemiology and the pervasiveness of industry funding, it's critical that the quality of the science applied in any particular study be subjected to intense scrutiny, the underlying methodology appraised for its ability to tease out the facts. The review methodology applied in the *Annals* research (GRADE) is widely thought to be the most rigorous, delivering outcomes that are most likely to be reliable and independent of bias. In the eyes of the many scientists who defended the *Annals* research, that rigorous methodology ultimately triumphed over doubts raised about transparency and conflicts of interest.

When individuals are targeted in the Wild West

In Chapter 11 I recounted the story of a medical practitioner in Tasmania whose advocation of low-sugar diets brought him into conflict with the Adventist church and those in the cereal and dietetics industries. Another story played out simultaneously, 10,000km away in South Africa; one that also demonstrates how the pursuit of commercial objectives by corporations can translate into influence over the debate about food and health in favour of plant-based diets.

Here is how the South African story ostensibly began. On 5 February 2014, an emeritus professor of sports science and nutrition, Professor Tim Noakes (whom we've met in this and previous chapters), tweeted the following to a woman who had enquired about whether it was OK for breastfeeding mums to eat a low carb, high-fat (LCHF) diet, and whether eating dairy and cauliflower might give a baby wind.

@ – @ – Baby doesn't eat the dairy and cauliflower. Just
very healthy high fat breast milk. Key is to ween (sic) baby
onto LCHF.[74]

On 6 February 2014, following a flurry of responding tweets
from other parties, including Johannesburg dietitian Claire
Julsing Strydom, then president of the ADSA (Association
for Dietetics in South Africa), Strydom reported Noakes to
the Health Professionals Council of South Africa (HPCSA),
complaining that his tweet was 'dangerous'. Her complaint led
to a formal hearing that set off what Noakes' lawyers called
the 'unprecedented prosecution and persecution of a world-
famous scientist simply for his opinions on nutrition'.[75] The
ordeal began in June 2015 and ended in June 2018 – after
the HPCSA's appeal committee confirmed in full its first
committee's ruling in April 2017, exonerating Noakes of any
wrongdoing. The story of Noakes' ordeal is recounted in the
book, *Real Food on Trial: How the Diet Dictators Tried to
Destroy a Distinguished Scientist*, which Noakes co-authored
with journalist Marika Sboros. (The book has been described
as 'an absolute jaw-dropping page turner',[76] an accolade for
which I can vouch.)

According to Noakes' lawyer, 'Dieticians brought the case
against Noakes because he disagreed with them.'[77] Dietitians
weren't the only ones who disagreed with Noakes. Those who
lined up against Noakes included not just Strydom and other
ADSA dietitians but others in the medical community who
objected to his views on LCHF diets and his challenge to the
medical orthodoxy linking saturated fat to heart disease. What
became clear during the course of the trial is that the reaction
to the tweet came in the wake of attempts to discredit Noakes
and his views about LCHF over a period of many years.

While Professor Noakes was the immediate target, it was
his unorthodox views about cholesterol (that the hypothesis

linking saturated fat and cholesterol to heart disease did not hold water) and diet (that LCHF was a safe and healthful diet) that his opponents seemed determined to discredit. In their attempt to discredit these views they were also indirectly giving credence to the plant-based cause.

How so? Because – as previously discussed – a real-food LCHF diet, which typically includes meat and other animal foods and excludes many of the carbohydrate-rich foods around which a plant-based diet is centred, poses an inherent challenge to a plant-based diet. If the LCHF diet and the plant-based diet were people, they would be natural adversaries. In attacking the former, as Noakes' opponents did, you are effectively giving credence to the latter.

The trial also revealed a spider's web of connections between corporations and those in the nutrition and medical community who are aligned around the anti-low-carb/pro-plant-based message. The case is littered with examples of medical practitioners and dietitians with potential competing interests, many of them documented in *Real Food on Trial*, and in Russ Greene's investigative piece for *Keep Fitness Legal*, 'Big food vs. Tim Noakes: The final crusade'.[78] Some were paid consultants to companies in the cereal and sugar industries.

Others were involved with ILSI. Russ Green summarised ILSI links as follows: 'A former ILSI South Africa president convinced the HPCSA to charge Noakes, another former ILSI South African president testified as an expert witness against him, and an ILSI-funded researcher consulted for the legal team prosecuting him.'[79]

Green also pointed out that ILSI and Big Sugar had given funding to the authors of a report that was used against Noakes (the Naudé Review), and that an ILSI trustee was involved in the Naudé Review, although her name never appeared in the published study. He asked, was this 'yet another example of hidden ILSI influence?'[80]

Based on Greene's analysis, Sboros hypothesised that the key drivers of the hearing against Noakes were likely those who were linked to ILSI.[81] Others involved included the former CEO of the Heart and Stroke Foundation of South Africa (HSFSA), who spoke out against Noakes and low-carb diets in the press before the hearing in 2013. The HSFSA's sponsorship by prominent firms within the food industry – producers of foods like polyunsaturated oils, confectionary, breakfast cereals, grains, sugar-sweetened beverages and ice cream[82] – would make it difficult for them to actively embrace any dietary approach that advises against the consumption of these foods. Heart Foundations around the world find themselves in a similarly awkward position. This is not to accuse them of intentional skulduggery, but merely to recognise the commercial realities underlying sponsorship arrangements.

Lessons from the battlefield

At the end of the four-year ordeal, which included an appeal when the HPCSA initially lost its case, Professor Noakes was declared not guilty. Like Gary Fettke, he was free to talk about real food and LCHF, and express whatever opinions he liked about conventional theories linked to the diet–heart hypothesis. How did Noakes come out the winner, when so many in the medical and nutritional establishment had seemed determined to discredit his ideas? Noakes and his witnesses used evidence to prove that he had not been negligent in talking about LCHF, whether in relation to breastfeeding mothers, babies or anyone else, and that his theories about the real causes of heart disease, obesity, diabetes and other chronic diseases are backed up by solid research. In contrast, the HPCSA's witnesses were unable to present sufficient convincing evidence to support their accusations against him.

Like the Fettke case, the Noakes case represents an extreme example of what happens when doctors, dietitians and academics take action to suppress messaging they disagree with. It also exemplifies a worrying level of interconnectedness between those same professionals and the corporate world, in the form of sponsorship arrangements, funding for studies, and consultancy agreements. It's impossible to say whether or to what extent that interconnectedness influenced the actions of those who stood against Noakes. But it's reasonable to ask whether biases – unconscious or otherwise – might have been a contributing factor. It's widely considered to be unwise to bite the hand that feeds you; failing to challenge the LCHF message might be seen as tantamount to biting the hand of those whose business it is to produce and promote high carbohydrate, plant-based foods.

Noakes had challenged not just establishment views about LCHF but the orthodoxy around LDL cholesterol. As such, he had struck at the heart of the ability of the medical establishment and the pharmaceutical industry to control the messaging around LDL. Control of that messaging is perhaps the single most important way that the pharmaceutical industry impacts the debate about food and health in favour of plant-based diets. We'll look at this now.

How Big Pharma stage manages the LDL show and fuels the fear of animal-sourced foods

Big Pharma's influence over the debate about cholesterol is really just part and parcel of its wider influence over medicine as a whole. I want to spend some time on this because it provides important context. Please bear with me while I take a short detour through the world of pharmaceutical influence over the medical establishment and medical opinion.

Dr Ben Goldacre explains exactly how pharmaceutical influence is wielded in his book, *Bad Pharma*.[83] He acknowledges all the good that the industry does – and there is much good – while exposing the ways in which the industry often manipulates and distorts science, and, with it, our perceptions of diseases and how best to treat them. He outlines the wide range of tactics deployed by pharmaceutical companies to influence research in their favour, including failing to publish studies with negative outcomes, summarising studies in such a way as to exaggerate or even distort results, designing trials in order to achieve a positive outcome, and withholding trial data, even from the researchers conducting the study. As Goldacre is at pains to point out, the problem is (most of the time)[84] not with individual researchers behaving improperly, but rather a system that allows, enables and even encourages industry to manage and manipulate the research process via what he calls 'elegant mischief at the margins of acceptability'.[85]

As a result of this elegant mischief, industry funded studies are far more likely to generate positive results for industry products. Goldacre cites a number of studies that show this to be true, including two systematic reviews which looked at all the studies ever published to see whether industry funding is associated with pro-industry results. Both found that industry funded trials were about four times more likely to report positive results.[86] 'There is no doubt on the issue,' says Goldacre. 'Industry sponsored trials give favourable results, and that is not just my opinion, or a hunch from the occasional passing study. This is a very well-documented problem and it has been researched extensively, without anybody stepping out to take effective action.'[87]

Others have painted a similar picture of industry influence over research, including Marcia Angell MD (former editor of the *NEJM* and author of *The Truth About the Drug Companies*), Jerome Kassirer (*On the Take: How Medicine's Complicity with Big Business Can Endanger Your Health*) and Dr Malcolm Kendrick (*Doctoring Data*). A 2005 feature in the *Journal of the American Board of Family Medicine* had this to say on the matter:

> The removal of research from academic centres also gives pharmaceutical companies greater control over the design of studies, analysis of data, and publication of results ... The end result: among even the highest quality research the odds are 5.3 times greater that commercially funded studies will support their sponsor's products than non-commercially funded studies.[88]

Another study, by *American Journal of Psychiatry* authors, found that 'in 90 per cent of the studies [analysed], the reported overall outcome was in favour of the sponsor's drug'.[89] And a 2008 article reported that drug studies are usually skewed towards study sponsors.[90]

Summing up the situation, Angell wrote, 'It is simply no longer possible to believe much of the clinical research that is published, or to rely on the judgement of trusted physicians or authoritative medical guidelines. I take no pleasure in this conclusion, which I reached slowly and reluctantly over my two decades as an editor of the *New England Journal of Medicine*.'[91]

If industry influence over the research process is well documented, so is the manner in which the industry sways both doctors and patients via its marketing activities. Marketing is a broad term which covers things like advertising in medical journals (and, in the US, direct to patients), sales visits to doctors, celebrity endorsements, medical conferences and the 'ghostwriting' of academic papers. (A practice whereby drug companies write academic papers then pay medical professionals to put their names to them.) According to both Goldacre and Angell, even many activities that are formally classified as 'education' for health professionals are in fact marketing efforts in disguise. Disclosures are made, of course, but not always in a way that registers with those on the receiving end of the education. One study of a pharmaceutical conference found that 89 per cent of presenters had COIs (conflicts of interest), and that there was an inverse correlation between the number of COIs of the presenter and the length of time that the disclosure information was displayed, resulting in a 'speed of delivery that almost always prevents adequate comprehension'.[92]

And of course, there are direct payments to health professionals, which are worth billions, says Angell:

> no one knows the total amount provided by drug companies to physicians, but I estimate from the annual reports of the top 9 U.S. based drug companies that it comes to tens of billions of dollars a year in North America alone ... this affects the results of research, the way medicine is practiced, and even the definition of what constitutes a disease.[93]

Other sources corroborate Angell's view that payments to medical professionals are common. A *BMJ* study found that 80 per cent of doctors on the boards of professional medical organisations in the US had financial ties to industry.[94] A 2017 investigation revealed that Australian nurses, dietitians, pharmacists and other health workers receive millions of dollars in payments (in the form of consulting and guest-speaking fees) from big pharmaceutical companies.[95] For the most part, this is completely legal and above board, just part of what Goldacre calls 'the banal, commercial reality of what these companies do'.

Above board and banal though they are, these funds have impact – evidence has shown that doctors who attend pharmaceutical company educational events, for example, do prescribe their products more.[96] Goldacre's book documents just how much impact other marketing activities have, influencing doctors' perceptions of different diseases and how to treat them. He acknowledges that while this influence can sometimes be helpful, it often leads to the prescription of a substandard or inappropriate drug.

A prescription mindset may be the more insidious outcome of these close links between industry and clinicians – the idea that pharmacotherapy, not nutrition, is the first line of intervention to treat and prevent chronic conditions. Innovation and dissent are other casualties of the system. Dr Kendrick writes that 'in the medical research world, those in positions of power do not take kindly to anyone daring to question the established order. Instead, they close ranks and retaliate.'[97] Harlan Krumholz MD, explains what retaliation means in practice:

> A hidden curriculum teaches us not to disturb the status quo. We are trained to defer to authority, not to question it. We depend on powerful individuals and organisations and are taught that success does not come often to those who ask uncomfortable questions or suggest new ways of providing care ... those who ask difficult questions or challenge conventional wisdom are often isolated. They may find few opportunities to speak and their writings may not be welcome. Compliance with normative behaviour may be forced by fear of recrimination. In some cases, junior faculty may fear that support from mentors will be withdrawn or promotions denied.[98]

Professor Noakes experienced the full force of the kind of retaliation that Krumholz describes when he was seen to be challenging the prevailing orthodoxy around cholesterol and diet. That orthodoxy is powerful indeed, and it is maintained by the same mechanisms that operate across the pharmaceutical industry as a whole – enormous industry influence over research and extensive marketing and 'education' efforts. And it's easy to see why so much effort is directed at maintaining the orthodoxy. If saturated fat and high LDL (on its own, and in the absence of other worrying indicators) ceased to be concerns, and it was universally acknowledged that high triglyceride levels and other symptoms of metabolic syndrome were the real culprits in heart-disease risk, and, moreover, that these symptoms could be treated with diet (in particular, a low carbohydrate, animal-food inclusive diet) – well, the writing would be on the wall for the statin makers.

Fortunately for the statin makers, they've managed to keep LDL at the top of the list of risk factors for heart disease. They've achieved this, in part, by controlling most of the research itself and by influencing the way research results are interpreted and communicated to medical professionals and the public, as well as by influencing the treatment protocols and guidelines issued by the AHA and the universities to whom it gives money.[99] If you're in any doubt about the extent of industry influence in this regard, I urge you to read Dr Kendrick's two books, *The Great Cholesterol Con* and *Doctoring Data*, or check out his blog at www.drmalcolmkendrick.org.

The result is a consensus surrounding LDL and statin treatment that Dr Kendrick has called a 'collective madness', and Dr Verner Wheelock has referred to as a bandwagon that rolls on, impervious to the reams of data that not only fail to support it but actually prove it to be false.[100] For Wheelock, the elephant in the room is all-cause mortality: even those studies that have shown some marginal benefit from lowering LDL cholesterol have demonstrated that the risk of death from other causes actually increases.[101]

The power of the consensus is so great that even where research is not funded by industry its results are often interpreted in a way that is favourable to the prevailing orthodoxy. Weak findings are amplified and any inconvenient, contradictory data is omitted. An example of the amplification of weak findings is represented by the 150-million-dollar LRC-CPPT study (Lipid Research Clinic's Coronary Primary Prevention Trial), funded by the NHLBI (National Heart, Lung and Blood Institute) and commencing in 1958, a study highlighted by Dr Wheelock. The study found that 1.6 per cent of those given the cholesterol-lowering drug suffered a fatal heart attack compared to 2 per cent of those in the control group. All-cause mortality (ACM) was virtually the same for both groups, 3.6 per cent versus 3.7 per cent. In absolute terms, says Wheelock, 'this was not exactly a profound difference'. This did not stop the trial director from proclaiming that the trial group (who had been given the cholesterol-lowering drug) had a 19 per cent reduction in risk, and that the study 'strongly indicates that the more you lower cholesterol and fat in your diet, the more you reduce your risk of heart disease'.[102] Note that, as is typical, it was the *relative* risk reduction (19 per cent) that was being highlighted, because the *actual* risk reduction was inconsequential (the trial group lost 1.6 people for every 100, whereas the control group lost 2 people). The trial director also failed to mention the ACM data, 'which would have destroyed the study's credibility'.[103]

As discussed briefly in Chapter 1, this and other studies have shown that the average life extension made possible by lowering cholesterol is minimal.[104] But in an environment where profits guide so many decisions, what incentive is there for statin makers to do anything other than downplay this reality? The lengths to which some will go to prioritise profits is evidenced by a story recounted by Professor Douglas Boyd, the inventor of the coronary artery scan (CAC scan). Boyd was keen to see widespread take up of the scan, which he believed would benefit both patients and doctors by providing more accurate assessments of heart disease risk. Boyd and his colleagues entered into discussions with the major pharmaceutical companies, offering to team up with them to use the scan to predict who might need to be prescribed statins. Every company turned him down, saying that they didn't want to encourage a take-up of CAC scans because 'that would mean we wouldn't get to sell our drugs to the people who don't need them'.[105]

Where does all this leave ordinary doctors and patients?

Thanks to food and drug industry power and influence – accepted and even encouraged by those at the top of health organisations, and part and parcel of customary funding arrangements – a skewed interpretation of the evidence (and in some cases, misinformation) drifts downwards to doctors who are too harried, too frightened or simply unwilling to question it. A worrying level of misinformation exists among doctors, with 92 per cent still believing, for example, that fat consumption could lead to cardiovascular issues. Fifty-four per cent of doctors and 40 per cent of nutritionists also believe that eating cholesterol-rich foods raises blood cholesterol and that statins definitely save lives.[106] All these views feed the plant-based message. The steady, drip-drip of messaging against saturated fats and animal foods, whether via official pronouncements or casual remarks by doctors, leads many to believe that they should fall in line with the plant-based zeitgeist.

Patients who do their own research often find that their GP disregards it (as we saw in Chapter 5). But as these patients take control of their health, preferring to use food as medicine rather than succumb to the lure of the statin or insulin solution, they contribute to an ever stronger body of evidence.

That evidence has caught the attention of the life insurance and reinsurance industries. Dr Eric Westman, who attended a conference called Food for Thought organised by a multinational life insurance company and the *BMJ* in 2018, explained why these industries have come on side: 'The life insurance industry is banking on people living longer, and people aren't living longer. These companies are looking for options for diabetes management other than the current standard medical treatment. They know that this [low-carb] works. So, they are the only ones who are aligned with us.'[107]

Professor Tim Spector writes, about the same meeting, that he 'sensed many different segments of the healthcare profession were openly contesting nutritional dogmas' and 'accepting that many of the cornerstones of our philosophy about eating well are based on flawed studies conducted many decades ago'. General practitioners were able to cite both clinical evidence and randomised trials showing that type-2 diabetes could be controlled without drugs with a low-carbohydrate, higher-fat diet, evidence that stood in stark contrast to 'official incentives that promote drugs first and guidelines recommending that diabetic patients should especially avoid fat'.[108]

UK doctors David and Jen Unwin, who have helped over one hundred of their own patients, and many more beyond their practice, to reverse their type-2 diabetes and address other medical conditions with a low-carb approach, have taken heart from this recognition from the life insurance industry, and from the power of grass-roots action to counterbalance official messaging. In the low-carb groups that they run, they witness patients sharing success stories, and in the global network of doctors with whom the Unwins are in regular contact, and the low-carb conferences that attract thousands, they see a grass-roots movement that will, eventually, foster a revolution in primary (GP) care. 'Seeing is believing,' says David Unwin: 'It's percolating up through primary care, then I predict that secondary care will be influenced. Whether or not it will overtake official advice in my lifetime, I don't know. But it's interesting that the American Diabetes Association now supports low carb and have said that it does work. The Scottish and Canadian organisations have done the same. Others will have to come on board or they'll look ridiculous, since so many people are improving their health by doing the exact opposite of what these organisations are saying.'[109]

For the Unwins, LCHF goes hand in hand with an appreciation of real food as medicine, and real food includes nutrient-dense animal foods. 'If people just ate local lamb, leeks and cabbages, the world would be a better place,' Jen says. The world is certainly a better place for the efforts of Drs Jen and David Unwin. Like other members of the grass-roots food-is-medicine movement, they are fighting for our health amidst the noise generated by the established voices within industry and nutritional science.

They're also battling the misinformation that is spread – wittingly or unwittingly – by the mainstream media, parts of which have ceased to investigate and report objectively on our behalf and have, instead, become akin to stage managers in the play that we see staged every day; a play that portrays a plant-based diet as the salvation of human and planetary health. We'll take a look at how media coverage can be misleading in the next chapter.

13

Headlines, Blurred Lines and Tricks of the Documentary Trade: How the Media Reflect and Reinforce the Plant-based Zeitgeist

A BBC news online feature in May 2020 offered up tips for individuals wanting to reduce their carbon footprint.[1] The article, based on research by Leeds University, concluded that living car-free or driving an electric car and making changes to energy use in the home would deliver more benefits than switching to a vegan diet; however, despite those findings, the photo beneath the headline was not of a car or a home, but of a burger.

Perhaps this was an innocent mistake. Maybe they didn't have a picture of a car or a house to hand. Maybe the burger just looked more attractive editorially. Or maybe the choice of photo was deliberate, the act of someone already biased against meat and towards a vegan diet; someone who thought the research *ought* to have shown that switching to a vegan diet was the single most impactful thing people could do. Whatever it was that led to the choice of photo, we can be reasonably sure that many will have read the headline and looked at the eye-catching picture[2] without registering the caption that said 'Switching to a vegan diet can help but doesn't quite have the impact of other measures', or without reading the entire article, and concluded that the number-one change they should make to their lifestyle is to stop eating meat. They would have heard this line of argument so many times before that they would have assumed that's what was being said or even ceased to question it.

The use of inappropriate photos, whether calculated or otherwise, is just one way in which the media can distort the public's perception and thus the debate about food, health and the environment. At the other extreme, bias has been found to be at play. In late 2020 the BBC was forced to admit that one of its programmes, *Meat: A Threat to Our Planet*, fronted by Liz Bonnin, had 'violated impartiality standards by giving viewers a partial analysis of the impact of global livestock farming on the global environment and biodiversity, based almost exclusively on intensive farming methods' in other countries, with limited relevance to UK consumers as the beef in the UK is not as intensively farmed.[3]

Like the BBC, *The Economist* gave readers a partial analysis when reporting on the conclusions of Marco Springmann's study, 'Multiple health and environmental impacts of foods', under the headline, 'How much would giving up meat help the environment?' and the subheading, 'Going vegan for two-thirds of meals could cut food-related carbon emissions by 60%'.[4] The study had many critics, but *The Economist* did not cite such criticisms or offer its own. Neither did it make readers aware that the study had been co-authored by a scientist with a record of advocating for plant-based diets and peer reviewed by an academic at an institution with a commitment to supporting the global mission of the Seventh-day Adventist Church, which, itself, advocates for plant-based diets for religious reasons.[5] (That, at the very least, would allow the reader to consider the influence of any unconscious biases.) To make matters worse, and as we saw in Chapter 7, *The Economist* got its own maths wrong by ten times, proclaiming, at the end of the article, that we could reduce our entire footprint by 85 per cent by becoming 'leaf eaters'.[6]

It's possible, as Professor Leroy suggests, that journalists do not fully understand the models on which they are expected to report.[7] If this is true in the case of *The Economist* what hope is there for how the facts are interpreted in a more populist publication? In July 2019, *Red* magazine featured an article titled 'Save the planet for the kids', in which it outlined the different ways that people could take action against climate change.[8] Suggestions included 'move your money', 'cut down on flying' and 'buy less stuff'. At the end of the article was a short section summarising '3 more ways you can flight climate change', one of which was 'Go Vegan(er)'. In the 'Go Vegan(er)' section, the founder of the non-profit project Environmentally Conscious was quoted as saying that livestock 'account for a quarter of negative emissions'. No one picked up on the fact that this claim was grossly inaccurate: as we saw in Chapter 7, livestock are responsible for 14 per cent of emissions globally, and for less than 6 per cent in places like the UK and the US. On reading the incorrect claim, thousands of *Red* readers might have walked away believing that 'going vegan' would make a much bigger difference than it actually would.

Of all the ways in which the media can misinform and distort, the use of misleading headlines is perhaps the most common. Four examples that I examined from early 2021 illustrate how easily this happens. The first pertains to the reporting on a study by Yangbo Sun, Buyan Liu and colleagues titled 'Association of major protein sources with all-cause and cause-specific mortality: prospective cohort study'.[9] (I discussed this study in the context of the evidence for meat and cancer in Chapter 1.) *The Times* reported on the study under the headline 'Vegans are full of beans in later years', with the lead sentence stating that 'A vegan-style diet high in plant proteins could almost halve older women's risk of an early grave.'[10] The *Daily Mail* (MailOnline) used the headline 'Time to ditch the meat? High protein vegan diet can slash the risk of early death by almost 50%, study reveals'.[11] It took a bit of digging around for me to locate the study to which both papers were referring, since most articles of this kind don't include details about or links to the studies in question. When I identified the correct study, I found that its conclusions did not in any way support the newspaper headlines. The data showed some extremely small, lower relative risks (note the word 'relative' here) associated with (note the word 'associated' here, meaning no causal link has been established) swapping out some animal proteins for some plant proteins. But the claimed 50 per cent reduction in mortality for older women was nowhere to be found. Moreover, on page seven of the study it was stated that 'animal protein intake was not associated with all-cause mortality, comparing the highest with the lowest quintile'. In other words, if you eat a little animal protein or a lot of it, it has no effect on the likelihood of your dying early.

There were many weaknesses in the study itself, including the fact that the FFQs (food frequency questionnaires) on which it was based had been found (by the authors' admission) to be less than 60 per cent accurate. (This is not unusual – the FFQs which serve as the basis of most epidemiological studies like this have been shown to be similarly unreliable.) These weaknesses aside, the newspaper headlines were not reflective of the data evidenced in the study. Sure enough, when I wrote to one of the authors of the study, he confirmed that the 50 per cent claim was not based on the conclusions of the study.

So what happened? It may be that the sub-editors who wrote the headlines simply expanded on one of the statements contained in the press release for the study, which was this: 'substitution of total red meat, eggs or dairy products with nuts was associated with a 12% to 47% lower risk of death from all causes depending on the type of protein replaced with nuts', seizing on the number 47 and rounding it up to 'almost 50'. Analysis of the data in the study itself reveals that there was a single data point (of many) showing that replacement of eggs with nuts was associated with as much as a 47 per cent reduction in CVD mortality. All other associations – and they are only associations after all, not evidence of causation – were significantly weaker (and even this one is a small relative risk in the context of the advice given by some scientists to discount any relative risks less than 100 per cent). One of the co-authors of the study, Yangbo Sun, warned (in the press release) that 'the interpretation of these findings could be challenging and should be based on consideration of the overall diet including different cooking methods'. But newspapers appear to have extrapolated from a single, challenging-to-interpret data point to produce dramatic headlines such as 'high protein vegan diet can slash the risk of early death by almost 50%'.

The headline of another article which appeared in the print edition of *The Times* less than a month later was similarly misleading. It proclaimed a 'Rasher of bacon a day linked to a 44% rise in dementia risk'.[12] In this instance, at least the text beneath the headline served to clarify matters. The supervisor of the research in question noted that 'this is a first step. We're not confirming anything here', adding that even if a link with processed meat were proven, the increase in absolute risk would be small. Other experts weighed in, one pointing to the relatively small sample size and warning us not to overinterpret the results. Another doctor who works with dementia patients said that the data 'wouldn't persuade me to give up the breakfast bacon'.[13]

What *The Times* headline might have said was that a recent observational study (which, by definition, cannot show causation) with a tiny sample size had shown a very small, and probably inconsequential, relative risk increase for dementia from eating bacon. But that doesn't make for a very exciting headline. On one level, you have to have some sympathy for those responsible for writing headlines interesting enough to generate the eyeballs and clicks that drive advertising revenues. Often, they have the unenviable job of trying to make silk purses out of sows' ears. This leaves us, as readers, with the unenviable job of making sure we can spot the sows' ears. The trouble is, most readers probably don't have the time to interrogate articles and the studies on which they are based, or even to read beyond the headlines. Which is why headlines should accurately reflect the content of both articles and source studies.

The experts interviewed for *The Times* article about bacon and dementia were able to qualify the headline. However, as is often the case, the qualifiers disappeared from subsequent coverage of the study. A week later, *The Times* published another article titled, 'Put down that bacon sandwich! It's bad for your brain'.[14] There was no mention of the fact that the association thrown up by the study was extremely small and relative, or of the reservations about the study's results that had been expressed by various experts.

In another case of mismatch between headline, story and study, both the print and online versions of *The Times* proclaimed that 'a plant-centred diet rich in leafy greens can reverse ageing by two years' under the headline, 'Fancy heading back in time? Eat your greens'.[15] It was reported that scientists from the Institute for Functional Medicine in Washington had discovered that 'eating mainly vegetables such as kale and Swiss chard helped to dramatically slow the rate of age-related biological processes'. But in the next paragraph, we discovered that the age-defying diet had included three weekly servings of liver and up to ten eggs a week. And yet the headline talked only of the benefits of eating greens. A more accurate headline would have proclaimed the benefits to longevity of eating highly nutritious foods such as greens, liver and eggs. But such is the power of the plant-based zeitgeist that headlines are almost invariably written to support it.

The media coverage of another study published in 2021 had the effect of exaggerating the benefits of eating a plant-based diet, not because of a mismatch between headline and study outcomes, but because the articles did not properly interrogate the study itself. The study, 'Plant-based diets, pescatarian diets and Covid-19 severity: a population-based case-control study in six countries', was originally published in *BMJ Nutrition Prevention and Health*.[16] Its abstract claimed that 'In six countries, plant-based diets were associated with lower odds of moderate-to-severe COVID 19. These dietary patterns may be considered for protection against severe Covid-19.' Headlines pertaining to the study included 'Vegans or pescatarian diet may reduce Covid severity, study finds' (*Evening Standard*); 'Vegans "much less likely to get severe Covid-19 than meat eaters", study suggests' (the *Independent*); and 'Vegetarians "three quarters less likely to get severe Covid than meat eaters"' (the *Telegraph*).[17]

These were spectacular claims. But those who appraised them with a critical eye – or were inclined to seek out the appraisals of independent experts – would soon find that, while the headlines *did* reflect the study's claims, the claims themselves were open to question. Experts came forward to point out various flaws in the original study: like all observational studies, it could show association but not causation; it had been based on self-reported data about dietary intake, which tends to be unreliable; the definitions of plant-based diets likely differed widely among the countries studied; the results for the self-professed plant-based eaters were likely confounded by other aspects of their lifestyle; the conclusions were based on a very small sample of cases; the diet categories chosen by respondents were not closely related to the actual diets they reported eating. (For that last one, read: those who claimed to eat a plant-based diet actually ate meat, fish and dairy several times a week.) One expert, Gunter Kuhnle (professor of nutrition and food science at the University of Reading), concluded that the study was interesting 'but does not provide much new information'. Another, Dr Carmen Pernas, a nutrition scientist at the University of Oxford, warned that 'the conclusions needs (sic) to be drawn cautiously in the context of several methodological issues'.

Dr Zoë Harcombe exposed those methodological issues with her customary precision. Her extensive critique is too lengthy to be included here, but I encourage you to seek it out at www.zoeharcombe.com (Plant-based diets & Covid-19). The stand-out fact, in the context of the bold claims being made by the study's authors and subsequent media headlines, is that (as pointed out above) those who claimed to eat a plant-based diet (and therefore, supposedly experienced less severe cases of Covid-19 as a result) did not actually eat a plant-based diet; they consumed meat, fish and dairy several times a week, and did not eat many more servings of vegetables than those who claimed not to eat a plant-based diet. Another point worth dwelling on is the following: there were four self-reported moderate to severe cases of Covid among those on (self-reported, and not very accurately) plant-based diets (representing 1.6 per cent of the total in this category), compared to thirty of those on (self-reported, and not very accurately) low-carbohydrate or high-protein diets (representing 6.2 per cent of the total). This led the study's authors to claim that those on low-carbohydrate or high-protein diets were four times more likely to experience moderate to severe symptoms. (6.2/1.6 = 3.9). But with such a small comparator group (four self-reported cases in the plant-based group), the result is bound to be exaggerated to the point of being meaningless. Dr Harcombe explains this using another example: 'if 20 children go skiing – 2 of them with autism – and 2 children die in an avalanche – 1 with autism and 1 without – the death rate for the non-autistic children is 1 in 18 (5.5%) and the death rate for the autistic children is 1 in 2 (50%). Can you see how bad (or good?) you can make things look with a small comparator group?'[18]

The many methodological flaws in this study led Dr Harcombe to label it 'misleading at best and disingenuous at worst'. So who's answerable for the propagation of misleading claims like these? Certainly, the authors of the study must bear some of the responsibility, as should the editors of the journal that published it. I would argue that those media that reported on the study under headlines such as those noted above must also bear some responsibility, their mistake being to proclaim the study's findings without properly interrogating the study itself. Experts like Dr Harcombe and those from the Science Media Centre came forward to conduct a proper interrogation, but their views were not covered in the mainstream media upon which so many rely for their information.

And this is how it happens. This is how relatively weak and unpersuasive studies achieve persuasive power, moving the public's consciousness towards the acceptance of the view that meat is harmful and plants are the way to go. It happens one headline, photograph, press release and citation at a time, with the result being that the cumulative message achieves the status of incontrovertible truth. Within the media industry, most of the participants probably think that they are doing the right thing, or at least doing their jobs. And to an extent, they are. Sadly, gross distortions of the truth are often the consequence.

If we should be alert to the cumulative effect of misleading headlines and repeated assertions about relatively weak studies, we should also be concerned about instances where media organisations publish or broadcast material that promotes the plant-based cause while also having a financial interest in the success of that cause.

Beyond the headlines: when financial and editorial interests become entangled

In 2019, Channel 4, through its commercial growth fund, made a seven-figure investment in The Meatless Farm, a company that makes plant-based alternatives to meat products that are sold in leading supermarkets.[19] The exchange of advertising time for equity would enable The Meatless Farm to create a major TV campaign, which would be aired across Channel 4 and its All 4 streaming service.[20] The Meatless Farm's founder, Morten Toft Bech, said that the company's mission is 'to make it easy for people to reduce their red meat consumption by switching to plant-based alternatives' and that 'Channel 4's audience, and environmental and ethical values, align strongly with ours'.

A few months later, in January 2020 (and timed to coincide with Veganuary), Channel 4 aired three programmes that dealt with the topic of meat-eating versus veganism in different ways. *Meat the Family* followed four families as they cared for farm animals at home for three weeks before deciding whether or not to send them to slaughter or save them and commit to becoming vegetarians. *How to Steal Pigs and Influence People* featured vegan activists who staged heists to rescue factory-farmed pigs (including one large-scale event called 'meat the victims'), as well as ex-vegans devouring raw meat at their raw carnivore picnic. *Apocalypse Cow*, discussed in previous chapters, depicted modern livestock farming as a cause of environmental destruction, and offered the radical proposition that it should be abolished and our meat created in labs made in solar-powered factories.

Apocalypse Cow was unashamedly pro-plant based, and *How to Steal Pigs and Influence People* seemed designed to put people off eating animal foods, even if it did interrogate the motives of the vegan activists. Scenes of ex-vegans chomping down on raw lambs' legs and hearts, blood dripping from their chins, would have appalled many an omnivore. Tom Calvert, head of legal for Dragonfly, the company that produced the programme for Channel 4, nevertheless defended the programme as being balanced: 'We believe that the programme gives a fair and balanced view of the "Meat the Victims" event from both sides, as well as presenting a fair reflection of vegan activism in the UK.'[21]

Meat the Family came down less heavily on the side of veganism. Families were forced to confront not only their affection for the farm animals in their care but the realities of some of the systems that moved animals from farm to table, with viewers being shown both factory-farming operations and higher welfare, free-range operations. And, having given thoughtful consideration to the realities to which they'd been exposed, some of the families opted to continue eating meat. The take-away message was not exclusively 'don't eat meat' but sometimes, 'think more carefully about the meat you do eat'.

While each of these programmes took a slightly different approach to exploring the topic of meat-eating versus veganism, another type of programme was missing in action altogether: Channel 4 did not air any programmes that might have advanced counter arguments to veganism in any meaningful way – a look at how regenerative farming can help us tackle climate change, for example, or an examination of animal foods as the unsung heroes of human nutrition. And those programmes that it did air, taken as a group, likely served both to raise the profile of veganism and to nudge viewers towards a greater level of acceptance of plant-based arguments. Some viewers might even have come away with a commitment to eat less meat, or to give it up altogether. This, of course, would be good news for a company like The Meatless Farm, whose stated mission, as we've seen, is 'to make it easy for people to reduce their red meat consumption by switching to plant-based meat alternatives'.[22]

And therein lies the rub. If Channel 4 and The Meatless Farm were unrelated entities, this confluence of editorial message and commercial benefit would not be a problem. But Channel 4 has invested in The Meatless Farm (shares being exchanged for advertising airtime) and therefore stands to gain from an uplift in The Meatless Farm's commercial prospects.

The MailOnline reported that 'Channel 4 has been accused of a massive conflict of interest for screening two films attacking the meat industry after making such a large investment in a vegan food company,[23] citing Stuart Roberts of the NFU as saying that the broadcaster's investment 'significantly undermines trust in journalism'. Some Channel 4 staff were also said to be concerned, one telling the *Mail on Sunday*: 'Whatever happened to us making programmes rather than doing these kinds of deals? It's one big conflict of interest.'[24]

A spokesperson for Channel 4 played down the potential conflict of interest, saying that both programmes complied with Ofcom's broadcasting code and that 'Channel 4 maintains clear separation between its editorial decisions and commercial activity. There is no conflict of interest.'[25]

However clear that separation may be in principle, it may be less clear in practice. It remains true that Channel 4 as a commercial entity is in a position to profit from an investment that could increase in value as a result of the programmes the channel chooses to air, and that it chose to air programmes favouring plant-based arguments but did not air any programmes that could be said to give fair hearing to the counter arguments.

Channel 4 viewers might reasonably ask whether it is ideal or even acceptable for a media company to be invested in a commercial operation that stands to make financial gains as a result of that media company's airing of content that takes sides in such an important debate.

The *Guardian*'s philanthropic partnerships: open journalism or a loudspeaker for one side of the argument?

Like Channel 4, the *Guardian* is financially linked to the producers of plant-based meats, albeit indirectly and via a different mechanism. The *Guardian* has received almost two million dollars (in two separate payments) from a US non-profit organisation called the Open Philanthropy Project (OPP).[26] The OPP has also donated an eye-watering 120 million dollars to animal rights activism, vegan activism and plant-based alternatives,[27] making a significant investment in Impossible Foods (the plant-based meat company founded by a man whose stated mission is to eradicate animal agriculture from the earth).[28] The OPP grant to the *Guardian* helps to fund 'Animals Farmed', announced in February 2018 and billed as a series that would 'look at how the animals that feed us live, and how the business of feeding us works. What happens in the factory farming system? And what does that mean for our planet?'[29] The OPP's payments to the newspaper are acknowledged on an information page on the *Guardian*'s website alongside that of other current philanthropic partnerships, such as that with the Bill and Melinda Gates Foundation (which is also invested in plant-based meat substitutes).[30]

Since 2018, the 'Animals Farmed' series has covered hundreds of topics related to farming and food production.[31] Important issues have been unearthed and discussed, such as the deforestation linked to the soya destined for livestock feed,[32] the overuse of antibiotics on some pig farms,[33] and the threat to small farms from mega dairies in the US.[34] The work of farmers who are providing an alternative to factory farming has occasionally been featured.[35] But a trawl through all the titles in the series listed on the *Guardian*'s website reveals that most of articles have painted a negative view of animal agriculture. (A group called AdaptNation[36] asserts that, of the more than 200 articles published in the two and a half years after the initiation of the series, all feature 'emotional imagery on animal husbandry and aerial shots of plant devastation', alongside 'worrying headlines, grave concerns' and the idea that a plant-based lifestyle is 'the only viable solution'.[37]) That negative view runs through much (though not all) of the *Guardian* coverage that is not part of the 'Animals Farmed' series and not sponsored by the OPP. Typical headlines include 'Why eating less meat is the best thing you can do for the planet' (December 2018), 'Reach peak meat by 2030 to tackle climate crisis' (December 2019), 'What we eat matters ... the biggest problem is livestock' (October 2019), and 'Why you should go animal free' (June 2020). In September 2020, the paper featured a piece titled 'EU's farm animals "produce more emissions than cars and vans combined"', using Greenpeace data that had been shown to be incorrect years before. Frank Mitloehner was forced to point out that 'not only is this an apples to oranges comparison but it unfairly and deliberately omits key data to skew favour one way while vilifying the other'.[38]

Given that the *Guardian* sometimes publishes content that is supportive of livestock farmers' perspective,[39] or raises questions about plant-based meats, for example,[40] should we still be concerned about the impact of content funded by the OPP or otherwise influenced by the OPP connection? Should we worry that the OPP-funded content might serve to create an imbalance in the paper's overall coverage? Might that content, when combined with the weight of pro plant-based coverage found elsewhere, tip the scales in favour of plant-based foods and plant-based advocacy in a way that detracts from our ability to appreciate alternative arguments, and alternative solutions to our environmental problems?

If you answered yes to these questions, you are not alone. Some journalists and scientists are concerned about the OPP connection and the *Guardian*'s impact on the overall debate. When I asked investigative food journalist Joanna Blythman why she thought that the plant-based message was so loud and insistent in the UK, compared to some other countries, she said that she thought the *Guardian* had a lot to do with it:

'Most millennials get their news online, and the *Guardian* is a free site whereas many others are behind a paywall. So, the *Guardian* prints this anti-livestock-farming content, and there's no paywall, so people pick it up. Many science correspondents for other papers see the *Guardian* getting all these hits so they just repeat the story. It's cut-and-paste journalism. If you took the *Guardian* out of it, you'd have a different debate. You have to remember, too, that a lot of Americans who want an alternative to the right-wing media read the *Guardian*. The spread of influence is huge.'[41]

Others have questioned the *Guardian*'s claim to espouse 'open, independent journalism' in the context of the OPP funding. The paper states that funding from readers safeguards their editorial work and maintains openness, enabling more people across the world to 'access accurate information with integrity at its heart'. Where ordinary readers are concerned, this is undoubtedly true. But, as Frank Mitloehner points out, the OPP is no ordinary reader. 'Its resources are significant, and it stands to gain financially and otherwise from furthering its anti-livestock agenda.'[42] Note that the OPP officer overseeing the *Guardian* investment is Lewis Bollard, a former operative of the Humane Society of the United States (HSUS), and recall that the OPP has donated large sums to animal rights and vegan activism and is also an investor in Impossible Foods. 'The OPP pays the *Guardian* to write anti-livestock pieces while being a major investor in plant-based meat alternatives,' says Mitloehner. 'You tell me if this is a conflict of interest or not.'[43]

As I've said, the OPP connection is acknowledged by the *Guardian* and it is always clearly noted that 'Animals Farmed' articles are supported by the OPP. In the online version of the publication, more information is provided via a link to 'About this content'. But how many readers have the time or the inclination to interrogate content that closely? How many bother to follow the links to discover that the OPP is a powerful organisation that has donated millions to animal rights and vegan activism and made a financial investment in Impossible Foods – a company whose founder professes to want to rid the world of all animal agriculture? How many then stop to consider that another of the *Guardian*'s philanthropic partners, the Bill and Melinda Gates Foundation, is also heavily invested in the development of plant-based meat alternatives, and that, via these relationships, the *Guardian*'s reporting pertaining to livestock farming and meat-eating is open to influence from those who stand to gain financially from the elimination of both?

My guess is very few.

Duped by documentaries

When it comes to dealing blows to the omnivore diet, none of the UK-based media organisations we've considered here can hold a candle to the makers of two US documentaries: *The Game Changers* and *Cowspiracy*. These two films have influenced the debate about food, health and the environment more than most of us realise, and much more than they should have. One of them is mostly about health, whereas the other one is mostly about the environment, so they make a good double act, furnishing plant-based advocates with everything they need to support their world view and recruit others to it.

After watching *The Game Changers*, young people, and indeed entire families, report 'giving veganism a go'. The *Cowspiracy* Facebook page is replete with evidence that young people were particularly persuaded by *Cowspiracy*'s claims, with this sort of declaration being common: 'The film is so convincing, well-researched and shocking that I knew instantly I could never eat meat or dairy products again.'[44]

Rancher Trent Loos recalls that *Cowspiracy* found its way into US schools and says that to this day he still gets calls from worried parents whose children are watching the film in school. And we know that *Cowspiracy* remains influential in the UK, five years after it first hit our screens, because the Edinburgh students protesting against meat being served on campus in 2019 carried placards emblazoned with the (entirely and spectacularly) false claim, likely plucked straight from the film, that cows cause 51 per cent of emissions.

There's a lot else wrong with *Cowspiracy* besides this outlandish claim about emissions. In fact, there's so much that's misleading and factually incorrect in both *Cowspiracy* and *The Game Changers* that a full critique could fill an entire book. Here, I'll alert you to the worst offences perpetrated by these two films and point you in the direction of more extensive critiques.

The Game Changers: plant-based propaganda masquerading as science

The Game Changers was released on Netflix to great fanfare in the autumn of 2019. It had already been released on iTunes, where it had become the best-selling documentary of all time. The big names attached to the film had undoubtedly played a role in stirring up interest and sales. Executive producers included Oscar-winning director James Cameron, Arnold Schwarzenegger, Jackie Chan, Lewis Hamilton, Novak Djokovic and NBA star Chris Paul. The presenter was Ultimate Fighting Championship fighter James Wilks. Promotional material described the film thus: 'A UFC fighter's world is turned upside down when he discovers an elite group of world-renowned athletes and scientists who prove that everything he had been taught about protein was a lie.'

Herein lies the first disingenuous aspect of the film. James Wilks plays the role of a guy who's become confused by conflicting advice on diet who 'goes off on an odyssey of discovery and kindly brings us along'.[45] But the film seems to be based on an agenda that was there at the beginning and all the way through the seven years it took to make it, and that agenda has little to do with exploration and everything to do with moving audiences towards the predetermined conclusion that plant-based is the way to go.

How could the film ever have reached any other conclusion, given the established views and potential conflicts of interest of the characters involved in its making? Several of the executive producers are heavily invested in the vegan cause: James Cameron, executive producer, as we saw in Chapter 12, is a vegan activist and founder/CEO of Verdient Foods, in which he has a 140-million-dollar investment. His wife, Suzy Amis Cameron, executive producer, is also a vegan activist and founder of Verdient Foods. Jackie Chan is an actor and vegan. Arnold Schwarzenegger is part owner of a supplement company that sells vegan products. Of the thirteen experts with a food or medical specialism interviewed in the film, the vast majority are well-known promoters of plant-based diets or have previously written books about or taken part in films promoting the plant-based cause.[46]

Of course, an expert line-up like this is exactly what you'd expect in a film with a plant-based agenda. Contrary perspectives mess with the singular narrative, so it's just clever film-making to ensure a consistent point of view. The trouble is, unless viewers do their research, they won't know that they are listening to experts who came to the film with a pre-determined inclination towards plant-based diets. They'll likely think that the experts are making an objective appraisal of the new evidence presented, rather than confirming long-held views, and they could see the nutritional claims presented as incontrovertible facts rather than highly contestable opinions that are based on some questionable interpretations of nutrition research.

Those with an understanding of nutrition saw through the disingenuous premise underlying the film and recognised everything else that was wrong with it. Human-nutrition scientist Stephan van Vliet said, 'I watched it on a plane, and I was shaking my head all the way through. It's propaganda dressed up as science.'[47] Journalist and author Marika Sboros called the film 'vegan hype of titanic proportions'.[48] Dr Jay Wrigley called it 'a bunch of manipulated bullshit propaganda with zero science to support any of it'.[49] Comedian and podcaster Joe Rogan might have put it most succinctly when he said, 'There's a lot of f***ery in this movie, man.'[50]

The debunking of *The Game Changers* became a mini industry. Nutritionist Tim Rees and nutrition research scientist Chris Masterjohn dissected the documentary with razor-like precision, pointing out its many flaws;[51] film maker

Brian Sanders produced a film about the many untruths and half-truths put forward by the documentary;[52] YouTube videos popped up to demonstrate why *The Game Changers* experiments were misleading;[53] a vegan even made a video declaring the documentary 'unconvincing'; and Joe Rogan hosted a two-hour interview with functional-medicine specialist Chris Kresser, in which Kresser debunked every argument put forward by the film.[54] The Rogan–Kresser interview spawned a cascade of further debate: Rogan hosted a one-on-one debate between Wilks and Kresser, during which Wilks shouted and hectored his way to a form of triumph, obfuscating the data at every turn. Kresser then wrote about his reflections on this debate, and his reaction to the personal attacks to which Wilks had subjected him. Kresser demonstrated that Wilks got a lot wrong and had cited studies that didn't actually support his points. Paul Saladino MD asked, 'did James Wilks get anything right against Chris Kresser?'[55]

Wilks didn't get much right in either the debate against Kresser or the film itself, as Tim Rees discovered when he subjected the film to a fine-tooth-comb analysis. He found the film to be misleading on a grand scale: 'One thing I've discovered is that nobody really checks the references that people put in. This is true of the WHO piece on cancer – people refer to that authority and that paper like it's some definitive, end-of-argument, seminal piece of work, which it absolutely is not. It's also true of *The Game Changers*. Not a single piece of the evidence cited by the film actually supports its claim that a completely plant-based diet is best for health. Not a single one.'[56]

Tim has an interesting relationship with the film. He went to school with James Wilks and was contacted by a third classmate just as he started researching the film. That classmate said, 'Mate, have you seen Wilko's documentary? It's great! I'm going to give it a go!' Tim explained why he felt he had to do the hard work of proving why the film was not, in fact, 'great' and why it was a bad idea for people to 'give it a go': 'I'm a registered nutritionist who's worried about the plant-based/vegan movement because people are already struggling to nourish themselves with the inclusion of animal produce – the best sources of bioavailable nutrients. Removing them magnifies this problem and leaves the young and impressionable malnourished and sick ... this is why I'm willing to spend my time uncovering the nonsense that we're being sold.'[57]

I urge you to seek Tim's comprehensive analysis of the evidence presented in the film at www.tim-rees.com. It's a cracking read, not something that's often said about texts replete with references to scientific papers. At the end of his analysis (by which point you will have seen how little of the evidence presented in *The Game Changers* stacks up), Tim says, 'Thanks for reading.' I say, 'thanks for writing', because were it not for Tim and others like him who went to great lengths to challenge this risible film, it might have captured even more impressionable minds than it did.

Among the impressionable minds that it is set to capture, sadly, are those of the US medical establishment. Soon after the film aired, it was reported that US doctors were requesting *The Game Changers* DVDs to hand out to their patients. And, as noted in Chapter 11, the film has been accredited by the American College of Lifestyle Medicine (that Seventh-day Adventist institution with a strong plant-based bias), meaning that every doctor or nurse in the US can get further education credits just by watching the film and taking a quiz developed by Wilks and his team.[58] Medics in Europe might also have fallen under *The Game Changers*' spell. Tim spoke to a doctor who said that seven out of ten of her colleagues had decided to try a vegan diet after seeing the film.

This is truly terrifying and confirms that Dr Saladino

might have been right when he said that he feared *The Game Changers* movie would 'cause tons of suffering over the next five years'. If you've taken on board the message of this chapter, at least you won't be among the sufferers.

Cowspiracy: misrepresentation and exaggeration with a big factual error at its heart

There are a great many similarities between *The Game Changers* and *Cowspiracy*, not least the fact that their take-away message is 'go vegan'. *Cowspiracy* also comes with a Hollywood pedigree attached. The film was created by directors Kip Andersen and Keegan Kuhn and was later backed by none other than Leonardo DiCaprio. As in *The Game Changers*, all of those interviewed leaned towards vegetarianism or veganism. (Not a regenerative farmer or agricultural scientist among them.) Moreover, *Cowspiracy* is based on the same faux-naive premise. We are meant to believe that Kip Andersen came to a 'realisation' that he couldn't affect climate change by doing all the things he was supposed to do, like turning off the lights or reducing water consumption, because it was animal agriculture that was causing the problem. But both he and Kuhn were self-described animal-rights activists before making the film, and Kuhn has stated that he's been a vegan for decades.[59] Do we honestly believe that they set out on the making of this film with anything other than a vegan agenda and in pursuit of a predetermined, vegan-friendly conclusion?

Positioning Andersen as an innocent who gradually discovered the truth is not a reflection of reality. Rather, it's a highly effective film technique. Everyone loves the story of a journey, particularly when that journey is undertaken by an 'easy going, regular guy in a baseball cap'.[60]

Like the makers of *The Game Changers*, Andersen and

Kuhn relied on cherry-picking, exaggeration and misrepresentation in order to convince us that animal agriculture is the cause of all of our environmental ills. Farmer Garth Brown commented that the film's great weakness was 'its single-minded determination to prove that veganism is the only reasonable approach to feeding people, a proof that it pursues without regard for the facts or nuance'.[61] Agricultural scientist Karin Lindquist wrote that the film is 'undoubtedly one of the most inaccurate films' she had ever had to watch: 'If a film only has one ultimate solution to the world-wide problem of feeding the world and climate change, [and that is] a "plant-based diet" or veganism, then yes, it is a propaganda piece and not an open ended documentary.'[62] Another critic slated the film for the 'mountains of misinformation' it contains, and for its failure to grasp 'a simple environmental concept based on easily observed cycles in nature'.[63]

Writing for the online news outlet *Daily Kos*, agro-ecologist Joshua Finch lambasted *Cowspiracy* for its absolutist position: 'A panacea is offered: global adoption of a vegan lifestyle as "the only way to sustainably and ethically live on this planet with 7 billion other people" … the film's absolutist position runs roughshod over nuance, presenting an exclusionary world-view as the only viable option.'[64]

Finch detailed how *Cowspiracy*'s absolutist position was built on reductionism, selective observation and vilification, saying 'rarely do all three come together in such a blatant display'. By bringing these three things together, Andersen and Kuhn manage to reduce a very complex problem to a single, simple solution.

One specific beef with the film that Finch shares with all critics concerns its erroneous claim that livestock are responsible for 51 per cent of emissions. When challenged, Andersen and Kuhn revised that number down from 50 to 18 per cent.[65] While closer to the truth, this number is still much higher than the real figure, as we saw in Chapter 7 (14.5 per cent calculated on a life-cycle basis, but just 5 per cent if direct emissions are used). As one critic pointed out, 'this is not a full and honest retraction. They're not putting their hands up and saying "Guys, we were wrong and we're sorry for misleading you." However, it does clearly tell us that the filmmakers now acknowledge that the real impact of animal ag [agriculture] on the climate is at least 60 per cent lower than the film claims.'[66]

The other major flaw in the film is that it shows us the very worst of industrial animal agriculture while failing to mention that this is not representative of the whole. We're given shots of crowded feedlots and immense plots of bare soil dotted with stationary cows. But as Finch points out, 'animal agriculture takes place in many forms throughout the world. From CAFOs in the United States and Europe ... to the nomadic people of Central Asia, to complex integration of animals in agroecosystems ... the environmental impact of any specific practice can only be determined by examining the specific details of said practice.'[67] Where, in *Cowspiracy*, are the shots of cattle happily grazing in knee-high grasses in middle America? Where are the scenes of cattle clambering across the rocky grasslands of North Yorkshire? Where is Gabe Brown's farm, or Joel Salatin's, or Christine Page's, or any of the farms around the world that raise livestock in a humane and environmentally friendly way? Why was there no acknowledgement of the scientifically proven carbon sequestration benefits of cattle on pasture?

With a gross exaggeration of emissions and the reduction of the totality of animal agriculture to the worst of industrialised animal agriculture at the heart of *Cowspiracy*, can we really trust anything else it tells us? I would suggest not. The film makes misleading claims about land use and deforestation, water use, methane, biodiversity and manure. And it says precisely nothing about soil health. Nothing about how soil is the foundation of all life, or the fact that decades' worth of industrial agriculture have resulted in much of the world's soil being denuded of organic matter, eroded or washed away. Nothing about the fact that regenerative livestock agriculture represents the only means of rebuilding the soil and safeguarding our future. No reference to the fact that the UN, in recognition of the necessity of protecting and building our soils, is encouraging the uptake of agro-ecology throughout the world.[68] No mention of agro-ecology at all, in fact.

We should be incensed on behalf of the soil and all those who care about it. We should also be incensed on behalf of several individuals who were treated very shabbily indeed by Andersen and Kuhn. The work of environmentalist Allan Savory, and a family of farmers, the Markegards, was shamefully misrepresented. Thankfully, another film came along, five years later, to provide both Savory and the Markegards with some redress. In *Kiss the Ground*, first aired in September 2020, Savory's work is given the respect it deserves, and Doniga Markegard is granted the time to explain how her form of agriculture can feed people without depleting resources. We see the charts she uses to manage her grazing system, keeping cattle on the move so that no piece of land ever gets overgrazed. We see her kneeling on the ground to show us the root hairs in a chunk of soil, root hairs that are connected to other root hairs and microfungi below ground. Doniga holds the soil in her hand as if it were a golden egg while she explains how carbon goes from the atmosphere into the root system of plants, which is sloughed off and turns into humus in the soil. 'The form of agriculture we use creates billions of lives,' she says proudly, 'in the form of soil microbes, nematodes and grassland birds – all that wildlife flourishes under a holistic agricultural system, versus a tilled crop field which is devoid of life.'

Kiss the Ground is not without its blind spots, but it's an infinitely superior film to *Cowspiracy*. Other excellent films about farming and the environment include *The Biggest Little Farm*, *Sacred Cow* and *Sustenance*. If you've watched *Cowspiracy*, you owe it to yourself to watch these, too.

That documentary makers and mainstream media outlets sometimes mislead should not surprise us. As has been said many times, by many people, if you don't read the newspaper you're uninformed, but if you do read the paper you're misinformed.[69] To avoid being misinformed, we need to be what Malcolm Kendrick calls 'naive sceptics'.[70] This means taking each headline – whether it be in a newspaper or a documentary – as though it *might* be true but applying a critical eye to the content beneath the headline, questioning the motivations of those who are cited, thinking independently, and consulting a variety of sources (ideally with radically different perspectives) to establish the validity of the original claims. As naive sceptics we can equip ourselves to understand the real solutions to the environmental and health crises we face. Those solutions are complex and far reaching. They are certainly not represented by the endorsement by much of the mainstream media of the simplistic plea for us to go plant based.

Onwards. Next, we're going to look at NGOs (nongovernmental organisations) such as EAT-Lancet, the World Economic Forum and the World Health Organization to see how they have lined up in support of the plant-based cause.

14

Why the Global Elites are Pushing the Plant-based Diet

Errant thinking patterns, says Dr Malcolm Kendrick, are evidenced when we see three things happening: the belief that you need to do something/anything; grabbing the simple/easy hypothesis too early; and being so certain that your hypothesis is correct that you don't do any studies to prove that it is beneficial – you just get on with it.[1] Kendrick explains how these three factors have driven us towards many a health solution that later proved to have serious negative and even disastrous consequences. He doesn't get into the topic of the solutions being proposed for environmental crises, but, my goodness, I reckon he would have a field day if he did.

With climate change and its related environmental impacts upon us, we have the perfect conditions for errant thinking patterns to take hold: we must do something, anything; we need a simple solution (clearly, it's the cows, so obviously we must stop eating meat); this is so obvious that we don't need to investigate further. Let's all just go plant based.

The global elites – by which I mean non-governmental organisations (NGOs) such as the United Nations (UN), the

World Health Organization (WHO), the World Business Council for Sustainable Development (WBCSD) and the World Economic Forum (WEF) – appear to have latched on to this errant way of thinking in a big way. And they have rallied around the work of a new NGO on the block, the EAT-Lancet Commission, echoing its cry for us to eat much less meat, or ideally no meat at all.

Here's how *The Lancet* set the stage for our three-step journey towards errant thinking in January 2019:

> Civilisation is in crisis. We can no longer feed our population a healthy diet while balancing planetary resources. For the first time in 200,000 years of human history, we are severely out of synchronisation with the planet and nature. This crisis is accelerating, stretching the Earth to its limits, and threatening human and other species' sustained existence. The publication now of Food in the Anthropocene: the EAT-Lancet Commission on healthy diets from sustainable food systems could neither be more timely nor more urgent.[2]

There's a large amount of truth in this statement. We are 'severely out of synchronisation with the planet and nature'. But, as we saw in Chapter 10, the question of whether or not we can still feed our population remains a hotly debated one. And if the problem is that we are stretching the earth's resources to their limit, it's far from proven that the mandating of a global near-vegan diet is going to be the silver bullet that fixes it.

To pinch the title of a book by author Ben Goldacre, I think you'll find it's a bit more complicated than that.[3]

You might hope that we'd have learned something from two previous attempts to find silver-bullet-like solutions to complicated problems. We've had the Green Revolution (a response to real and anticipated food shortages) followed by the diet revolution (instigated by the 1977 McGovern Committee Report, Dietary Goals, in response to rising rates of heart disease). The first revolution ended up contributing to the destruction of our soils and the second one arguably sabotaged our health.

It's worth reminding ourselves of the language that was used by the McGovern Committee to justify immediate action in the face of what was considerable opposition to its Dietary Goals report from many prominent politicians and scientists: 'Senators don't have the luxury that a research scientist does of waiting until every last shred of evidence is in.'[4] In other words, and applying Dr Kendrick's framework: (1) We cannot afford to wait. We must do something, anything! (2) Reducing saturated fat and cholesterol, that seems like the obvious answer; and (3) We don't have all the data to tell us if it's the right answer, but that will take too long to gather, so let's just go!

In this manner, hysteria triumphed over evidence. Nina Teicholz wrote: 'Dietary Goals, compiled by one interested layperson, Mottern, without any formal review, became arguably the most influential document in the history of diet and disease. Following publication of Dietary Goals by the highest elective body in the land, an entire government and then a nation swivelled into gear behind its dietary advice.'[5]

Animal fats and foods were out, the low-fat high-carb diet was in; this situation would prevail for the next forty years. Reading EAT-Lancet's proposals for a new global diet, and witnessing the likes of the UN and UNICEF rush to endorse it, many people have had a troubling sense of déjà vu. By pushing us down the EAT-Lancet planetary-health route, might our elites be making the next 'big mistake'? And if they are, how are we, as ordinary citizens, going to stop this juggernaut?

One thing we can do is educate ourselves about the

organisations driving the change. If we can understand at least a little about who they are and how they are connected, we can decide for ourselves whether their proclamations represent the best or the only way forward, or just one view among many, and a view that warrants critique and challenge. We don't just have to fall into line, as the mayors of fourteen cities – including London, Toronto and São Paulo – did in 2019 when they signed up to encourage the implementation of EAT's recommendations within their cities by 2030.

EAT-Lancet under the microscope

In Chapter 2, I referenced some of the critical responses to the EAT-Lancet diet. Dr Zoë Harcombe and Dr Georgia Ede found the diet to be nutritionally deficient and not evidence based; nutrition researchers Adam Drewnowski and Will Masters pointed out that the diet was not affordable in most of the world; and researchers Zagmutt, Pouzou and Costard maintained that the EAT-Lancet researchers had made false assumptions leading to overblown claims about the diet's benefits and that the diet would only serve to fuel the global obesity and diabetes crises.

These critiques represent just the tip of a veritable iceberg of condemnation of the diet. To get an idea of just how big that iceberg is, you could check out the references listed at the end of a blog by Benjamin David Steele: the blog is a merciless exposition of the flawed thinking of the EAT-Lancet Commission and the diet that resulted.[6] Here's a flavour of what the critics had to say. Stanford professor John Ioannidis stated that the health claims in the EAT-Lancet diet are 'science fiction. I can't call it anything else.'[7] Frank Mitloehner wrote, 'EAT-Lancet's environmental claims are an epic fail. And the Commission knows it.'[8] Joanna Blythman asserted that the diet was 'a processed food diet reinvented'.[9] Frédéric Leroy and Martin Cohen accused Eat-Lancet of being 'the new kid on the block with all the latest gear' and said that 'the portrayal of meat as "intrinsically harmful" could lead to widespread malnutrition'.[10] Dr Mark Hyman said that the report failed to recognise that well-managed holistic farm and rangeland ecosystems rely on animals to sequester carbon, and, remarkably, seemed to be calling for the increased use of chemical agricultural inputs.[11]

So what do we know about the commission that came up with this near-vegan diet that, by the commission's own admission, is not appropriate for the young, the old, the sick, the frail, the malnourished or pregnant women, and which fails – in the eyes of so many – to take into account environmental and agricultural realities?

The who's who of EAT-Lancet

The EAT-Lancet Commission started life as the EAT initiative, founded in 2013 by the Stockholm Resilience Centre (SRC) in partnership with the Stordalen Foundation and boosted by a three-million-pound investment from the Wellcome Trust in 2016. The SRC is itself the joint initiative of three institutions, including the Beijer Institute and the Stockholm Environment Institute (SEI), the latter having been organised by Maurice Strong, an oil businessman and UN diplomat who believed in 'business solutions' to environmental problems. Strong was also instrumental in the foundation of the World Resources Institute (WRI) and the World Business Council for Sustainable Development (WBCSD) – an organisation that now boasts two hundred members in a wide range of industries, representing a global management elite that wishes to approach the environmental crisis as a profitable enterprise.[12]

This family tree is interesting because it highlights the

fact that the EAT initiative is very much part of a tradition of corporate-led global initiatives attempting to manage and control so-called 'great transitions'. As proponents of a great food transformation, EAT has garnered the support of its predecessors.[13] Recently, a Global Commons Alliance (GCA) was formed, consisting of the EAT foundation and several other global institutions (WBCSD, WEF, WRI and UNEP – the UN Environment Programme). The GCA is tightly associated with the Food and Land Use Coalition, which proposes a 90 per cent decrease in red meat intake for Australians by 2050, as well as the business-linked C40 Cities initiative. This initiative has dietary exclusion of meat and dairy as one of its key targets.[14]

Given the kind of company that EAT keeps, it's not surprising that it has ended up promoting a near vegan diet. But EAT's anti-meat bias is also underpinned by the philosophies of its founders, the Stordalen Foundation and the SRC. The Stordalen Foundation is the brainchild of Gunhild Stordalen, a doctor and environmentalist, and her husband at the time, Petter Stordalen, the millionaire owner of a Nordic hotel chain. Gunhild is a committed vegetarian. (Her husband was somewhat less committed, as we'll see later.) Therefore, even though the Stordalen Foundation positions EAT's objectives as being 'to expand the interdisciplinary scientific knowledge platform on the interconnections between food, health and environmental sustainability',[15] it's likely that the 'behavioural change at a population level' that the foundation would like to see is one that would nudge us all towards being vegetarians or vegans.

What about EAT's other founders? The SRC harbours a longstanding antipathy towards animal foods and has published numerous documents describing meat consumption as a major threat to the environment.[16] The Wellcome Trust seems to have similar underlying plant-based leanings. Importantly, the trust was founded by Henry Wellcome, who was raised as a Seventh-day Adventist.[17] (We saw how wedded the Seventh-day Adventists are to plant-based diets in Chapter 11.)

A post on The Wellcome Trust website makes its anti-meat leaning abundantly clear. Although there is some up-front talk about working with EAT to reform a food system that is destroying human and planetary health and bringing together 'policy makers, industry leaders, researchers and civil society to develop solutions that are practical and have support from all sides',[18] the trust sets out its stall pretty early, and it's not a stall that will be selling animal foods. To illustrate the kind of reform the trust would like to see, the following example is given: 'Eating too much red meat is a risk factor for obesity, for environmentalists who know that rearing animals for meat produces large amounts of greenhouse gases, for retailers who compete to sell meat at ever lower prices and for beef cattle farmers who frequently operate at a loss. If these communities could address these challenges in collaboration rather than in isolation, the potential benefits for both individual wellbeing and the global environment are great.'[19]

The links between red meat and obesity, and red meat and greenhouse gases, are positioned as incontrovertible facts. And for all the trust's talk of finding solutions that have support from all sides, we know that what eventually came out of EAT was the recommendation of a diet that virtually eliminates meat and other animal foods. It would seem that the farmers, ranchers, pastoralists and omnivores of the world did not qualify as any of the communities from whom support was required.

With Gunhild Stordalen's foundation, the SRC and the Wellcome Trust as its founders, it's hardly surprising – though, some would argue, not inevitable – that EAT would come up with a plant-based Planetary Health Diet. However, the membership of the EAT Commission itself also leaned towards vegetarianism and veganism. The co-chairs of the commission were Harvard professor Walter Willett, who, as discussed in previous chapters, has been discouraging meat consumption and promoting vegetarian diets since 1990,[20] and Professor Johan Rockström from the SRC. Fully 80 per cent (thirty-one out of thirty-seven) of the commissioners espoused vegetarian views before joining the EAT-Lancet project, many having written extensively about the need to reduce or eliminate meat consumption. Among the co-authors (who comprised eighteen of the commission's thirty-seven members) was known vegan advocate Marco Springmann and no less than ten employees of the SRC. The whole commission was drawn from a remarkably narrow cast. There were plenty of people with 'policy' and 'metrics' in their job titles, but just four with any nutrition specialism. And where were the farmers and the regenerative agriculture experts? Their sole representative was Dr Anna Lartey from the Food and Agriculture Organisation (FAO) of the UN. Nina Teicholz wrote, 'this was clearly a highly biased group, and the outcome of their report was therefore inevitably a forgone conclusion ... like-minded people talking to themselves is not a scientific debate, and the product of these inbred conversations cannot be considered a scientific product'.[21]

Teicholz notes that none of the authors disclosed their potential competing interests, whether intellectual or financial. In many cases, the authors' potential competing interests involve their place of employment, in think tanks that promote vegetarian diets and/or meat reduction. As Teichoz points out, if one's livelihood depends on supporting a certain point of view, this is arguably a very strong potential conflict of interest.[22] In light of that potential conflict, it's imperative that researchers make every effort to counter it by going back to first principles and giving serious consideration to research that challenges the view to which they might be inclined. That effort does not appear to have been made by the authors of the EAT-Lancet report. 'It does not cite a single clinical trial to support the idea that a vegan/vegetarian diet promotes good health and fights disease,' says Teicholz, but relies instead on epidemiology, a kind of science that 'has been shown to be accurate, when tested in rigorous clinical trials, only 0–20% of the time'.[23]

A compromised process

Let's take stock. Thus far, we have a commission largely comprised of plant-based advocates with multiple potential competing interests, chaired by two leading plant-based advocates, appointed via an opaque process and overseen by wealthy and influential founders who have a long-standing interest in converting the world to the plant-based cause. Add in the facts that their plant-based dietary recommendations are based on a subjective interpretation of the science, and that this science was comprised entirely of epidemiological research showing weak associations between diet and disease, and it wouldn't be unreasonable to think the process to be somewhat compromised.

It is also important to consider the fact that some thirty large corporations have aligned themselves with EAT via an amalgamation called FReSH (Food Reform for Sustainability and Health), a bridge to the WBCSD.[24] (This is the organisation founded by Maurice Strong that you'll recall from earlier in this chapter.) These corporations – mostly from the processed food, bio-tech, pharmaceutical and chemical industries – manufacture and sell products that will be more in demand as a result of the large-scale adoption of a plant-based diet. The EAT seal of approval, by allowing them to greenwash their brands and products, represents a gold-plated marketing opportunity. And the scapegoating of animal agriculture as a primary driver of global warming serves to divert attention away from any unhealthy and polluting activities that these companies might be involved in.

Think about what PepsiCo has to gain from its affiliation with EAT. For starters: a nice distraction from the war on sugar that would surely have taken a firmer hold of our collective consciousness were we not so caught up in the war on meat. In addition, there's the potential for an increase in demand for processed food and drink products, many of which will now qualify, if not as healthy options, then at least as acceptable ones, under the EAT dietary guidelines. PepsiCo has openly declared the future to be vegan.[25] Should we be surprised? After all, market expansion opportunities are the lifeblood of commercial organisations.

The same gains are likely for companies such as Unilever, Kellogg's and Nestlé, all part of FReSH. These companies are essentially already vegan, since most of their packaged foods are made up of the same basic ingredients: soya, corn, grains, sugars and salt.[26] Now, thanks to their alliance with FReSH and EAT, they can promote these products as 'healthy' and boost sales by slapping a vegan – or, at the very least, plant-based – label on all their packaging. Some are going further. Simultaneously with the EAT report being published, Nestlé announced that it had entered into a joint four-billion-dollar investment in The Future Food Initiative with Givaudan (a producer of flavours and fragrances) and Bühler (a process engineering company), with the goal of developing so-called healthy food products. Unsurprisingly, its first research is to focus on 'plant-based nutrition and ancient plants'. With these three companies as partners, how likely is it that the plant foods they produce will be fresh, whole or real, rather than the ultra-processed variety?

Stefan Scheiber, CEO of the Bühler Group, said that the initiative would 'help combat global hunger concerns and align perfectly with our ambition of addressing global challenges of hunger and malnutrition'.[27] Now, I'll admit the possibility that the Bühler Group and its partners do count the reduction of hunger and malnutrition among their genuine ambitions. But it's important to note just how well those words – hunger, malnutrition – serve what is almost certainly another ambition: to capitalise on a massive marketing opportunity by aligning themselves with the vegan message and those who promote it.

What of the chemical companies? They stand to gain from the boost in sales of their artificial fertilisers and pesticides that will result from EAT's plan. More plant-based foods like the Impossible Burger, and every other processed vegan food currently in development, will require vast amounts of corn and soya, most of it grown with the help of what EAT calls 'radical improvements in the efficiency of fertiliser',[28] which sounds to me like code for 'bring on the chemicals!' Chemicals, of course, would be a big part of the future envisioned by EAT, since animal agriculture would be minimised to the point where it could no longer serve to nourish and rebuild our soils.

For a company like Yara International, the FReSH/EAT connection is like a gift from the gods. Yara, a chemical company largely owned by the Norwegian government, is one of the world's largest producers of synthetic fertilisers, which are major contributors to soil degradation and climate change. Yara has invested millions in shaping the international agricultural agenda, recently targeting Africa, Brazil and India. It has also been involved in one of Norway's biggest corruption scandals, having been caught paying millions in bribes to Indian and Libyan officials.[29] Now, thanks to the greenwashing effect of its participation in FReSH, it has been given a fresh start and a route to more and bigger markets.

The plant-based revolution could be seen as a gift for

all large chemical companies. 'It has to be Monsanto's wet dream,' said Glen Burrows, the Ethical Butcher: 'whereas the concept of regenerative agriculture incorporating livestock has to terrify them. Hang on, people can produce nutrient-dense food and they don't need fertiliser or pesticides or any artificial inputs at all? It's easy to see why they back the plant-based message that the single biggest thing you need to do to reduce your footprint is to reduce meat consumption. That's just the message they need to drive their business forward.'[30]

Frédéric Leroy wrote that Big Ag's participation in FReSH was surely influenced by its discovery that the plant-based lifestyle market generates large profit margins, adding value through the ultra-processing of cheap materials such as protein extracts, starches and oils.[31] FReSH, it would seem, may not be exclusively or even primarily about sustainability, any more than ILSI is exclusively or primarily about health.

EAT's corporate partnerships are not confined to FReSH. EAT is also working closely with a campaigning group called the Barilla Center for Food and Nutrition (BCFN). (Both Gunhild Stordalen and Walter Willett have been keynote speakers at its International Forum on Food and Nutrition.) BCFN, established in 2009, describes itself as an 'independent think-tank', even though the owners of the pasta giant Barilla are on its board of directors and the organisation shares a name with the company. The authors of a study promoting BCFN's double food pyramid have declared that they acted 'in the absence of any commercial or financial relationships that could be construed as potential conflicts of interest'. Maybe so. But we know from the evidence presented in Chapter 12 that corporate sponsorship and funding often leads to research outcomes in favour of industry's products, and that sponsorship deals are entered into with the goal of enhancing brand value in mind. And the Barilla sponsored food pyramid – which discourages the eating of meat and recommends cereals – a subset of which is pasta – will undoubtedly enhance its own brand value. Something that is positioned as a scientific instrument for global policy (and, which might genuinely be viewed as such by some within the corporation) thus conveniently serves as a highly effective marketing tool.[32]

Other marketing tools deployed by Barilla include: the publication of a book, *Nourished Planet*, authored by BCFN and edited by Danielle Nierenberg, president of a think-tank dedicated to 'environmentally friendly ways of alleviating hunger, obesity and poverty' (note the clever deployment of those winning words again: 'hunger', 'obesity' and 'poverty'); the provision of funding to groups such as Boston-based Oldways, which promotes the use of whole grains; campaigning in Washington DC via sponsored newsletters to politicians; and exerting influence over nutrition science itself by funding more than ten studies with outcomes that favour increased consumption of grains and pasta, including one study that was reported as showing that eating pasta is 'linked to weight loss'.[33]

Barilla's management team might well count the prevention of hunger and obesity and the salvation of the planet among its goals. But it would be naive not to acknowledge that the company is also riding a highly lucrative zeitgeist all the way to the bank.

It's about the money, but that's not all it's about

If corporations are ultimately in it for the money (as they are obliged to be, by the way, given their responsibilities to shareholders), what motivates EAT itself, besides the plant-based leanings of its founders, funders and commissioners? Frank Mitloehner's email exchange with an EAT representative confirmed that the diet hadn't been designed with planetary health in mind, but to 'reduce the risk of premature mortality due to dietary related causes'. But the diet can't be entirely about human health either, because it is deemed (by EAT itself) to be nutritionally unsuitable for large segments of the population.[34] So, what is it all about, EAT?

Professor Leroy warns against thinking of EAT or any of the NGOs lined up behind it as entirely homogeneous, saying that 'there's internal friction in all of them'. This heterogeneity is what enables the UN to convey conflicting personas, allowing it, for example, to designate the years 2016–2025 as the Decade of Nutrition[35] while simultaneously promoting highly processed foods like the Impossible Burger and the nutritionally deficient Planetary Health Diet. Similarly, the UN's former executive secretary for climate change can insist that meat eaters should be treated like smokers, while its constituent organisations the IPCC and FAO publish reports which recognise the critical role of livestock within agroecological systems.

The motivations of these large organisations are likely as divergent as their actions and outputs. But, says Leroy, control – 'over resources, production, consumption and discourse' – emerges as a common theme. 'The entire Planetary Health Diet framework is about suppressing diversity and individual choice – diversity equals chaos ... and brings the unpredictability that these high-modernist, top-down planners detest.'[36]

Another commentator labelled the top-down plans coming out of organisations such as EAT as 'old-school social control and social engineering' with an underlying paternalism.[37]

The WBCSD's Vision 2050 document is a prime example of an attempt at social engineering.[38] Its aims are laudable enough. Who would argue with the following aspects of their stated vision for food: that everyone has access to nutritious and affordable food; food is consumed sustainably; diets become healthy and sustainable; and the world moves towards a circular food system with zero loss and waste? But the fine print attached to such goals is what's potentially worrying. Who will define what kind of diet is healthful and sustainable, for example? And if businesses are to be encouraged to 'develop and scale an array of new, healthy and sustainable protein sources' who will assure the actual healthfulness and sustainability of those sources? And how will we prevent all power and wealth in the food system from becoming concentrated in the hands of the corporate innovators, at the expense of local food suppliers and consumers?

The list of signatories to the Vision 2050 document offers little reassurance. The vast majority of the forty-two signatories are large corporations in the banking, finance, technology, vehicle manufacturing, chemical, cement, engineering and retail industries. Just six (including Unilever and Nestlé) are from the food industry, and these are all engaged in the production of processed foods. On one level, of course, the engagement of corporations in resolving the big issues of the day is a positive. Better to have them onboard than resisting change at the sidelines. But important questions present themselves. What *kind* of change will we get with those corporations onboard? And is it right that the design of a future food system should be influenced by companies so unconnected to real food, food culture and farming? Where are the representatives of regenerative agriculture and community food projects, and where is the deep understanding of human nutrition? And, looking at the bigger picture, is social control and social engineering of this type, involving large corporations, really what the world needs, or could it have grave unforeseen negative consequences, not least for freedom of speech and choice?

An organisation called IPES FOOD (International Panel

of Experts on Sustainable Food Systems) certainly views corporate-led social engineering as having negative consequences.[39] Its founder, Pat Mooney (winner of The Pearson Peace Prize in Canada), has spoken out against the 'corporate bamboozle on world food systems' and in favour of the long food movement (decentralising control, democratising food, using regenerative approaches) as an antidote to agri-business-led transformations. The language of multi-stakeholder systems sounds reasonable but is, he says, a 'most insidious and dangerous concept' and a 'complete falsity'. 'The real negotiation is not multi-stakeholder – it's really just a negotiation between governments and corporations' and 'it has to be rejected'.[40]

The global coalition driving The Great Food Transformation

Entities like the WBCSD, the WEF, EAT, the UN, the WHO, and FReSH represent a global coalition of influential, like-minded organisations united in several goals, one of which is increasing the uptake of a plant-based diet around the world. The coalition has amplified the plant-based message to such an extent that many of the world's governments and large swathes of the global population believe it to be the only way forward. And the message can only get louder as the ties between different members of the coalition become more extensive. In 2020, the UN named Impossible Foods one of its Climate Action Award winners and provided what amounts to advertising for the brand via a tweet about its having won the award. The WEF and the UN signed a Strategic Partnership Framework to 'accelerate the implementation of the 2030 Agenda for Sustainable Development', a move that was condemned as a WEF takeover of the UN.[41] The UN also placed

EAT at the heart of its own food strategy, naming Gunhild Stordalen as chair of the 'Sustainable diets' work track of its 2021 Food Summit, and appointing the WHO as the 'anchoring agency'. WEF and WRI representatives were involved in the various work tracks for the summit, alongside others known to be involved in plant-based advocacy (The Good Food Institute, a well-funded lobby group for vegan tech; the president of Good Food Fund in China, a vegan activist; and a representative of the Cool Food Pledge, a pro-plant-based organisation, also a member of the WRI).[42] Ajay Vir Jakhar, chairman of the Farmers Forum in India, may have been there to emphasise the important role of farmers in the shift to sustainable consumption, but his voice was likely to be drowned out by the voices of those with different views. We probably shouldn't expect much in the way of balanced, evidenced-based outcomes from this summit, but, as Frédéric Leroy pointed out, we are likely to see a lot more 'high profile bashing of livestock farming and meat and dairy'.[43]

At the time of writing, early indications of specific outcomes from the summit were not encouraging. A Science Reader (a publication documenting research by the scientific group and its global partners in support of summit action agendas) bearing the stamp of the summit was, according to one commentator, 'in complete denial of recent discoveries in soil science' and 'driven to sustain the status quo industries'.[44] Additionally, several attendees I spoke to reported having been immensely frustrated by the singular plant-based message running through some of the summit's workstreams.

The organisations in the global coalition are powerful and espouse strong views that often stand in contradiction to the behaviour of individuals within them. Although Gunhild Storladen has a stated passion for addressing climate change, she was reported as travelling around the world in a 26-million-dollar private jet. The commissioners and authors of the EAT-Lancet report also clocked up some spectacular emissions-generating air miles as they travelled around the world to multiple workshops and meetings. Stordalen's (now ex) husband, Petter, doesn't appear to be a fan of the commission's dietary recommendations – during a trip to Las Vegas, he posted a photo of himself eating a giant burger at the Heart Attack Grill.[45]

In the face of such immense influence and inconsistency, we would be wise to maintain a healthy scepticism towards pronouncements made by EAT and global organisations of its ilk. The power of scepticism came to the rescue in 2019, when the EAT report was first published. Scientists, nutritionists, doctors and others came together on social media around the hashtag #Yes2meat, generating an avalanche of critiques of the EAT report. EAT's own analysis of the social media campaign revealed how successful it had been, and the extent to which it had scuppered EAT's plans to amass immediate global support for their diet.[46] Rather than take the feedback as a prompt to have a rethink, EAT complained about content pollution and the spread of disinformation.

#Yes2meat may have led EAT and other global institutions to feel temporarily down, but they are certainly not out. Gunhild Stordalen's comments prior to the UN Food Summit were chilling: 'Our goal is therefore to take full advantage of the Summit to build an *unstoppable* global movement for change that we can keep growing well beyond the Summit, to *force* the kinds of far-reaching changes that the world now desperately needs.'[47] (Italics mine.)

Stordalen followed up this statement by claiming to be 'humbled' by the opportunity. But it's difficult to see Stordalen, EAT or any of their corporate or institutional partners as entirely humble. Even if they are well intentioned, and believe wholeheartedly in their cause, the result of their combined efforts is a movement that short-changes objective science, enhances and concentrates power and profits, and will be more likely to fail both human and planetary health than save them.

Dr Harcombe has urged us to wake up and 'understand the global agenda threatening our diet and thus health'. Real food, she says 'is simply not that lucrative and we are pawns in an increasingly scary world'.[48] Joanna Blythman has issued similar counsel:

> Watch out for increasingly ubiquitous phrases popping up in the public realm of food – 'The Great Food Transformation', 'Food Systems Shift', 'The Planetary Health Diet' – and recognise them for what they are, a well-resourced, co-ordinated, top-down attempt to reshape what we eat. Unchallenged, such ideas would largely remove food production from the natural sphere and fill our plates with ultra-processed, multi-component foods that could generate massive profits for their makers.[49]

The Great Reset

The latest variation on these ubiquitous phrases is The Great Reset, the plans for which are captured in a diagram on the WEF website.[50] The diagram, best described as a wheel with many spokes, depicts some fifty aspects of global life that need to be reset, including Corporate Governance, Justice and Law, Financial and Monetary Systems, and, of course, The Future of Food. This is social control and engineering on a grand and truly terrifying scale.

Joanna Blythman has called the reset 'an extreme form of globalisation, a fourth industrial revolution, if you like, that would centralise control of society in a few hands'. It has emerged from a 'Davos based set of uber-wealthy individuals and corporates'. Its influence can already be detected in a report by the UK Health Alliance on Climate Change, a coalition of health professionals who have called for a tax on meat to force a 50 per cent reduction in consumption and for mandatory food labelling based on crude assessments of the emissions cost of foods. Their report, like many of its kind, was replete with flawed analysis, cherry-picked studies and untenable assumptions, but that didn't stop the media from trumpeting its headline conclusions.[51] Is the UK Health Alliance one of what Blythman calls the many 'foot soldiers' of the orchestrated agenda that will take the Great Reset into our schools, hospitals and homes? Her warning about the Great Reset is stark:

> This technocratic push will soon impinge on all our lives. Your child's school will be told to run meat-free days. The hospital will drop beef for vegan 'sausages'. Public health messaging, seeping into school education, will seek to persuade you and your children that all meat, even the grass-fed, outdoor reared meat that the UK is so good at producing, is to be shunned. First we will be 'nudged' to abandon food habits that have sustained omnivore populations around the globe for millennia, next we will be forced through fiscal measures. Be aware of this orchestrated agenda. Its foot soldiers are already out and about.[52]

Dr Marcia Angell wrote, about the pharmaceutical industry, that it 'is taking us for a ride, and there will be no real reform without an aroused and determined public to make it happen'.[53] The architects of the Great Reset are taking us for a ride, too. We must be that 'aroused and determined public' if we are to avoid the damage to human and environmental health that would result from the wholesale adoption of their recommendations.

Part Four

How Should We Eat?

'Eat fresh, local, seasonal whole food, based on your environment and cultural beliefs, avoiding added sugars and processed foods.'

DR GARY FETTKE,
Orthopaedic surgeon

'The need to amend foods, and to take nutrient supplèments, could be reduced by creating phytochemically rich plants and herbivores and by creating cultures that know how to combine foods into meals that nourish and satiate.'

FRED PROVENZA, MICHEL MEURET, PABLO GREGORINI,
'Our Landscapes, Our Livestock, Ourselves: Restoring broken linkages among plants, herbivores, and humans with diets that nourish and satiate', *Appetite*

'I have come to understand that even good farmers cannot single-handedly determine the fate of their farms. They have to rely on the shopping and voting choices of the rest of us to support and protect nature-friendly, sustainable agriculture.'

JAMES REBANKS,
English Pastoral: An Inheritance

15

How to Eat to Optimise Human and Planetary Health: The Real Food Solution

The public debate about food, health and the environment has become centred on a single question: should we eliminate animal foods from our diet? This question has pitted plant-based advocates against omnivores in a battle characterised by heated argument, malicious attacks, an absence of nuance, and a failure to grasp and address the complex relationships that define our ecosystem.

This question – should we eliminate animal foods from our diet? – is surely the wrong one to be asking, however. The right question is this: what foods are essential to human health and longevity, and can these foods now be produced in a way that minimises environmental harm and maximises environmental benefits?

If you've reached this point in the book, you'll know that the evidence does not support the eating of a plants-only diet. What diet, therefore, *does* the evidence support? How should we eat? I've used the word 'how' intentionally here because it captures the idea that it is not just what we put on our tables and in our mouths that's important, but *how* it is grown or raised, *how* we choose and obtain it, *how* it's prepared. Raising, choosing, buying, preparing – these are all important parts of the process.

To answer this question – how should we eat? – we might take a cue from those farmers who have concluded that the key to the future lies in the past. Talking to his young son about his own farm, James Rebanks said: 'I try to explain why I care about muck, and beetles and peat bogs, and fungi and worms. I try to explain that the future of the farm lies in replicating as best we can the habitats (and natural processes) of this once-wild valley, thousands of years ago.'[1]

Just as the past can be a guide to farmers, it can also be a guide to the consumers of their produce. To eat in a way that nourishes and sustains us we need to re-familiarise ourselves with forgotten principles. There's no better way to understand what that means than to revisit the work of Dr Weston A. Price, the crux of which is summarised in the prologue to the 2008 edition of his seminal work, *Nutrition and Physical Degeneration,* first published in 1939.

> The implication of the Price research is profound: if civilised man is to survive, he must somehow incorporate the fundamentals of primitive nutritional wisdom into his modern lifestyle. He must turn his back on the allure of civilised foodstuffs that line his supermarket shelves and return to the whole, nutrient dense foods of his ancestors. He must restore the soil to health through nontoxic and biological farming methods. And he must repair the 'greatest breakdown in our modern civilized diet', which is the gradual replacement of foods rich in fat-soluble activators with substitutes and imitations compounded of vegetable oils, fillers, stabilisers and additives.[2]

Dr Price articulated the dietary principles that would repair the 'breakdown in our modern civilised diet' in a letter to his nephews and nieces.[3] In it he talked about the 'tragic mistake' that society had made in 'getting away from the natural foods that are low in energy and high in minerals', and the importance of eating foods that are rich in phosphorus, calcium and vitamins, particularly fat-soluble vitamins. Fish, eggs, meat and cooked vegetables were to be consumed in abundance, as were milk, cheese and butter 'made from cows that have been on a rapidly growing young wheat, either fresh or stored grass', and 'butter made in June' and eaten chiefly for its vitamin content. Intake of sugars and starches was to be avoided, with consumption of white flour products and pastries kept 'to a minimum'. Dr Price deemed fruits 'desirable as an adjunct' but warned that most are very low in minerals.

Some seventy years later, Michael Pollan (*In Defence of Food*) reminded us that Dr Price had found the common denominator of good health to be eating 'a traditional diet consisting of fresh foods from animals and plants grown on soils that were themselves rich in nutrients'.[4] He urged us to eat 'food' rather than 'edible food-like substances', by which he meant the packaged, processed stuff so denuded of nutrients that lines the shelves in the middle of a supermarket.[5]

Dr Gary Fettke's prescription for a healthy diet captures the essence of Dr Price's principles in a single sentence: 'Eat fresh, local, seasonal whole food, based on your environment and cultural beliefs, avoiding added sugars and processed foods.' Dr Fettke's emphasis on the importance of 'environment and cultural beliefs' harks back to Dr Price's observation that each of the healthy traditional populations ate the plant and animal foods that they could obtain from their local environment and as prescribed by their cultural traditions. The foods eaten by the Inuit of Alaska were not the same as those eaten by the Gaels in the Outer and Inner Hebrides or the Polynesians, but all the diets were rich in nutrients and devoid of processed, or de-natured, foods, and all contained animal fats and foods.

Each of the doctors and nutrition experts I consulted when writing this book has their own concise credo that is consistent with Dr Price's principles. Dr Zoë Harcombe, for example, advises people to eat real food and choose food for the nutrients it provides.[6] Emphasising the importance of nutrients, dietitian Diana Rodgers asks us to 'eat like a nutrivore'.[7] Researcher and biochemical engineer Ivor Cummins suggests that we avoid sugar, seed oils and refined carbohydrates while eating plenty of meat, fish and eggs. Bariatric surgeon and author Dr Andrew Jenkinson favours the 'greengrocer, butcher, fishmonger diet' full of fresh, whole foods and devoid of vegetable oils.[8] The Public Health Collaboration tells us simply to eat real food, avoid fake food and be active every day. Cardiologist Aseem Malhotra, nutritionist Izabella Natrins, and the Real Food Campaign UK[9] promote similar, real-food credos.

Dr Malcolm Kendrick summed up the real food message nicely in his book about heart disease and how to prevent it (*The Clot Thickens*):

> rather than creating endless lists [of foods to eat] here is a more general rule to follow. Eat food that looks like food. Real food, natural food. Food without a list of ingredients 10-feet long on the side. Fish, meat, vegetables, fruit, cream, eggs. You should be able to get everything that you require from 'natural' food. All the vitamins, minerals, potassium, and things that boost your nitric oxide.[10]

Food that nourishes

Real food is where it's at. Price's traditional populations seemed to have an instinctive sense of what real, nutrient-dense food was in the context of their own environment. Some among our older generations seemed to have that instinct, too. But for many, that instinctive knowledge about what constitutes good food, and which particular foods the body needs at any point in time, has been lost. To regain the 'wisdom of the body', we can learn from animals, says Fred Provenza. Provenza and fellow researchers Pablo Gregorini and Cindi Anderson, contend that animals meet their own needs for nutrients and self-medication through three interrelated processes.[11] First, they must have access to a variety of wholesome foods – the more they are restricted (for instance to a feedlot ration) the less they can maintain health. Second, a mother's knowledge – of what and what not to eat and where and where not to forage – is essential for helping her offspring get a start in life. Third, liking for food (that is, the foods an animal wants to eat at any point in time) is influenced by feedback from cells and organ systems in response to nutritional and medicinal needs, which are met by nutrients and thousands of other compounds produced by plants.

Animals in confined systems are unable to meet their own nutritional and medicinal needs by selecting the foods they need. Humans have ended up in a version of a confined system, in which our ability to select foods that meet our own nutritional and medicinal needs has been weakened by the combination of a food environment replete with ultra-processed foods and a barrage of conflicting advice from the media and the authorities. 'We stopped listening to the wisdom of the body and yielded to the advice from authorities,' says Provenza. To regain access to that wisdom, we need to give ourselves access to a wide variety of whole foods and restrict access to the ultra-processed foods that are the 'noise' corrupting our tastes, our minds and our instincts for nutrition and drowning out the wise words from the body.

It's arguable, says Provenza, that if everyone had access to a wide variety of whole foods and was encouraged to eat them, we would have no need for national dietary guidelines.

Simply sticking to real food will get many people most of the way there with healthy eating. But those who are in suboptimal metabolic health, or who suffer from particular conditions, or 'fatten easily' (to use Gary Taubes' term), a simple commitment to eating real food might not be enough. Taubes cites physician Jennifer Hendrix, who said that 'just eat real food' is excellent advice for preventative medicine, but insufficient for those who are not in good health: 'Once a person has obesity, and particularly obesity with comorbidities like diabetes and hypertension, it's much more complicated. I've never seen anyone who had a weight problem their whole life have the weight go away merely by changing to a real food diet, because some of those real foods are still fattening.'[12]

The foods that are fattening, particularly to those who fatten easily, are carbohydrate-rich foods, says Taubes, making a convincing case for why this is so in his book *The Case for Keto*. This is a simple truth that has been so hard to understand because we've been trapped in what he calls 'a context of naive conventional wisdom – eat less or not too much, avoid fat and saturated fat, eat mostly plants'.

If the real food guidelines are not specific enough for some, official guidelines (of the Eatwell variety) are almost completely useless. They are written for the lean and the already healthy, and they don't even take the unhealthy into account, as Taubes points out, and as Nina Teicholz, in her capacity as director of the Nutrition Coalition, has consistently argued. These guidelines are blind to the evidence that many, if not most people, could benefit from dramatically reducing their intake of carbohydrates – and refined carbohydrates in particular.

The carbohydrate question

The advice to avoid refined grains and sugars is something that almost all dietary approaches, from Paleo to Weight Watchers, have in common, and there is plenty of evidence to support that advice. Remember that the traditional diets of the healthiest people studied by Dr Price contained no refined carbohydrates whatsoever. The benefits of controlling the intake of refined carbohydrates have been seen in studies of Western populations, too, and include a reduced risk of heart disease, better blood pressure control, reproductive health and neurological health, and the elimination of those irritations of middle age: heartburn and snoring.[13] A ketogenic diet, which removes not just carbohydrates of the refined variety but virtually all carbohydrates, has been shown to be effective against a range of medical conditions including epilepsy and cancer, as we saw in Chapter 5.

The extent to which carbohydrates should be avoided, however, can really only be determined at the level of the individual. Izabella Natrins writes that 'depending on our state of health, what we want to achieve with dietary adjustments, our lifestyle and energy needs, our ability to store and use glycogen and the quality of the carbs we consume, they can be great for us, or they can give us grief'.[14]

Vinnie Tortorich's message – *no* sugar, *no* grains, or NSNG – works for his clients, and it has helped to keep his cancer at bay. But Tortorich recognises that not everyone can be, or needs to be, quite as strict. Even Vinnie will eat a slice of birthday cake or drink a few glasses of red wine when the occasion calls for it. His advice: if you want the benefits of eating a low-carb diet but you also love carbs, don't say 'never', just say 'rarely'. Cheat sometimes but be a conscious cheater.[15]

This advice will work for some people. For others, argues

Gary Taubes, and particularly for those who 'fatten easily', are addicted to carbohydrates or have severe cases of type-2 diabetes, cheating can be the road to ruin. Their diet must consistently be not just low carb (meaning none of the obvious culprits such as pasta, bread, rice, sweets, cakes or desserts) but *very* low carb/ketogenic (excluding starchy vegetables and many fruits too). Debra Scott, whose type-2 diabetes is in remission, knows that a slice of wholegrain bread will send her blood sugars soaring. Professor Tim Noakes has concluded that he must eat virtually no carbohydrates at all if he wants to control his diabetes – even a handful of blueberries will cause his blood sugar levels to go haywire.

For some, however, a diet without any carbohydrates is the definition of dietary hell. And are you going to tell an Italian not to eat pasta? I'm certainly not. Besides, some people can eat all the pasta they want and suffer no health consequences. If you are not one of these people, you might take heart from Vinnie Tortorich's reminder that the Italians (of which he is one) have never eaten giant bowls of pasta on a daily basis, in any case. Pasta was always a side attraction, there to soak up the sauce or accompany the meat or fish. It can be enjoyed, just not in huge quantities at every meal.

The same could be said about bread: eat it sparingly and make sure it's the right kind. As we saw in Chapter 4, bread isn't what it used to be, and most modern bread is devoid of nutrients. Your best option, says Izabella Natrins, is a high-quality, authentically produced sourdough loaf.[16] Read the ingredients, there should be just three: flour, salt and water. Better still, make your own.

As we saw in Chapter 4, conditions such as eczema, leaky gut, IBS and autoimmune conditions can be exacerbated by grains. If you suffer from any of these conditions, you might benefit from cutting out bread altogether. And if you're trying to lose weight, bread and other carbohydrates are not your friends. (See Chapter 5 for a review of this evidence.) If you are diabetic or in poor metabolic health, bread and other carbs are your number-one enemy.

For further guidance on answering the 'how much carbohydrate?' question, you might refer to Ben Bikman's guidelines about metabolic health and carbohydrates and his insulin resistance quiz (found in *Why We Get Sick*). The quiz includes questions about belly fat, blood pressure and triglyceride levels, with answers determining how many grams of carbohydrate are appropriate for you to consume on a daily basis.[17] (Remember, grams of carbohydrate do not equate to the grams of food on your plate. You can easily find out the grams of carbohydrate in any given weight of food by searching online, reading food labels, or using an app such as Carb Manager.) Other lifestyle factors can also help you to reduce insulin resistance: for example, improving the quality of your sleep, getting regular exercise, lowering stress levels, practising time-restricted eating and stopping smoking.

The question 'how much carbohydrate' is just one of the questions you might have about how to apply real-food principles in your own life. Other questions might pertain to calories (do they matter?), fruits and vegetables (what's the right number?), meat (how much?), fat (how much and what type?), and meal frequency. Let's look at each of these questions in turn.

Do calories matter?

Calories don't matter as much as you might have been led to believe. Certainly, if you consistently eat many more calories than is right for your body, you will gain weight. And if you reduce calorie intake enough, you will lose weight. But that weight probably won't stay off unless you continue to deprive yourself, because the body fights against long-term deprivation by reducing its metabolic rate. And there is no straight, mathematical line between calorie intake and weight loss (or weight gain). In short, and as argued by the physicians and obesity experts we met in Chapter 5, the CICO (calories-in, calories-out) theory is overly simplistic, some say wrong.

To appreciate how off-the-mark the CICO theory is, you might want to go back to Chapter 5 and remind yourself of PHC founder Sam Feltham's personal experiment involving three different diets (see page 182). Sam tried three periods of consuming 3,000 more calories than he was used to eating, but he did it on three different diets: a low-carb, real-food diet; a low-fat, fake-food diet; and a low-fat vegan diet. On the low-carb, real-food diet he gained just 1.3kg, when the CICO formula would have predicted a gain of 6.1kg. Clearly, the type of food you eat matters more than the number of calories, and real-food diets that are low in carbohydrates have been shown to be most effective for weight loss and control.

Fruit and vegetables – what's the right number?

As we saw on page 71, the number five was plucked from the air and the five-a-day rule has no basis in evidence. That said, fruit and vegetables grown in good soil can contain valuable vitamins, minerals and phytochemicals, and they add colour, taste and texture to meals, so it's best to eat a wide variety every day. Variety is beneficial, not only for maximising nutrient and phytochemical intake but also for encouraging a more diverse bacterial population in the gut.[18] Just as diverse mixes of plant species create what Fred Provenza calls 'homes, grocery stores and pharmacies' for creatures residing in and above the soil, diversity is key for the health of our microbiome.[19]

But not everyone can tolerate fruit and vegetables in large quantities. You might be fine following Michael Pollan's policy (Eat food. Not too much. Mostly plants) but, if you suffer from an autoimmune condition, you could be better off following Amber O'Hearn's advice (Eat meat. Not too little. Mostly fat). (I discussed O'Hearn's research in Chapter 6.) You be the judge. Pay attention to what different fruits and vegetables do to you. Tap into that wisdom of the body. And remember that everything is a potential toxin, depending on the dose.[20] My mother's digestive system screams for help when she eats salad three days in a row. My husband – whose chronic indigestion and equally chronic snoring habit disappeared when he cut most of the carbs from his diet – thought he could tolerate cauliflower until he ate two bowls of homemade cauliflower soup for dinner and was kept awake by the first bout of chronic indigestion he had experienced in months. And we have the salutary lesson provided by Liam Hemsworth, whose green smoothie habit gave him kidney stones from oxalate poisoning.

If you can't tolerate many plant foods, you can get almost a full complement of nutrients from animal foods, provided you eat a wide variety and include foods like pasture-raised meat and eggs, cheese, oily fish, liver and bone broth. And don't forget the herbs and spices, which are not just optional extras but are also good for health, providing phytochemicals while enhancing palatability and satiation.[21]

How much meat should you eat?

As with many aspects of diet, the answer to this question is 'it depends'. People's protein needs vary widely, being determined by age, gender, weight, and metabolic and general health. The WHO recommends that adults should consume a minimum of

0.83g of protein per 1kg of bodyweight (about 54g of protein per day for a 65kg/10st 4lb adult). But we know that many protein experts consider the protein RDA to be too low for optimal health and would prefer that people consumed at least 1g of protein for every 1kg of bodyweight (therefore: 65g for a 65kg/10st 4lb adult). You could obtain this amount of protein with a menu such as this:[22]

Breakfast: one egg and half an avocado (8g of protein)
Lunch: tuna salad made with 100g tuna and a handful of lettuce (28.5g of protein)
Dinner: 100g steak or chicken and 100g broccoli (27.8g of protein, of which 2.8g comes from the broccoli)

I am not suggesting that you eat only these foods (which deliver too few calories and insufficient fat and nutrients), but that your protein needs would be met by such a combination of foods. It's also a good idea to include some protein in every meal – registered dietitian Valeria Burnazov recommends a minimum of 30g – to stave off hunger and the desire to snack, particularly in the evenings.[23]

If you choose not to eat meat on a daily basis, or at all, you can ensure that you consume your daily requirement of all the EAAs by including some animal-sourced foods, such as fish or cheese, in some of your daily meals. If, after reading this book, you still prefer to get all your protein from plant sources, you will need to think carefully about which ones are complementary in terms of amino acid profile and make sure that you eat these within a few hours of one another. You also need to be cognisant of the fact that the protein from plant foods is less digestible (and therefore less bioavailable) than that from animal foods. Your absolute protein intake will need to be significantly higher to compensate for this. (That is, higher than 1g per 1kg of bodyweight.)

In the context of these facts about protein, you would have to say that most people should be eating some meat, fish and/or eggs every day. EAT-Lancet's recommendation that we consume a maximum of 16g of meat per day, or *Lancet* editor Richard Horton's suggestion that we think about eating meat once or twice a *month*, is misguided in this context. For those with type-2 diabetes, those who gain weight easily, or those who rely on ketogenic diets to control conditions such as epilepsy, and must therefore make meat more central to their diet, such recommendations could be detrimental in the extreme.

This is why the incantation that 'we should all be eating less meat' is something of a nonsense. How much meat do you already eat? How much do you need to eat to meet your specific protein needs, optimise your health or control a medical condition? The incantation is not just nonsensical but unjust and injurious when applied to those in the developing world, where malnourishment and stunting is common, and more, not less, meat is called for.[24] If you are consistently eating less than the 100g a day of meat suggested in the sample menu noted earlier, it's arguable that you, too, would benefit from eating more meat. A hundred grams of meat a day translates into 37kg of meat per year, still a good deal less than the current average per capita consumption in either North America or Europe: about 97kg and 70kg respectively.[25]

Balancing health and environmental considerations

Of course, human health is not the only consideration here (though it is a very important one); there's also the important question of how much quality protein the food system can reasonably and sustainably supply. As Robert Barbour of the Sustainable Food Trust put it to me, the right way to look at the 'how much meat?' question is to ask how much meat can be supplied by production systems that are fully sustainable.[26] An individual can't possibly know the macro-level answer to that question, but they can commit to eating meat only from sustainable systems. That means eating the best meat you can find, pasture raised in regenerative farming systems and without grain inputs. (Regenuary, a movement initiated by The Ethical Butcher as an alternative to Veganuary, aims to recruit people to eating foods that are 'local, seasonal and farmed using regenerative methods'.) Ironically, given all the brouhaha around red meat, that probably means that those of us who eat a lot of chicken will need to add some red meat back into the diet. The evidence suggests, in any case, that eating two to four moderate servings of red meat a week can be beneficial to health.[27] That red meat could be beef, lamb, duck or liver, and the more variety in the diet, the better.

The argument for 'better meat' (that is, meat from sustainable systems) is made by Diana Rodgers and Robb Wolf in their book, *Sacred Cow*, and their film of the same name. As we saw in Part Two of this book, meat from regenerative farming systems comes not at a cost to the environment, but with benefits. There is an increasing amount of evidence that meat from regenerative farming systems also benefits human health. According to researchers Provenza, Anderson and Gregorini, eating meat from animals foraging on phytochemically rich diets can have positive metabolic effects above and beyond any increased intake of omega-3 fatty acids:

> The benefits to humans of eating phytochemically and biochemically rich meat accrue as livestock assimilate some phytochemicals and convert others into metabolites that become muscle and fat, which become biochemicals that improve health. That is similar to, but distinct from, benefits realized by eating phytochemically rich herbs, spices, vegetables, and fruits ... the metabolic effects of eating

meat from animals foraging on phytochemically rich diets are due in part to the ability of phytochemicals to modulate inflammation.[28]

If the widespread consumption of phytochemically rich meat is where we want to get to, we need to be cognisant of the fact that we can't get there all at once, and that parts of society can't even begin to get there now. Both health campaigner Brian Sanders and Dr Eric Westman were at pains to emphasise this point to me. They have helped thousands of Americans reverse chronic health conditions via low-carb diets that include work-a-day meat like that from McDonald's (without the bun, fries and soda). For people with chronic health conditions and living on very low incomes, some meat – whatever the quality – is better than no meat.

As regenerative livestock farming becomes more common, and industrial systems are phased out, even fast-food burgers could one day be labelled 'sustainable'. That's certainly the aim of Greenpeace's campaign to persuade retailers and fast-food chains to stop sourcing industrially produced meat. There are already signs that this is happening. In 2020, Canadian fast-food chain A&W stopped promoting plant-based meat substitutes and began highlighting their commitment to serving meat from regenerative farming systems.

As we consider the different ways to reduce our individual food-related carbon footprints, it's also important to remember that choosing the right meat (or reducing meat intake) is not the only or the best option open to us. Recall the data produced by Sarah Bridle in *Food and Climate Change: Without the Hot Air* (discussed in Chapter 9) – you could reduce your food footprint by more than a third[29] (without any nutritional downside) by cutting out the carbs (bread, pasta, cereal, rice, sugar, sweets, desserts, soft drinks and alcohol) and eliminating personal food waste.

As consumers aiming to balance nutritional and environmental considerations, we also have to be aware that any labelling schemes that are introduced will give us only part of the picture. As discussed in Chapter 10, the new scheme being developed for the UK (by Foundation Earth) aims to capture more than just carbon emissions, but may not reflect the full complexity of any individual food's environmental footprint, or its nutritional value.

Can you really eat fat, and if so, how much?

The bias against saturated fat will likely be with us for some time. Despite the fact that the limit on saturated fats is not, and never has been, supported by evidence, and notwithstanding the efforts by many in the nutrition field to have the saturated fat limits in dietary guidelines lifted,[30] it could be years before the medical and media establishments stop trying to terrify us with imagery of arteries clogged with saturated fat.

But, hopefully, the evidence presented in this book has convinced you not to fear fat. It's good for us, and we cannot live without it.[31] But we must eat the right kinds of fats – natural fats such as olive oil, coconut oil, butter, lard, goose fat and the fat in avocados and meat – not unnatural fats such as those in industrialised seed oils. If you must include some seed oils in your diet, opt for a high-oleic sunflower oil or rapeseed (canola), which has a much lower PUFA content and is lower in linoleic acid than regular sunflower, soybean or corn oil.[32] (Around 20 per cent as opposed to more than 50 per cent.)[33] Rapeseed oil used for cooking in your kitchen is also far less likely to be damaging than rapeseed oil consumed as part of ultra-processed food.

If using olive oil, be aware that adulteration is a widespread problem (that is, mixing olive oil with seed oils), particularly in the US.[34] There are a number of ways to mitigate against the risk of getting a big dose of PUFAs with your olive oil: buy only 'Extra Virgin' olive oil; check for a harvest date on the label; look for third party certification seals (such as the Extra Virgin Alliance mark in Europe); and look for olive oil in darker coloured glass (which protects against degradation, and is therefore a sign of a quality supplier). You could also try putting your olive oil in a (very cold) fridge – if it contains mostly monounsaturated fats it should become more viscous and a bit cloudy. While this is not a fool-proof test, 'if your olive oil doesn't thicken at all, that's a pretty good sign that it's a fake'.[35] Alternatively, you could email the supplier for confirmation that their olive oil is pure. (I did this once when a new brand of olive oil I'd bought didn't thicken in my fridge. I was rewarded with a long reply detailing extensive photographic evidence that the oil was pure and did in fact thicken if the fridge temperature was cold enough.)

There are two other things to note about fats. First, animal fats from pasture-raised animals deliver many more nutrients than those from factory-raised animals, so seek out butter, lard and fatty meat from pasture-raised animals. Second, it's best to avoid the high-fat–high-carb combination. Fats and carbs are rarely found together in nature, but they tend to be found a great deal in processed foods. Dr Ted Naiman warns that fat–carb combinations, such as are found in a cupcake, can drive overeating and weight gain: 'Foods that are simultaneously high in carbohydrates and fat, with a high energy density, are rarely found in nature and they are highly palatable and addictive. These foods completely hijack our satiety and mercilessly drive overeating.'[36]

Natural fats, in the absence of carbs, are unlikely to cause overeating. They are satiating and self-limiting. One of the joys of being on a low-carb, high-fat diet is that you are rarely hungry, rarely tempted to snack. And remember Dr Weston Price's advice to 'eat butter chiefly for its vitamin content': natural fats provide nutrients, too.

How often should you eat?

Dr Naiman also advises reducing carbohydrate frequency. Carbohydrates cause blood sugars to rise and fall, and insulin to be produced, and the less often this happens, the better. Reducing the frequency with which you eat carbohydrates forces your body to become 'fat adapted', or able to function using stored body fat.[37]

Most experts recommend reducing not just the frequency of *carbohydrate* intake but also the frequency of *food* intake, full stop. Dr Harcombe advises people to eat a maximum of three times a day, a regime that precludes snacking. Other doctors, such as Dr Jason Fung, have shown that confining our eating to a window of eight hours a day (say, between noon and 8pm) has benefits for weight loss and overall metabolic health. Time-restricted eating is a useful discipline for those who are used to endless snacking. By definition, it means that you won't reach for that bag of crisps or bowl of ice cream while watching TV.

Adapting to perfection

Dr Natasha Campbell-McBride stresses that 'we are all different; every one of us is a unique individual'.[38] Each of us has a different heredity and constitution, acid–alkaline balance, water–electrolyte balance, and different anabolic–catabolic cycles (the daily, seasonal and one-off cycles of building and cleansing within the body).[39] Genetic epidemiologist Tim

Spector also contends that our response to food is highly individualised.[40] Normal people can vary tenfold in their blood sugar responses to identical foods, for example.[41] Consequently, there is no such thing as a diet that works for everyone.

In 1956, Dr Roger Williams coined the term 'biochemical individuality' in recognition of the fact that different people have different nutritional needs, a concept that he explored in his book of the same name. William Wolcott and Trish Fahey have captured this idea of the 'one and only you' in their recently published book, *The Metabolic Typing Diet*. They maintain that 'any food or nutrient can have virtually opposite biochemical influences in different people'[42] and that diets need to be specifically tailored to the individual. They use metabolic typing (based on a simple questionnaire) to customise a diet to a person's unique body chemistry. The book is a useful tool for those who want to understand their own needs at a granular level and could be of particular benefit to those with health problems that conventional nutrition advice has failed to resolve.

Nutrigenomics – the study of the effects of food and food constituents on gene expression, and of how genetic variations affect the nutritional environment in the body – is a burgeoning field. It may eventually be commonplace for people to eat diets that have been carefully designed to suit their particular genome. For the time being our best option is to eat real, nutrient-dense food and to pay attention to the effects of different foods on our own physical and mental health. Paying attention, being conscious consumers of food, taking responsibility for our health, listening to the wisdom of the body – these are the goals. But we face some significant practical challenges in achieving these goals, particularly as we attempt to eat in a way that is good for us as individuals while also minimising harm to the environment. Shopping for the most nutrient-dense, sustainably produced foods is not an uncomplicated business. Affordability is an issue, and we face imperfect choices, not to mention having families who won't always eat as we'd like them to. Plus, there's cooking involved, which suits some very well and others not at all.

Shopping

The most nutrient-dense food comes from systems that are also best for the environment and for animal welfare. But finding these foods in the modern food system is not always easy. The free-range eggs on sale at most supermarkets are better than factory-farmed eggs, but hens who lay them do not actually have much space; organic eggs come from hens with a little more freedom and space, but not as much as we like to think. The best, most nutritious eggs from fully pasture-raised chickens are hard to come by, unless you live in close proximity to a farm that sells them.

The same applies to meat. Grass-fed beef doesn't necessarily mean grass-finished. Meat can be labelled grass-fed if more than 50 per cent of the animal's feed is grass (as opposed to grain). Therefore, much of the grass-fed beef in supermarkets and some butchers will come from cows for which up to 49 per cent of the diet could be grain-based feed. The label 'organic chicken' doesn't mean that the chicken has spent its life in a field scratching around for grubs and worms, but simply that its cereal feed was grown organically. And most pasture-raised pork is still fed a diet based largely on soya.

If you're serious about obtaining the best-quality produce, your best option is to shop at farms, farmers' markets, butchers and fishmongers who are willing to vouch for the provenance of their produce. (Sheila Cooke from 3LM, the UK hub of the Savory network, advises anyone interested in eating well and sustainably to 'make friends with a farmer', although if you live in a city, you may have to do this via a farmers' market or online ordering.) Ask questions: if they're proud of what they're selling they should answer. In the UK, you can also look for meat that is certified by the PFLA (Pasture-Fed Livestock Association)[43] or the growing Land to Market programme managed by the Savory Institute.[44] Another option is to buy your meat from an online specialist in produce from organic and grass-fed systems. For ideas as to where to buy sustainably produced real food, nutritionist Izabella Natrins has some useful resources at www.izabellanatrins.com and in her book, *The Real Food Solution*.[45] Online suppliers such as Farm2Fork deliver sustainably sourced food, including grass-fed beef. A UK-based organisation called Farms to Feed Us (www.farmstofeedus.org) aims to 'connect people with farmers, fishers and food producers during the Covid-19 crisis and beyond' and provides access to an extensive database of producers of high-quality food produced in organic and/or regenerative systems. The Ethical Butcher sources meat from farms that are PFLA standard or certified, meaning that it is from animals that are 100 per cent grass fed. These farmers have taken a pledge not to feed any grains at all to animals, and to use antibiotics only for essential medical treatment. Ethical Butcher farms also employ regenerative agriculture techniques such as holistic grazing and silvopasture.

In the US, the Weston A. Price Foundation produces an annual guide to 'the healthiest foods' in supermarkets, health-food stores and directly purchased from farms and by mail order.[46] Also in the US, a website called EatWild, founded by Jo Robinson, provides links to producers of meat, eggs and dairy from grass-fed animals.

If you want to understand more about meat itself – what makes for sustainable and nutritious meat, why you should eat it and where to find it – you might start with Diana

Rodgers and Robb Wolf's online course, Meat Curious.[47] For a more UK-specific focus, many consumers have taken 3LM's Holistic Management Fundamentals course, where you can learn about regenerative agriculture and what to look for as a conscious consumer. Or simply visit www.ethicalbutcher. co.uk or www.pastureforlife.org/trace-your-meat/ and watch the videos about the farms with which they partner.

Ideally, we'd all eat meat only from regenerative farming systems. As more of us demand better meat, more farms will be incentivised to improve production methods so that they can supply it. And as more of us move our custom to those producing and selling better quality meat, supermarkets will be incentivised to up their game. Whatever meat you choose to buy – from a company like The Ethical Butcher, your local butcher, or a farmers' market – you know that it will be a darn sight better for you and for the environment than buying the lowest price, factory-farmed meat you can find in the supermarket. If we don't like the system that produces our food, we can stop buying food from that system. As shoppers, that's our super-power.

As shoppers, we also have the power to impact one of the biggest sources of carbon emissions – food waste. Some common themes emerge. A recent study covered by *New Scientist* showed that one of the biggest causes of in-home food waste is shopping without a list and buying things you don't need. Another study showed that buying in smaller quantities results in people throwing out far less.[48] The message is clear. We need to make lists and stick to them, buy fresh produce in smaller quantities, but more often, and only buy in bulk (taking advantage of those tempting BOGOF deals, for example) when we're certain we can use or freeze the produce. Learning how to cook with leftovers is also really valuable.

Affordability

There is no doubt that quality produce from sustainable farming systems tends to be more expensive than ordinary fare. When Glen Burrows started selling his large, soya-free chickens, they were around £30 each. (They now retail for significantly less.) 'We got some flack for that,' he says. 'But instead of asking why our chicken is selling for £30, people should be asking why there are chickens on sale in supermarkets for £5. The narrative is all wrong.'

Glen is right. Chickens shouldn't be on sale for £5 each, because that price doesn't reflect the harm that industrial farming and production methods cause to the animals, to human health and to the environment. The quest for ever-cheaper food has got us into the mess in which we find ourselves today. Consider that in the 1970s people spent around 25 per cent of their income on food, whereas today they spend 15 per cent.[49] Is that progress? Not if it means industrially farmed animals raised on soya shipped from Brazil, soil stripped of its nutrients, rivers polluted with manure and run off from fields doused in chemicals, farmers deprived of a decent living, and substandard food on our tables. If we want a better system, we need to pay for that system.

Some people can easily afford to pay for better produce from a better system and will be able to eat as much meat as they always have (and enough to meet the bulk of their protein needs from meat). Others can afford to pay for better produce if they make it the priority in their household budgets, over and above other items. Many of us can also afford better quality, real food if we cut our spending on fake food and skip the packaged nonsense foods in the middle of the supermarket. Is a soya-free, pasture-raised chicken really unaffordable if it takes the place of all the cereals, crisps, sugary drinks, biscuits and oven-ready pizzas you might have bought instead?

Addressing the affordability question, Diana Rodgers looked at ten foods that might be found in a typical American shopping basket, including a Snickers bar, a packet of cookies, a packet of doughnuts, a blackbean burger, Beyond Meat Beefy Crumbles, strawberries and Vegan Pure protein powder. She compared these products with grass-fed beef from Walmart, looking at both cost and nutritional value. Not only did the beef come in at a lower cost per ounce ($0.34) than all ten of the other products, but it also delivered vastly greater amounts of nutrition. Rodgers concluded that 'suggesting that people eat grass-fed beef is not an elitist suggestion at all, it's just a matter of choices'.[50]

Processed vegan foods are generally more expensive than their non-vegan counterparts, making animal-sourced foods (even the regenerative kind) look relatively affordable. A recent analysis found that the plant-based versions of a host of products were more expensive in four out of five cases. M&S's Plant Kitchen No Pork Sausage Rolls, for instance, sell for £2.25 versus 80p for the pork version. Waitrose's own brand oat milk is priced at £1.55, versus 89p for the same amount of dairy milk. Explaining such price differences, supermarkets argue that vegan foods often have higher production costs because of the complex processes used to create them.[51] (Another reason to avoid them.)

Glen's advice for those who don't think they can afford to eat good meat is to learn to cook like their grandmothers. Buy less, but make it stretch: 'That means using the whole chicken to make several meals. It also means learning to cook cheaper cuts. Sure, not everyone can afford to eat grass-fed fillet steak three times a week. But they can buy shin, or stewing beef, or liver, and cook delicious meals with these.'[52]

Glen worked with a top chef to show that three main meals for a family of four could be made from one of his largest soya-free chickens. The last of these was a nutritious soup made with all the parts of the chicken that most people throw away. I did the same experiment at home, using one of The Ethical Butcher's chickens (the meatiest, most delicious chicken I had ever eaten) to make a roast chicken dinner for two, a chicken curry for four, and a chicken and vegetable soup for three. That's nine delicious, nutritious main meals for the price of a high-welfare chicken (£25) and some vegetables and spices (around £8), or just over £3.50 per person per meal.[53] Many of us might spend the same on a takeaway or high-end ready meal without even thinking about it.[54]

If nine meals are made from one sustainably raised chicken, the amount of chicken in each meal will admittedly be relatively small. If more people eat this way – because they want to eat meat from sustainable systems – per capita meat consumption will likely decrease overall, as I noted in Chapter 10. The shortfall in quality protein will have to be made up by protein from other animal foods – eggs, fish and dairy – as well as from plant sources. But plant proteins can never – and *should* never – be considered to be complete replacements for animal proteins, for all the reasons discussed in Chapter 2.

Over time, however, sustainably raised meat will likely become less expensive to buy. Several of the farmers to whom I spoke said that while their product currently sells at a premium, that premium will shrink as more and more producers start offering regeneratively farmed meat and supply chains deliver it to consumers more effectively. The laws of supply and demand will kick in, as they always do. In some places, regeneratively produced meat is already available at competitive prices: in May 2021, a US branch of Costco was offering four grass-raised, grass-finished sirloins for under sixteen dollars – less than the price of the frozen plant-based burgers in the next aisle.

No matter how much the price of regeneratively farmed meat comes down, those living on extremely low incomes or relying on benefits will not be able to afford it. They haven't the money for cooking like their grandmothers, and will struggle to get any quality protein, let alone enough. But this reality should not distract us, and our government, from the goal of giving everyone access to quality food. Joanna Blythman warns against making poverty an excuse for bad food, or a bad food system. 'It's scandalous that in a country like ours people do not have enough money to buy good, wholesome food. But that means some people need more money. You don't address the problem of food poverty by promoting bad food. You don't need a tin of boiled potatoes to eat in your bedsit; you need more money. Poverty is used as an excuse for bad food.'[55]

In the run up to Brexit and the implementation of the UK's new Agriculture Bill, Jamie Oliver wrote extensively about the fact that high food standards shouldn't be the preserve of the well off. He cited a Which? poll showing that people from lower-income families feel most strongly about the need to protect UK food standards. He also stressed the importance of standards, since the cheaper, lower quality food would end up in schools and hospitals, where people have no choice but to eat it.[56]

Imperfect choices

Most people are trying to fit food shopping into busy lives. They run from work to home, or from one job to another, squeezing in a quick stop at the supermarket on the way. They might not have time to seek out organic vegetables or pasture-raised chicken; they're forced to take what's on offer.

Even those with the time to browse can be confronted with imperfect choices. You can buy vegetables from your local greengrocer, but they might not be organic or even terribly fresh. In a supermarket, you may be faced with the choice between organic blueberries from Peru and non-organic ones from Kent. Another dilemma arises if you buy boxes of vegetables from a supplier that specialises in scooping up vegetables rejected by other retailers for being the wrong size or shape. Sometimes the produce is not organic, so you will have to grapple with the question of whether it is better to be eating vegetables that would otherwise have gone into a waste mountain (better in terms of emissions from landfill), or to seek out produce that had been grown without pesticides and chemical fertilisers (better for you and the soil).

Each choice we make affects the environment in a different way. Eating local fruit and vegetables, for example, might not actually reduce your carbon footprint in terms of emissions from transport, since transport generally represents a relatively small part of the emissions load. (This is true for many, but not all, plants: those that are often flown by plane, such as asparagus or out of season fruits and vegetables, are exceptions.) But eating locally produced food can deliver other environmental benefits. It reduces pressure on water-stressed countries and forces us to eat according to the seasons. (Those strawberries you're eating in February might be grown in energy-hogging greenhouses, which farmer Andrew Owens likens to 'eating pure fossil fuels'.) By eating locally grown produce you are also providing invaluable support for local farmers, whose survival is critical to national food security. And, with a little effort, you are better able to trace the farming system that your food comes from and to understand whether or not it is truly regenerative.

Provenza, Anderson and Gregorini argue that a revival of local food systems – driven, in part, by a need to reduce reliance on fossil fuels – will have multiple benefits, creating 'opportunities for communities to produce food locally in ways that nurture relationships among soil, water, plants, herbivores, farmers/ranchers and consumers' and placing agriculture 'at the heart of communities'.⁵⁷

Joanna Blythman argued for a return to 'locavorism' in a *Times* editorial, 'It would be feast, not famine, if we only learnt to love our own food.'⁵⁸ 'We needn't rely on big chains selling produce from half a world away,' she wrote. 'This land is a larder of local and seasonal fare.' As for the fashion for eating more plant foods, she said, 'while any sane person would applaud an ecologically sensitive expansion of our fruit and vegetable and arable sectors, an increased reliance on solely plant food would make us more dependent on imports.'

Because we shop in an imperfect retail environment, even the most conscientious of shoppers will face difficult choices sometimes: terms like 'locally sourced', 'organic', 'free-range' and 'sustainably produced' jostling for priority in the mind. Blythman offers this advice: 'People should just do the best they can in their circumstances. Keep in mind what goals you're trying to achieve overall, but don't make it a hierarchy, and don't beat yourself up, just do what you can. There's more choice available than you might think. You don't have to use supermarkets. And if you can get broccoli that's local but not organic, or high-welfare free-range meat that's not organic, then choose what's available. Whatever you do, it's better than choosing feedlot beef, and better than not thinking about it at all.'⁵⁹

Farmer Andrew Owens takes a similar view, believing that simply thinking about our choices makes a difference: 'Anybody doing anything is a major step. If someone walks into a butcher one day and decides to buy the more expensive but organic chicken or whatever, then they decide to do this once or twice a month, that's doing something. Or if everyone decided to buy loose onions rather than the ones in plastic. That's something. Everyone is waiting to hear what the right thing is. But, actually, the right thing can be lots of individuals making one good decision at a time.'[60]

Feeding children

As adults, we can discipline ourselves to make good food choices. But what parent hasn't been faced with the challenge of feeding a child who refuses to eat certain (or any) vegetables or insists on having pasta with tomato sauce for dinner every day? Many children are extraordinarily fussy, and most would happily consume their own bodyweight in sugar every day if we let them.

If one or more of your children is both extremely fussy and doggedly determined to remain so, my sympathies go out to you. I've been there, and wish you all the patience and persistence you'll need to set your child on a path to healthy eating. As for the averagely reluctant child who we want to persuade to eat well, we might take some pointers from an experiment conducted by Dr Clara Davis in the 1920s. Over the course of several years, Dr Davis gathered together groups of babies aged from six to eleven months and placed them on a special 'self-selection diet'. The children, who had never tasted solid food, were offered a selection of whole, natural foods (including fruit, vegetables, fish and meat) and given free rein, every day, to eat only what they wished. Each child chose differently; however, the likes and dislikes of the children generally served them well. While the children started out in generally poor health, within a few months, 'all the children were pink-cheeked and optimally nourished'.[61] It seems that Fred Provenza's 'wisdom of the body' might have been at work.

For Bee Wilson, author of *First Bite: How We Learn to Eat*, the most significant finding from these experiments was not that children's likes and dislikes varied so much and seemed to be a matter of nature rather than nurture, but that children could benefit from a radically restructured food environment. The real secret, says Wilson, was that all the foods on offer were unprocessed whole foods, so it didn't matter which ones the children were drawn to, they 'could not help but eat a diet of an excellent standard of nutrition'.[62]

If modern parents can restructure their children's food environment so that it is largely devoid of processed foods and full of a wide variety of whole plant and animal foods, perhaps it doesn't matter which of those whole foods children choose to eat. And provided children get their essential nutrients first, from whatever combination of whole foods they prefer (or that you can encourage them to eat), treats in moderation won't do them any harm.

Cooking

In June 2020, Dr Michael Eades, co-author of the book *Protein Power*, and low-carb advocate, tweeted this: 'In my 35+ years of taking care of patients and preaching the virtues of a low-carb diet, I've come to the conclusion that the single best thing you can do for your health is to spend more time in your own kitchen.'[63]

Dr Andrew Jenkinson pressed home the same point in his book, *Why We Eat (Too Much)*: 'If most of the food you consume is made up of fresh vegetables, meat, fish and dairy products, *and is home cooked* (without vegetable oil), you will be on the right track to improving your cellular metabolic health' (italics mine).[64]

There's no getting away from the fact that if you want to eat real food and cut down on your consumption of refined sugars, grains and oils, you will have to cook. But cooking needn't be difficult or complicated. There's nothing simpler than shoving a chicken in the oven, then serving it with steamed, buttered broccoli and new potatoes. Or making a slow-cooked casserole with chopped beef shin, carrots and onions. Dishes like these are works of moments, or at least works of under 15 minutes, even if they spend an hour or two in the oven.

For those who are daunted by the challenge of making a wholesale swap to sourcing and cooking real food, I'd say to start small and take it one day or one week at a time. I love the seventy-two small steps to a real-food lifestyle contained in Joel Salatin and Sina McCullough's book, *Beyond Labels: A Doctor and a Farmer Conquer Food Confusion One Bite at a Time*, a book that is 'dedicated to anyone who wants to eat better and doesn't know how'.[65] The book is written in the context of the US farming and retail system, but the ideas and practical steps it lays out are equally relevant to people living in other countries.

... and not cooking

Even the most enthusiastic of home cooks can't cook every meal, however. When time runs short and life gets a bit crazy, a ready-prepared meal might be the only option. If you do eat commercially prepared food sometimes, do yourself a favour and check the ingredients list carefully and choose something with the fewest artificial ingredients and no added sugar. This will require some sleuthing on your part, since most ready meals come laden with additives, chemicals and seed oils. Even the providers of upmarket, home-cooked-style meals invariably use seed oils in their products.

When eating in restaurants, we are entitled to ask about the kinds of oils used to prepare the foods, and about the provenance of the meat in any dish. Farmer Matthew Evans recommends that you ask your waiter questions about where their meat comes from and how it was farmed: if they can't answer the question, or you didn't like the answer they give, he says choose the vegetarian option instead.[66]

Beyond our shopping baskets and kitchens: the bigger picture

As consumers, we do have some power to influence the food system, and farmers are relying on us to use it. Farmer and author James Rebanks says that 'even good farmers cannot single-handedly determine the fate of their farms. They have to rely on the shopping and voting choices of the rest of us to support and protect nature-friendly, sustainable agriculture.'[67]

Consumers are not all powerful, however. And retailers are constrained by the fact that most people's choice of meat is based on price, and most are only prepared to pay a small premium for what they perceive to be high-quality, high-welfare meat.[68] We need our government and policy makers to act to preserve the best of our food system while moving it in a direction that serves both our health and the health of the environment. Everyone I spoke to during the course of writing this book had a wish list for government policy. At the top of the list is better protection and support for our farmers. Farming incomes have been consistently squeezed by pressure from large retailers within the supply chain, with their survival dependent on agricultural subsidies. With the UK's exit from the European Union that support is due to end. Many farmers will struggle to make ends meet, let alone invest in regenerative farming methods that capture carbon, preserve soil and enhance biodiversity. At the time of writing, the new UK Agricultural Bill has been passed. There has been much talk about supporting farmers as they transition to a post-Brexit world, and about incentivising farmers to care for the environment. But, as discussed in Chapter 10, the proof will be in the pudding, and it isn't yet clear that the pudding is rich enough in financial support and incentives. Moreover, trade deals like the one agreed with New Zealand in late 2021 have raised fears of competition from abroad leading to a flood of cheap imports that may move our own farming system in the wrong direction.[69]

Neither is it clear that the UK government has fully embraced the message about the power of regenerative agriculture to transform landscapes and address environmental challenges. There has been more talk about persuading farmers to give up their land and turn it over to rewilding schemes than there has about supporting farmers in transitioning to regenerative farming practices.

A group called The Vegan Conservatives seem to have missed the regenerative message altogether. At the start of Veganuary 2021, their spokesperson said that he was thrilled that so many Conservative MPs would be going vegan for January and claimed that 'moving towards a plant-based food system is critical if we are to prevent dangerous climate change, reduce pandemic risk, and protect animals'. Farmer and writer Jamie Blackett responded, pointing out the fallacies underlying this stance. 'We should not be afraid to point out,' he said, 'that livestock grazing is a vital part of the planet's carbon cycle,' and that British grassland sequesters 'megatons of carbon in our soil each year'. Moreover, 'this stands in stark contrast to the rainforest burning, wildlife destroying monoculturalists who deplete soils and expend irreplaceable water supplies to supply Big Food with the raw materials to supply ... soya burgers and almond milk lattes.'[70]

In October 2021, however, a glimmer of hope emerged in the form of UK environment secretary George Eustice's nuanced take on the call for lower meat intake. Interviewed in the *Daily Telegraph*, he claimed to support the principle of eat less, and eat better, and to have embraced the growing movement around regenerative agriculture.[71] Tony Juniper, head of Natural England, also commented that the meat from animals grazed as part of conservation or rewilding projects could be sustainable in comparison to meat from intensively reared animals fed crops grown on deforested land on the other side of the world.[72] Also encouraging was the announcement, in late 2021, that UK farmers would be paid to take basic measures, such as using cover cropping, to restore soil health, although many felt that this programme did not go nearly far enough.[73]

There was also much to applaud in the UK's National Food Strategy, published in June 2021. It provided some support for the idea of investing in farmers, reducing pesticide use and transferring some land to low-intensity mixed farming, while highlighting the need to help the UK break free from the 'junk food cycle'.[74] But the report could have provided much stronger advocacy for a shift towards the regenerative farming systems that protect our soils, build nutrient density into our food and, ultimately, benefit farmers' incomes and balance sheets. Rather than build the case for regeneratively farmed meat, the report dismissed its potential to provide enough meat[75] and emphasised the need to consume more alternative (plant-based) proteins, with no recognition of the nutritional cost of doing so. The concept of nutrition was dealt with inadequately throughout the report, sometimes being described in terms of a limited set of factors ('unhealthy' being equated to saturated fat, sugar and salt content, for example, rather than the absence of vitamins and minerals).[76] And the report fell into the usual trap of deeming land use to be inefficient on the basis of calories/land and protein/land ratios, with no consideration given to the quality of the calories or the protein.[77]

One welcome aspect of the Food Strategy report was the call for better food education, from early years through A level and other qualifications, with cookery and nutrition lessons inspected by Ofsted with the same rigour as maths or English lessons.[78] The work of the charitable initiative Chefs in Schools[79] could be a good model to work from. Farmer George Young stressed that agricultural college curriculums also need to be fully adapted to the new reality, teaching students less about the benefits of efficient, chemical-input-driven industrial methods and more about the benefits of regenerative methods.

Young would like to see the education system teaching about and valuing not just food and cooking skills but also other essential life skills: 'What are the three things that are essential to life? Food, clothing and shelter. Yet those courses are either non-existent or undervalued in schools. If you really teach kids about food, clothing and shelter, imagine the community effect when the kids who are good at these things – building and making stuff – are truly valued, and when those courses that are about making things are given equal status to the more academic subjects. Imagine the benefit if everyone knew their worth in the community.'[80]

The danger with education about health and nutrition is that education programmes could get hijacked by vested interests backing politically correct advice of the Eatwell variety. But let's imagine an education system in which children were taught, not about the corporate-backed Eatwell Guide, but about basic nutrition (macronutrients, vitamins and minerals), and about the kind of ancestral eating principles discovered by Weston A. Price. By teaching about food in a historical context we could give children a sense of what it means to be human and healthy and equip them to withstand the barrage of marketing and propaganda to which they are subjected by the food industry.

Let's imagine, also, a world in which the government didn't just talk about the need for people to lose weight, as the UK government did in the midst of the Covid-19 pandemic.

Imagine if, instead, they helped people to understand *why* they get fat, and what 'fat' means in the context of metabolic health. Imagine, also, the UK government taking a leaf out of the Brazilian government's books and focusing on driving home a simple 'avoid processed food, eat real food' message, and putting in place the education and community programmes to back it up.

'To counter obesity and other diet-related diseases,' wrote Fred Provenza, 'legislators would have to prioritise the well-being of the public over that of corporations by changing the laws that incentivise corporations to create harmful foods.'[81] The UK's National Food Strategy document also recognised the need to put in place an appropriate regulatory environment to incentivise food companies to produce more healthful foods. The UK government took a small step towards doing this in November 2020 when it proposed a ban on all online advertising for processed foods aimed at children. Predictably, the manufacturers of those foods reacted with outrage. The government held the line, announcing in June 2021 that junk food adverts will be subject to a near total online ban and that a 9pm television watershed would be in place by early 2023.

Low-carb, real-food enthusiast Chris Rooney proposed a wider set of actions for the government to take, which he called a 'Metabolic Manifesto':

- Replace the food traffic-light system with something that doesn't pretend carbohydrates are not sugar.
- Food labels to quote the number of whole food ingredients and number of refined, processed ingredients.
- Incentivise GP surgeries based on type-2 diabetic and prediabetes remission rates. Equip them with the tools to achieve this.
- Scrap the Eatwell Guide/food pyramid guidelines.

Launch a public health campaign based on the importance of whole, unprocessed foods.

- Use the benefit system to help people in poverty access whole foods rather than processed foods (e.g. vouchers, discounts).
- Use planning laws to restrict the number/propensity of fast-food outlets.
- Add fasting insulin test to the standard panel of blood tests – educate doctors to interpret the results.
- Apply the same restrictions on sports/events sponsorship by junk food/sugary brands as applies to tobacco.
- Glucose testing (CGM or strips) to be offered to all type-2 diabetics and prediabetics for six months post diagnosis.
- Use the tax system to incentivise small independent producers and retailers of healthy whole foods.
- Ask advocates of different weight loss/diabetes management strategies to each devise a twenty-week plan – then run a fully medically supervised randomised controlled trial to test the effectiveness of each strategy (on weight loss, HbA1c [blood glucose], fasting insulin and ratio of HDL cholesterol to triglycerides. Publish the results.[82]

Chris's proposed manifesto, which he put forward as a means of starting a debate about the policies required to improve public health, is more ambitious than anything I've seen from government or health advocacy groups. The government's diabetes prevention programme, which it says resulted in 18,000 fewer people in England being diagnosed with type-2 diabetes between 2018 and 2019, addresses some of the challenges covered by the manifesto. But how can we nudge the government to be more ambitious still?

One thing we can do is write to our MPs, making it clear that we want better support for farmers, a more sustainable food system, and health policies and practices that recognise the real causes of chronic ill health. Once an MP receives a few hundred letters on the same subject, they are obliged to act. We can also give support to organisations such as Farms to Feed Us, the Savory Institute, the Pasture for Life organisation, the Soil Association, the Sustainable Food Trust, the Real Food Campaign and the Public Health Collaboration, all of which are fighting for a future in which nutrient-dense, real food is produced in a way that aligns with our goal of healing the environment.

We might take the opportunity to express to our representatives how we feel about proposals for a meat tax, about which there was much discussion in and around the Cop26 meeting in Glasgow in November 2021. As Alice Thompson wrote, 'a tax on meat is bad solution to climate change' for it 'would penalise small-scale, ecologically friendly UK farmers while encouraging cheap imports and intensive methods'.[83] A tax would also harm those on low incomes, whose access to nutrient-dense foods like meat and other animal-sourced foods would be further diminished. Moreover, it would send entirely the wrong message, which is that meat, in itself, is bad for health, when the very opposite is true.

We might also ask of our schools that they take a more intelligent and far-reaching approach than is represented by a knee-jerk commitment to serve more vegetarian meals. What if, instead of banning meat from school cafeterias, head teachers banned all junk such as soft drinks and processed sugary foods, and committed to sourcing meat from local, pasture-based farms? What if they committed to programmes that enhance children's understanding of where food comes from and how it's grown? Small market-garden projects, farm visits and in-school education sessions provided by farmers could all be part of that process.

On a personal level, each of us can equip ourselves for the fight. And, make no mistake, we *are* in a fight. We are in a fight for our own health and for the future of the food and farming system, and the environment in which it sits. If we allow the conversation to continue to be about how we can shift both our diets and the farming system towards a plant-based model, we will be trampled on, and ultimately controlled, by all those who stand to gain from that model. And, as Professor Leroy has warned, such a situation would be difficult if not impossible to reverse.

What does it mean to equip ourselves? I believe it means being that naive sceptic, so that the next time you read a headline telling you that eating red meat gives you an 'x' per cent higher risk of getting cancer, or that eating a plant-based diet will make you live longer and save the planet, you stop, take a breath and ask questions. Who produced the study and who paid for it? What might they have to gain from the published result? Is the study observational (epidemiological)? Is the risk they are talking about relative (almost certainly) and small (less than 100 per cent)? Then refresh your memory of the studies covered in Chapter 13, and recall how the published conclusions were not supported by the data and findings within the studies themselves. Could the study you're now reading about be one of those? Would epidemiology expert John Ioannidis count it among the vast majority of published research findings that are false?

If you don't feel equipped – or don't have the time – to interrogate studies yourself, you can consult the work of others who've done the interrogation for you. People who I rely upon to provide regular, layperson friendly analyses of studies are Drs Zoë Harcombe, Georgia Ede, Peter Attia and Malcolm Kendrick (website addresses are provided in the resources section).

And if you don't like what you learn when you've asked your own questions or consulted the reliable analyses of others, do as Dr Malcolm Kendrick does. Crumple. Throw. Bin.[84]

As you discard studies that aren't worth the paper they're printed on, aim to develop a healthy mistrust of the top-down advice coming from those who produce industry-backed dietary guidelines. Do as Professor Tim Spector insists we all must do, which is to 'learn more ourselves about the food we eat and the science behind it so that we can avoid the smokescreens and make informed individual choices'.[85] Seek out information from those who do not have close ties to Big Pharma or Big Food or the NGOs intent on controlling the entire food system and us within it. Instead, pick any of the experts mentioned in this book and listen to their podcasts or read something they've written. (A list of my favourite podcasts, websites, books and films is provided at the end of this book.) They are independent thinkers, and their advice is the best that's out there. It has already transformed the health and lives of many thousands of people.

Knowledge is power. Seek it out. Use it. Resist the plant-based con and become an advocate for your own health and the health of our planet.

Abbreviations

Numerous abbreviations feature throughout this book. The following list is not exhaustive but includes those that are used most often.

ABCMF: Australian Breakfast Cereal Manufacturers Forum
ACLM: American College of Lifestyle Medicine
ACSM: American College of Sports Medicine
ACTH: adrenocorticotropic hormone
ADA: American Diabetes Association (also, American Dietetics Association, now called the Academy of Nutrition and Dietetics)
ADSA: Association for Dietetics in South Africa
AHA: American Heart Association
AHPRA: Australian Health Practitioners Regulatory Agency
AIC: American Institute of Cancer
ALA: a short-chain fatty acid that's a precursor to DHA and EPA
AMA: American Medical Association
AMP: adaptive, multi-paddock grazing
AND: Academy of Nutrition and Dietetics
BCFN: Barilla Center for Food and Nutrition
BMI: body mass index
BMJ: *British Medical Journal*
BSLM: British Society of Lifestyle Medicine

CAC: coronary artery calcium

CAD: coronary artery disease

CAFO: confined animal feed operation

CALM: Christian Association of Lifestyle Medicine

CCC: Committee on Climate Change

CGM: continuous glucose monitor

CH4: methane

CHIP: complete health improvement programme

CICO: calories-in, calories-out

CIWF: Compassion in World Farming

CO2: carbon dioxide

CO2e: carbon dioxide equivalents

COIs: conflicts of interest

CSS: Centre for Sustainable Systems

CVD: cardiovascular disease

DAA: Dietitians Association of Australia

DALYs: disability-adjusted life years

DHA: docosahexoenoic acid, a long-chain omega-3 fatty acid

DIAAS: digestible indispensable amino acid score

DiRECT: DIabetes REmission Clinical Trial

DRIs: US Dietary Reference Intakes

DV: daily value

EAAs: essential amino acids

EASD: European Association for the Study of Diabetes

EIM: Exercise is Medicine

ELMS: Environmental Land Management Scheme

EPA: Environmental Protection Agency

EPA: eicosapentaenoic acid, a long-chain omega 3-fatty acid

ESV: end-stage veganism

FAO: Food and Agriculture Organization

FDA: Food and Drug Administration

FFQs: Food Frequency Questionnaires

FL: feedlot, or confined feed yard

FNCE: Food and Nutrition Conference and Expo

FoTE: Friends of the Earth

FReSH: Food Reform for Sustainability and Health
GAIN: Global Alliance for Improved Nutrition
GBD: Global Burden of Disease
GCA: Global Commons Alliance
GEBN: Global Energy Balance Network
GFHGNP: French Paediatric Hepatology, Gastroenterology and Nutrition Group
GHGs: greenhouse gas emissions
GI: glycaemic index
GL: glycaemic load
GWP: Global Warming Potential
HDL: high-density lipoprotein
holoTC: holotranscobalamin
HPCSA: Health Professionals Council of South Africa
HPS: Heart Protection Study
HSFSA: Heart and Stroke Foundation of South Africa
HSUS: Humane Society of the United States
IARC: International Agency for Research on Cancer
IBS: irritable bowel syndrome
ICT: information and communications technology
IFBA: International Food and Beverage Alliance
IFF: International Flavours and Fragrances
IFIC: International Food Information Council
ILSI: International Life Sciences Institute
IPCC: Intergovernmental Panel on Climate Change
IR: insulin resistance
JAMA: Journal of the American Medical Association
JRA: juvenile rheumatoid arthritis
LCHF: low carbohydrate, high fat
LCA: life cycle assessment
LDL: low-density lipoprotein
LMEd: Lifestyle Medicine Education Collaborative
LRC-CPPT: Lipid Research Clinic's Coronary Primary Prevention Trial
MMA: methylmalonic acid

MSPR: multispecies pasture rotation
N2O: nitrous oxide
NACNE: National Advisory Committee for Nutrition Education
NAFLD: non-alcoholic fatty liver disease
NCI: National Cancer Institute
NCD: non-communicable disease
NEJM: New England Journal of Medicine
NFU: National Farmers Union
NGOs: non-governmental organisations
NHLBI: National Heart, Lung and Blood Institute
NHMRC: National Health and Medical Research Council
NICE: National Institute for Health and Care Excellence
NIH: National Institutes of Health
NPA: National Pig Association
NRCS: National Resources Conservation Service
NSNG: no sugar, no grains
NRF: nutrient-rich foods
OPP: Open Philanthropy Project
OWiD: Our World in Data
P&G: Procter & Gamble
PAHO: Pan American Health Organization
PCOS: polycystic ovarian syndrome
PCRM: Physicians' Committee for Responsible Medicine
PET: positron emission tomography
PFLA: Pasture-Fed Livestock Association
PHA and PNA: types of lectins
PHC: Public Health Collaboration
PHE: Public Health England
PPG: Patient Participation Group
PUFAs: polyunsaturated fatty acids
PURE: Prospective Urban Rural Epidemiology study
RCT: randomised controlled trial
RSPCA: Royal Society for the Prevention of Cruelty to Animals
SAD: standard American diet

SDA: Seventh-day Adventist Church

sdLDL: small, dense form of low-density lipoprotein

SEI: Stockholm Environment Institute

SRC: Stockholm Resilience Centre

THI: True Health Initiative

THINCS: The International Network of Cholesterol Skeptics

TOFI: thin on the outside, fat on the inside

UN: United Nations

UNEP: UN Environment Programme

UPFs: ultra-processed foods

USDA: United States Department of Agriculture

VLCD: very low-calorie diet

WBCSD: World Business Council for Sustainable Development

WCRF: World Cancer Research Fund

WEF: World Economic Forum

WFN: Water Footprint Network

WHIRCDMT, sometimes referred to simply as
WHI: Women's Health Initiative Randomized Controlled Dietary Modification Study

WHO: World Health Organization

WRI: World Resources Institute

WWF: Worldwide Fund for Nature

Sources of reference

Extensive research has gone into writing this book, and over 1,000 sources of reference have been examined. These sources are acknowledged with a number in the relevant position in the text. In order to keep the book to a manageable size, the corresponding details of those studies have been placed on the website www.thegreatplantbasedcon.com so that you can delve deeper if you wish.

Resources

Podcasts

There are many excellent podcasts featuring discussions with thought leaders in the fields of human and environmental health. These are my favourites, each one with a different slant and tone, but all accessible, entertaining and informative.

The Drive, with Peter Attia, MD www.peterattiamd.com

The Fat Emperor, with Ivor Cummins www.thefatemperor.com

Fitness Confidential, with Vinnie Tortorich https://vinnietortorich.com/category/podcast/

Human Performance Outliers, with Dr Shawn Baker www.humanperformanceoutliers.libsyn.com

Low Carb MD, with Dr Jason Fung, Dr Brian Lenzkes, Dr Tro Kalayjan and Megan Ramos www.lowcarbmd.com

Peak Human Podcast, with Brian Sanders www.peak-human.com

The Doctor's Farmacy, with Dr Mark Hyman www.drhyman.com/blog/category/podcasts/

UK Low Carb Podcast, with Dan Greef

Blogs and websites

For high-quality information about health, nutrition and nutrition research, I rely on Dr Georgia Ede's www.diagnosisdiet.com, Dr Zoë Harcombe's www.zoeharcombe.com and Chris Kresser's www.chriskresser.com. All can help you to get to grips with your own health challenges and guide you through the morass of confusing nutrition research that makes the headlines every day.

Others providing excellent advice and articles on aspects of nutrition are Mark Hyman MD (www.drhyman.com), Lucinda Miller (www.naturedoc.co.uk), Izabella Natrins (www.izabella-natrins.com) and Tim Rees (www.tim-rees.com). For intelligent analysis of current debates pertaining to cholesterol, heart health, statins and more, visit Dr Malcolm Kendrick's website and blog (www.drmalcolmkendrick.org). If you want to deepen your understanding of cholesterol (and particularly if you are what is known as a hyper-responder), Dave Feldman's https://cholesterolcode.com is also an excellent resource.

Diet Doctor (www.dietdoctor.com) is an excellent resource for those interested in low-carb and ketogenic diets, providing recipes, meal-plans and articles about the science behind low-carb eating. The six hundred success stories featured on the site will inspire you, and some will make you weep. The Public Health Collaboration (https://phcuk.org) also provides access to research about the low-carb route to health and access to an extensive ambassador network. Other quality resources include www.lowcarbusa.org, www.lowcarbdownunder.com.au and https://ketomaria.com. For those with diabetes, www.diabetes.co.uk has proved to be an invaluable source of information and support. The Charlie Foundation (https://charliefoundation.org) provides information and resources for those interested in using ketogenic diets as therapy.

If you're interested in the wider debate about food, health and the environment, visit https://aleph-2020.blogspot.com, a website launched by a group of more than thirty scientists, including Professor Frédéric Leroy, in late 2020, and Dr Frank Mitloehner's blog, at https://ghgguru.faculty.ucdavis.edu. These two resources will help you cut through the misinformation about the impact of livestock farming on the environment, and give you a more balanced, nuanced understanding of the issues and the debate.

For the latest on the US dietary guidelines process, as well as excellent articles about aspects of the nutrition debate, visit https://www.nutritioncoalition.us. And for research about the influence of the Seventh-day Adventist Church on dietary guidelines, go to Belinda Fettke's www. isupportgary.com.

For accessible information about regenerative agriculture and stories about the people who are practising it, Diana Rodger's Instagram feed is fantastic (@sustainabledish). Follow @globalfoodjustice to learn about sustainability in the context of the challenges of nourishing the world. For snapshots of what regenerative agriculture looks like in the UK, visit www.ethicalbutcher.co.uk or follow @ethicalbutcher on Instagram. Other websites showcasing the regenerative agriculture story are www.pastureforlife.org, www.3lm.network, www. eatwild.com, soil4climate.org and www.savory.global. To stay informed about the challenges we face in creating more sustainable agriculture, stay connected to www.sustainablefoodtrust.org. And for discussions about real food in the context of sustainability, go to www.realfoodcampaign.org.uk.

Recommended reading

Health and nutrition

The Big Fat Surprise by Nina Teicholz
The Carnivore Code: Unlocking the Secrets to Optimal Health by Returning to Our Ancestral Diet by Paul Saladino, MD
The Carnivore Diet by Shawn Baker, MD
The Case Against Sugar by Gary Taubes
The Case For Keto: The Truth About Low-Carb, High-Fat Eating by Gary Taubes
The Clot Thickens: The Enduring Mystery of Heart Disease by Dr Malcolm Kendrick
Doctoring Data by Dr Malcolm Kendrick

Eat Rich, Live Long by Ivor Cummins and Jeffry Gerber, MD

Fat Chance: The Hidden Truth About Sugar, Obesity and Disease by Dr Robert Lustig

First Bite: How We Learn to Eat by Bee Wilson

Fitness Confidential: Adventures in the Weight Loss Game by Vinnie Tortorich

Fork in the Road by Dr Jen Unwin

Good Calories, Bad Calories by Gary Taubes

Grain Brain: The Surprising Truth About Wheat, Carbs, and Sugar – Your Brain's Silent Killers by Dr David Perlmutter

The Great Cholesterol Con: The Truth about What Really Causes Heart Disease and How to Avoid It by Dr Malcolm Kendrick

Healthy Eating: The Big Mistake by Dr Verner Wheelock and Marika Sboros

How Statin Drugs Really Lower Cholesterol and Kill You One Cell At A Time by James B. Yoseph and Hannah Yoseph, MD

Lies My Doctor Told Me: Medical Myths That Can Harm Your Health by Dr Ken Berry

The Metabolic Approach to Cancer by Dr Nasha Winters and Jess Higgins Kelley

The Mineral Fix by James DiNicolantonio and Siim Land

Nourishing Traditions: The Cookbook that Challenges Politically Correct Nutrition and the Diet Dictocrats by Sally Fallon with Mary G. Enig, PhD

Nutrition and Physical Degeneration by Weston A. Price, DDS

The Obesity Code: Unlocking the Secrets Of Weight Loss by Dr Jason Fung

The Obesity Epidemic: What Caused It, How We Can Stop It by Dr Zoë Harcombe

The Pioppi Diet: A 21-Day Lifestyle Plan by Dr Aseem Malhotra and Donal O'Neill

The P:E Diet: Leverage Your Biology to Achieve Optimal Health by Ted Naiman, MD, and William Shewfelt

*The Plant Paradox: The Hidden Dangers in 'Healthy' Foods
    That Cause Disease and Weight Gain*, by Steven R.
    Gundry, MD

*Protein Power: The High Protein, Low Carbohydrate Way
    to Lose Weight, Feel Fit, and Boost Your Health* by Dr
    Michael Eades and Dr Mary Dan Eades

Pure, White and Deadly by John Yudkin

*Real Food for Pregnancy: The Science and Wisdom
    of Optimal Prenatal Nutrition* by Lily
    Nichols, RDN, CDE

*The Real Meal Revolution: The Radical, Sustainable
    Approach to Healthy Eating* by Professor Tim Noakes,
    Jonno Proudfoot and Sally-Ann Creed

A Statin Free Life by Dr Aseem Malhotra

Stop Feeding Us Lies by Charlie Spedding

*Tripping Over the Truth: How the Metabolic Theory
    of Cancer Is Overturning One of Medicine's Most
    Entrenched Paradigms* by Travis Christofferson

Vegetarianism Explained: Making Informed Decisions by Dr
    Natasha Campbell-McBride

*What to Eat: Food That's Good for Your Health, Pocket and
    Plate* by Joanna Blythman

*Wheat Belly: Lose the Wheat, Lose the Weight, and Find Your
    Path Back to Health* by William Davis, MD

Why We Eat (Too Much): The New Science of Appetite by Dr
    Andrew Jenkinson

Why We Get Fat, and What to Do About It by Gary Taubes

*Why We get Sick: The Hidden Epidemic at the Root of
    Most Chronic Disease – and How to Fight It* by Ben
    Bikman, PhD

Food, health, farming, regenerative agriculture and environment

*Beyond Labels: A Doctor and a Farmer Conquer Food
    Confusion One Bite at a Time* by Sina McCullough,
    PhD, and Joel Salatin, farmer

Defending Beef: The Case for Sustainable Meat Production by
Nicolette Hahn Niman

Dire Predictions: Understanding Climate Change by Michael
E. Mann and Lee R. Kump

Dirt: The Erosion of Civilisations by David R. Montgomery

*Dirt to Soil: One Family's Journey into Regenerative
Agriculture* by Gabe Brown

The Dirty Life: On Farming, Food and Love by Kristin Kimball

*Drawdown: The Most Comprehensive Plan Ever Proposed to
Reverse Global Warming* edited by Paul Hawken

English Pastoral: An Inheritance by James Rebanks

*Farm to Fork: The Challenge of Sustainable Farming in 21st
Century Britain* by Joe Stanley

*For the Love of the Land: A Cookbook to Celebrate British
Farmers and Their Food* compiled by Jenny Jefferies

*Holistic Management: A Commonsense Revolution to Restore
Our Environment* by Allan Savory with Jody Butterfield

*Nourishment: What Animals Can Teach Us About
Rediscovering Our Nutritional Wisdom* by Fred Provenza

*On Eating Meat: The Truth About its Production and the
Ethics of Eating It* by Matthew Evans

*The Real Food Solution: A Treasury of Wisdom for Energy,
Vitality and Better Health for You and Your Planet* by
Izabella Natrins

Sacred Cow: The Case for Better Meat by Diana Rodgers
and Robb Wolf

So We Shall Reap by Colin Tudge

The Vegetarian Myth: Food, Justice and Sustainability by
Lierre Keith

Influences on our food system and our health

*Billion Dollar Burger: Inside Big Tech's Race for The Future
of Food* by Chase Purdy

*Bad Pharma: How Medicine Is Broken and How We Can Fix
It* by Ben Goldacre

The Dorito Effect: The Surprising New Truth About Food and Flavor by Mark Schatzker

Food Fix: How to Save Our Health, Our Economy, Our Communities and Our Planet – One Bite at a Time by Dr Mark Hyman

The Hacking of the American Mind: The Science Behind the Corporate Takeover of our Bodies and Brains by Dr Robert Lustig

In Defence of Food by Michael Pollan

Real Food On Trial: How the Diet Dictators Tried to Destroy a Top Scientist by Dr Tim Noakes and Marika Sboros

Shopped: The Shocking Power of Britain's Supermarkets by Joanna Blythman

Spoon-Fed: Why Almost Everything We've Been told About Food is Wrong by Tim Spector

Swallow This: Serving Up the Food Industry's Darkest Secrets by Joanna Blythman

The Truth About Drug Companies by Dr Marcia Angell, MD

Films

The Biggest Little Farm (www.biggestlittlefarmmovie.com, Amazon Prime), *Kiss the Ground* (www.kisstheground.com, Netflix) and *Sacred Cow* (www.access.sacredcow.info) are excellent and inspiring films about the power of regenerative agriculture to heal our environment. *Fat: A Documentary (1 & 2)* and *Fat Fiction* (both on Amazon Prime) are eye-opening documentaries examining how the US dietary guidelines shaped our views about what constitutes a healthy diet and led to a damaging and unfounded bias against saturated fat. *Beyond Impossible* challenges the claims made by the fake meat industry. *The Cereal Killers Movie* (www.cerealkillersmovie.com) reveals the myths underlying traditional nutrition advice. *The Extra Time Movie* (www.exratimemovie.com) is a film about achieving better heart health, with a very powerful human story at its own heart. *Statin Nation* (available on Amazon Prime) reveals the story behind the mass prescription of cholesterol medications, and *The Widowmaker* (also on Prime), tells the story of the development of both preventionist and interventionist technology in the cardiology world, highlighting the ongoing battles between the parties involved.

Acknowledgements

This book had its beginnings in long talks with my sister, a Canadian vet. We were deeply frustrated by the debate about food, health and the environment, which seemed to exist in a parallel universe to the facts as we understood them. She suggested that I write a book providing an alternative to the dominant narrative promoting the widespread adoption of a plant-based diet. Thus began more than two years of researching and writing, a process that has been invigorating and exhausting. Thank you, Cal, for the experience and for your unwavering support throughout.

I am also deeply indebted to the following individuals (listed here in alphabetical order), who gave so generously of their time and expertise via interviews and/or extensive email correspondence. It is no exaggeration to say that I could not have written this book without their input.

Dr Shawn Baker, orthopaedic surgeon, health and nutrition podcaster, CEO of Meat R/X; **Robert Barbour**, researcher with the Sustainable Food Trust; **Joanna Blythman**, award-winning investigative food journalist and author; **Gabe Brown**, farmer, author and founding partner of Understanding Ag; **Valeria Burnazov**, registered dietician; **Glen Burrows**, The Ethical Butcher; **John Cherry**, farmer and founder of the Groundswell Regenerative Agriculture Conference; **Sheila Cooke**, co-founder of 3LM, the UK and Ireland hub of the Savory Institute Network; **Ivor Cummins**, bio-chemical engineer turned lipid and chronic disease specialist, author, health and nutrition pod-caster; **Henry Edmunds**, farmer; **Sally Fallon Morell**, author of *Nourishing Traditions* and founding president of the Weston A. Price Foundation; **Dave Feldman**, software engineer, entre-preneur, founder of the cholesterolcode.com; **Sam Feltham**, founder of the Public Health Collaboration; **Belinda Fettke**, trained nurse and researcher/writer; **Dr Gary Fettke**, orthopaedic surgeon and low-carb advocate; **Tucker Goodrich**, risk manage-ment specialist and Pub-Med warrior; **Dr Zoë Harcombe PhD**, researcher, author, blogger and public speaker; **Paul Hart**, plant protein specialist; **Pete Huff**, co-director of the Pasture Project, an initiative of the Wallace Center at Winrock International; **Lierre Keith**, former vegan, author and environmental activist; **Professor Frédéric Leroy**, professor in the field of food science and bio-technology at the Vrije University, Brussels; **Trent Loos**, Nebraskan rancher and broadcaster; **Lucinda Miller**, family naturopath; **Dr Frank Mitloehner**, UC Davis professor and air quality specialist, director of the CLEAR Center; **Izabella Natrins**, author and real food nutrition and lifestyle medicine coach; **Professor Tim Noakes**, exercise and sports medicine sci-entist and founder of The Noakes Foundation; **Andrew Owens**, farmer; **Fred Provenza**, author and professor emeritus of behav-ioural ecology in the Department of Wildland Resources at Utah State University; **Tim Rees**, registered nutritionist, health and lifestyle coach and writer; **Brian Sanders**, health and nutri-tion advocate, filmmaker, and CEO of Sapien; **Marika Sboros**, investigative journalist and author; **Joe Stanley**, award- winning farmer and columnist; **Professor Alice Stanton**, professor in cardiovascular pharmacology at the Royal College of Surgeons in Ireland, and director of human health at Devenish Nutrition; **Nina Teicholz**, science journalist, author, and executive director of The Nutrition Coalition; **Karl Thiddemann** of Soil4Climate; **Vinnie Tortorich**, health and fitness expert, author, podcaster and filmmaker; **Dr David Unwin**, award-winning general prac-titioner in the UK; **Dr Jen Unwin** consultant clinical health psychologist; **Stephan van Vliet,** human physiologist at the Duke Molecular Physiology Institute at Duke University; **Dr Eric Westman,** associate professor of medicine at Duke University, and co-founder of the Duke Keto Medicine Clinic; **Dr Allen Williams,** farmer, researcher, author and founding partner of Grass Fed Insights, Understanding Ag, and the Soil Health Academy; **George Young,** farmer and agroecology advocate.

Particular thanks must go to Belinda Fettke, Tucker Goodrich, Paul Hart, Fred Provenza, Marika Sboros, Nina Teicholz and Stephan van Vliet, all of whom provided extensive feedback regarding critical sections of the book and took the time to unearth important sources.

Profound thanks also to those who shared both their personal experiences and their astute observations with me, including Mark G., Rob Halliday, Natasha Hodge, Marion Holman, Andy Reynolds, Chris Rooney, Debra Scott, Ravi, and my old friends David, Jim and Lianne.

My work was also greatly informed by the published work of: Professor Myles Allen; Cindi Anderson; Dr Marcia Angell; Ty Beal; Mike Berners-Lee; Dr Ken Berry; Dr Ben Bikman; Jamie Blackett; Sarah Bridle; Dr Natasha Campbell-McBride; John and Molly Chester; Travis Kristofferson; Nathan Cofnas; Maria Cross; Dr Dominique D'Agostino; Dr William Davis; Dr James DiNicolantonio; Adam Drenowski; Dr Michael Eades; Dr Georgia Ede; Dr Andreas Eenfeldt; Matthew Evans; Joshua Finch; Dr Jason Fung; Dr Jeremy Gerber; Dr Ben Goldacre; Russ Greene; Pablo Gregorini; Dr Steven Gundry; Nicolette Hahn Niman; Dr David Harper; Will Harris; Paul Hawken; Patrick Holden; Dr Mark Hyman; Dr Joan Ifland; Seth Itzkan; Dr Andrew Jenkinson; Dr Malcolm Kendrick; Sara Keough; Chris Kresser; Scott Kronberg; Dr Robert Lustig; Dr Aseem Malhotra; Professor Michael Mann; Chris Masterjohn; David Montgomery; Pat Mooney; Dr Ted Naiman; Marion Nestle; Lily Nichols RDN; Professor Tim Noakes; Sally Norton; L. Amber O'Hearn; Christine Page; Dr David Perlmutter; Michael Pollan;

Chase Purdy; James Rebanks; Diana Rodgers; Dr Paul Saladino; Joel Salatin; Allan Savory; Dr Brett Scher; Dr Jamie Seaman; Professor Tim Spector; Charlie Spedding; Benjamin David Steel; Gary Taubes; Colin Tudge; Alison Van Eenennaam; Dr Verner Wheelock; Bee Wilson; Dr Nasha Winters; Robb Wolf; James Wong; Dr Jay Wrigley; Richard Young; Peter Ballerstedt.

The extensive endnotes bear testimony to the contribution of the many hundreds of authors, farmers, journalists, medical professionals, researchers and scientists whose work I consulted. I am deeply indebted to them all.

Huge thanks go to my agent, Euan Thorneycroft, who glimpsed the potential in an early proposal and helped shape it, and to my publisher at Piatkus, Zoe Bohm, who gave me the opportunity to contribute to the debate and provided unequivocal support through a process that was not without its complications. I'd particularly like to thank my editor, Jillian Stewart, whose devotion to the book matched my own; Meryl Evans, for her detailed and constructive feedback; Matthew Crossey, for helping me to put across the book's essential messages; and Holly Harley, for picking up the reins from Zoe so enthusiastically. Thanks also to the wider team at Little, Brown – design, production, ops, publicity and sales – for all their hard work.

I am beyond grateful to my husband and children, who never wavered in their support for me and for this project, even as they were hearing arguments to the contrary on a daily basis. My eldest daughter provided editorial guidance which was of immense value (any error in reflecting that guidance is entirely my own) and my husband bent over backwards to give me the support I needed, taking up all domestic slack and graciously relinquishing the use of our shared home-office. My sister and her family – a very 'sciency' lot – have been cheerleaders, sounding boards and consultant statisticians from afar. My parents have been, as ever, unflagging in their encouragement and enthusiasm. This kind of support is what makes writing possible.

Index